Bone Tumor Pathology

Editor

JUDITH V.M.G. BOVÉE

SURGICAL PATHOLOGY CLINICS

www.surgpath.theclinics.com

Consulting Editor
JASON L. HORNICK

September 2017 • Volume 10 • Number 3

ELSEVIER

1600 John F. Kennedy Boulevard • Suite 1800 • Philadelphia, Pennsylvania, 19103-2899

http://www.theclinics.com

SURGICAL PATHOLOGY CLINICS Volume 10, Number 3
September 2017 ISSN 1875-9181, ISBN-13: 978-0-323-54574-7

Editor: Stacy Eastman
Developmental Editor: Donald Mumford

Surgical Pathology Clinics (ISSN 1875-9181) is published quarterly by Elsevier Inc., 360 Park Avenue South, New York, NY 10010. Months of issue are March, June, September, and December. Business and Editorial Office: Elsevier Inc., 1600 John F. Kennedy Blvd., Ste. 1800, Philadelphia, PA 19103-2899. Accounting and Circulation Offices: Elsevier Inc., 3251 Riverport Lane, Maryland Heights, MO 63043. Periodicals postage paid at New York, NY and at additional mailing offices. Subscription prices are $206.00 per year (US individuals), $274.00 per year (US institutions), $100.00 per year (US students/residents), $258.00 per year (Canadian individuals), $312.00 per year (Canadian Institutions), $258.00 per year (foreign individuals), $312.00 per year (foreign institutions), and $120.00 per year (international & Canadian students/residents). Foreign air speed delivery is included in all *Clinics'* subscription prices. All prices are subject to change without notice. **POSTMASTER:** Send address changes to *Surgical Pathology Clinics*, Elsevier, 3251 Riverport Lane, Maryland Heights, MO 63043. **Customer Service: 1-800-654-2452 (US). From outside the United States, call 1-314-447-8871. Fax: 1-314-447-8029. E-mail: JournalsCustomerServiceusa@elsevier.com (for print support) and JournalsOnlineSupport-usa@elsevier.com (for online support).**

Reprints. For copies of 100 or more, of articles in this publication, please contact the Commercial Reprints Department, Elsevier Inc., 360 Park Avenue South, New York, NY 10010-1710. Tel. 212-633-3874; Fax: 212-633-3820; E-mail: reprints@elsevier.com.

Surgical Pathology Clinics of North America is covered in *MEDLINE/PubMed (Index Medicus)*.

Contributors

CONSULTING EDITOR

JASON L. HORNICK, MD, PhD
Director of Surgical Pathology, Director, Immunohistochemistry Laboratory, Brigham and Women's Hospital, Associate Professor of Pathology, Harvard Medical School, Boston, Massachusetts, USA

EDITOR

JUDITH V.M.G. BOVÉE, MD, PhD
Professor, Department of Pathology, Leiden University Medical Center, Leiden, The Netherlands

AUTHORS

NICHOLAS A. ATHANASOU, MD, PhD, MRCP, FRCPath
Nuffield Department of Orthopaedics, Rheumatology and Musculoskeletal Sciences, Nuffield Orthopaedic Centre, University of Oxford, Oxford, United Kingdom

DANIEL BAUMHOER, MD
Consultant Pathologist and Head of the Bone Tumour Reference Centre, Institute of Pathology, University of Basel, Basel, Switzerland

JUDITH V.M.G. BOVÉE, MD, PhD
Professor, Department of Pathology, Leiden University Medical Center, Leiden, The Netherlands

JODI M. CARTER, MD, PhD
Assistant Professor, Department of Laboratory Medicine and Pathology, Mayo Clinic, Rochester, Minnesota, USA

ARJEN H.G. CLEVEN, MD, PhD
Department of Pathology, Leiden University Medical Center, Leiden, The Netherlands

JEAN MICHEL COINDRE, MD
Professor, Institut Bergonie, Université de Bordeaux, Bordeaux, France

ENRIQUE DE ALAVA, MD, PhD
Chairman, Unidad de Anatomía Patológica, Department of Pathology, University Hospital Virgen del Rocío-Biomedical Institute of Seville, CSIC-University of Seville-CIBERONC, Seville, Spain

CARLOS E. DE ANDREA, MD, PhD
Assistant Professor, Department of Histology and Pathology, University of Navarra, Navarra, Pamplona, Spain

ANGELO P. DEI TOS, MD
Department of Pathology, Azienda ULSS2 Marca Trevigiana, Treviso, Italy; Department of Medicine, School of Medicine, University of Padova, Padova, Italy

UTA FLUCKE, MD, PhD
Department of Pathology, Nijmegen Medical Center, Radboud University, Nijmegen, The Netherlands

MARCO GAMBAROTTI, MD
Department of Pathology, Rizzoli Orthopaedic
Institute, Bologna, Italy

MARIA GNOLI, MD
Medical Geneticist, Department of Medical
Genetics and Skeletal Rare Diseases, Rizzoli
Orthopaedic Institute, Bologna, Italy

PANCRAS C.W. HOGENDOORN, MD, PhD
Department of Pathology, Leiden University
Medical Center, Leiden, The Netherlands

BENJAMIN MATTHEW HOWE, MD
Assistant Professor, Department of Radiology,
Mayo Clinic, Rochester, Minnesota, USA

SHUN IIDA, MD
Senior Resident, Department of Pathology,
Koshigaya Hospital, Dokkyo Medical
University, Koshigaya, Saitama, Japan

HIROKI IMADA, MD
Research Associate, Department of Pathology,
Koshigaya Hospital, Dokkyo Medical
University, Koshigaya, Saitama, Japan

CARRIE Y. INWARDS, MD
Professor, Department of Laboratory Medicine
and Pathology, Mayo Clinic, Rochester,
Minnesota, USA

FRANCOIS LE LOARER, MD, PhD
Department of Pathology, Institut Bergonie,
Université de Bordeaux, Bordeaux, France

ZSOLT OROSZ, MD, PhD
Nuffield Department of Orthopaedics,
Rheumatology and Musculoskeletal Sciences,
Nuffield Orthopaedic Centre, University of
Oxford, Oxford, United Kingdom

PIERO PICCI, MD
Department of Pathology, Rizzoli Orthopaedic
Institute, Bologna, Italy

DANIEL PISSALOUX, PhD
Departement de Biopathologie, Centre Leon
Berard, Lyon, France

FRANCESCA PONTI, BSB
Department of Medical Genetics and Skeletal
Rare Diseases, Rizzoli Orthopaedic Institute,
Bologna, Italy

ALBERTO RIGHI, MD
Department of Pathology, Rizzoli Orthopaedic
Institute, Bologna, Italy

ANDREW E. ROSENBERG, MD
Professor of Pathology, University of Miami
Miller School of Medicine, Miami, Florida, USA

MIKEL SAN-JULIAN, MD, PhD
Assistant Professor, Department of
Orthopaedic Surgery and Traumatology,
University Clinic of Navarra, Navarra,
Pamplona, Spain

**LUCA SANGIORGI, MD, PhD (Clinical
Genetics)**
Head of Medical Genetics Department of
Rizzoli Orthopaedic Institute, Department of
Medical Genetics and Skeletal Rare Diseases,
Rizzoli Orthopaedic Institute, Bologna, Italy

MARTA SBARAGLIA, MD
Department of Pathology, Azienda ULSS2
Marca Trevigiana, Treviso, Italy

WANGZHAO SONG, MD
Department of Pathology and Medical Biology,
University Medical Center Groningen,
University of Groningen, Groningen, The
Netherlands

ALBERT J.H. SUURMEIJER, MD, PhD
Professor of Pathology, Department of
Pathology and Medical Biology, University
Medical Center Groningen, University of
Groningen, Groningen, The Netherlands

KAROLY SZUHAI, MD, PhD
Associate Professor, Department of Molecular
Cell Biology, Leiden University Medical Center,
Leiden, The Netherlands

FRANCK TIRODE, PhD
Cancer Research Center of Lyon, Laboratoire
de recherche translationnelle, Centre Leon
Berard, Lyon, France

DAVID G.P. VAN IJZENDOORN, BSc
Department of Pathology, Leiden University
Medical Center, Leiden, The Netherlands

DANIEL VANEL, MD
Department of Pathology, Rizzoli Orthopaedic
Institute, Bologna, Italy

DOMINIQUE RANCHERE VINCE, MD
Departement de Biopathologie, Centre Leon
Berard, Lyon, France

TAKEHIKO YAMAGUCHI, MD, PhD
Professor, Department of
Pathology, Koshigaya Hospital,
Dokkyo Medical University, Koshigaya,
Saitama, Japan

YAXIA ZHANG, MD, PhD
Assistant Professor of Pathology, Lerner
College of Medicine, Robert J. Tomsich
Pathology & Laboratory Medicine Institute,
Cleveland Clinic, Cleveland, Ohio, USA

Contents

Bone-Forming Tumors   513

Yaxia Zhang and Andrew E. Rosenberg

> Bone-forming tumors are defined by neoplastic cells that differentiate along the lines of osteoblasts that deposit neoplastic bone. The morphology and biological spectrum of bone-forming tumors is broad, and their accurate diagnosis requires the careful correlation of their clinical, morphologic, and radiologic characteristics. Immunohistochemical and molecular analyses have an important role in select instances. At present, the identification of neoplastic bone largely depends on histologic analysis, which can be subjective. The major types of osteosarcoma are defined according to their morphology, origin within or on the surface of the bone, and their histologic grade.

Integrating Morphology and Genetics in the Diagnosis of Cartilage Tumors   537

Carlos E. de Andrea, Mikel San-Julian, and Judith V.M.G. Bovée

> Cartilage-forming tumors of bone are a heterogeneous group of tumors with different molecular mechanisms involved. Enchondromas are benign hyaline cartilage–forming tumors of medullary bone caused by mutations in *IDH1* or *IDH2*. Osteochondromas are benign cartilage-capped bony projections at the surface of bone. *IDH* mutations are also found in dedifferentiated and periosteal chondrosarcoma. A recurrent *HEY1-NCOA2* fusion characterizes mesenchymal chondrosarcoma. Molecular changes are increasingly used to improve diagnostic accuracy in chondrosarcomas. Detection of *IDH* mutations or *HEY1-NCOA2* fusions has already proved their immense value, especially on small biopsy specimens or in case of unusual presentation.

Giant Cell–Containing Tumors of Bone   553

Zsolt Orosz and Nicholas A. Athanasou

> Giant cell–containing tumors of bone are characterized morphologically by the presence of numerous osteoclastic giant cells. Correlation of clinical, radiologic, and laboratory findings is required for accurate histopathologic diagnosis and treatment of a giant cell–containing tumor of bone. In differential diagnosis, it is particularly important to note the age of the patient and the skeletal location of the lesion. This article considers the range of neoplastic and nonneoplastic lesions, which histologically contain numerous osteoclastic giant cells, and focuses on several lesions that frequently enter into the differential diagnosis.

Ewing Sarcoma, an Update on Molecular Pathology with Therapeutic Implications   575

Enrique de Alava

> Ewing sarcoma is a developmental tumor characterized by balanced chromosomal translocations and formation of new fusion genes. Despite the large amount of

knowledge regarding the molecular aspects obtained in the last few years, many questions still remain. This article focuses on research on the molecular pathology and possible developments in targeted therapies in this malignancy and discusses some related bottlenecks, as well as the possible role of pathologists, the availability of samples, the lack of appropriate animal models, and the resources needed to carry out preclinical and clinical research.

This article focuses on families of round cell sarcomas other than classical Ewing sarcomas. Until recently, these tumors were referred to as so-called Ewing-like tumors, as they morphologically resemble Ewing sarcomas but are negative for canonical fusion transcripts of Ewing sarcomas involving gene members of the ETS family of transcription factors. Clinicopathologic and molecular evidence has dramatically influenced the diagnostic approach of these tumors in recent years. Molecular data that support these sarcoma subtypes are biologically distinct from those of Ewing sarcomas, thereby advocating discarding the all-embracing and confusing terminology of "Ewing-like tumors."

The classification of vascular tumors of bone has been under debate over time. Vascular tumors in bone are rare, display highly overlapping morphology, and, therefore, are considered difficult by pathologists. Compared with their soft tissue counterparts, they are more often multifocal and sometimes behave more aggressively. Over the past decade, with the advent of next-generation sequencing, recurrent molecular alterations have been found in some of the entities. The integration of morphology and molecular changes has led to a better characterization of these separate entities.

Recent molecular investigations of chordoma show common expression of various receptor tyrosine kinases and activation of downstream signaling pathways contributing to tumor growth and progression. The transcription factor brachyury (also known as T) is important in notochord differentiation, and germline duplication of the gene is often found in familial chordomas. Nuclear expression of brachyury is consistent in chordoma and in benign notochordal cell tumor. Based on the molecular evidence, targeting of several kinds of molecular agents has been attempted for the treatment of uncontrolled chordomas and achieved partial response or stable condition in many cases.

Myoepithelial tumors (METs) of bone (BMETs) are a rare but distinct tumor entity. METs that are cytologically benign are termed myoepitheliomas; METs with malignant histologic features are called myoepithelial carcinomas. BMETs have a wide age range, may involve any part of the skeleton, and have a variable spindle cell and epithelioid morphology. Bone tumors to be considered in the differential diagnosis are discussed. Additional techniques are indispensable to correctly diagnose BMETs. By immunohistochemistry, BMETs often express cytokeratins and/or EMA together with S100, GFAP, or calponin. Half of BMETs harbor EWSR1 (or rare FUS) gene rearrangements with different gene partners.

Hematologic neoplasms that primarily present in bone are rare; this article describes the most common examples of hematologic tumors primarily presenting in bone, including plasma cell myeloma, solitary plasmacytoma of bone, primary non-Hodgkin lymphoma of bone, acute lymphoblastic leukemia/lymphoma, and Langerhans cell histiocytosis. The macroscopic and microscopic features, differential diagnosis, diagnostic workup, and prognosis of all these different entities are discussed, with special emphasis on common differential diagnosis.

The jaws combine several unique properties that mainly result from their distinct embryonic development and their role in providing anchorage for the teeth and their supporting structures. As a consequence, several bone-related lesions almost exclusively develop in the jaws (eg, osseous dysplasias, ossifying fibromas), have distinct clinical features (eg, osteosarcoma), or hardly ever occur at this location (eg, osteochondroma, enchondroma). The specific characteristics of these tumors and tumorlike lesions are outlined in this article.

Primary bone sarcomas represent extremely rare entities. The use of now abolished labels, such as malignant fibrous histiocytoma and hemangiopericytoma, has significantly hampered the chance of identifying specific entities. It is now accepted that a broad variety of mesenchymal malignancies most often arising on the soft tissue may actually present as primary bone lesions. A more accurate morphologic partition is justified based on availability of distinct therapeutic options. An integrated diagnostic approach represents the only way to achieve a correct classification. In consideration of the significant complexity, primary bone sarcomas should ideally be handled in the context of expert centers.

A number of nonneoplastic conditions can mimic tumors of bone. Some of the more common mimics of primary bone tumors include infectious, inflammatory, periosteal, and degenerative joint disease-associated lesions that produce tumorlike bone surface-based or intraosseous lesions. This article considers a spectrum of reactive and nonreactive processes including stress fracture, subchondral cysts, osteonecrosis, heterotopic ossification, osteomyelitis, sarcoidosis, and amyloidoma that can present in such a way that they are mistaken for a tumor arising primary in bone.

Maria Gnoli, Francesca Ponti, and Luca Sangiorgi

Tumor syndromes, including bone neoplasias, are genetic predisposing conditions characterized by the development of a pattern of malignancies within a family at an early age of onset. Occurrence of bilateral, multifocal, or metachronous neoplasias and specific histopathologic findings suggest a genetic predisposition syndrome. Additional clinical features not related to the neoplasia can be a hallmark of specific genetic syndromes. Mostly, those diseases have an autosomal dominant pattern of inheritance with variable percentage of penetrance. Some syndromic disorders with an increased tumor risk may show an autosomal recessive transmission or are related to somatic mosaicism. Many genetic tumor syndromes are known. This update is specifically focused on syndromes predisposing to osteosarcoma and chondrosarcoma.

SURGICAL PATHOLOGY CLINICS

THE CLINICS ARE AVAILABLE ONLINE!
Access your subscription at:
www.theclinics.com

Preface

Molecular Pathology of Bone Tumors: What Have We Learned and How Does It Affect Daily Practice?

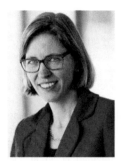

Judith V.M.G. Bovée, MD, PhD
Editor

Bone tumors are often found to be difficult by pathologists, because they are rare, and in total, almost 60 entities are recognized with considerable morphologic overlap. Similar to the classification of soft tissue tumors, the World Health Organization 2013 recognizes different categories: benign (n = 20), intermediate locally aggressive or rarely metastasizing (n = 10), and malignant (n = 28), and as such, the different bone tumor entities differ widely in treatment and outcome. In contrast to soft tissue tumors, immunohistochemistry is often of limited value, although in recent years some novel immunohistochemical markers have proven their value. On the other hand, radiologic information is imperative, as for some bone tumors it is not possible to render a definitive diagnosis without taking the exact localization in bone into account. The diagnosis of bone tumors, even more so than in soft tissue, therefore needs to be established in a multidisciplinary team.

Over the past two decades, an increasing amount of genetic data has become available, educating us about the mechanisms involved in the development of bone tumors. For instance, the recent discovery of *isocitrate dehydrogenase* gene mutations in enchondroma,[1,2] or *histone*

H3.3 gene mutations in giant cell tumor of bone and chondroblastoma,[3] has not only increased our knowledge on the role of epigenetic changes affecting differentiation in the development of bone tumors[4] but also provided us with novel molecular and surrogate immunohistochemical tools that can help us in the differential diagnosis.[5,6] As such, these molecular data are increasingly important for diagnosis and clinical decision making.

The routine decalcification of bone tumor specimens, which is essential for proper morphology that still remains the cornerstone of the diagnosis, poses a severe limitation when implementing routine molecular testing for bone tumors. Acid-based decalcification methods degrade the nucleic acids and thereby severely compromise molecular testing of bone tumors, causing a very high failure rate. It is therefore imperative that bone tumor labs keep part of the tissue frozen, or use EDTA-based decalcification methods.

This issue of *Surgical Pathology Clinics* is devoted to bone tumors and addresses diagnostic bone tumor subgroups that often pose difficulties to pathologists (ie, cartilage-forming, bone-forming, giant cell–containing, vascular,

Surgical Pathology 10 (2017) xiii–xiv
http://dx.doi.org/10.1016/j.path.2017.06.001
1875-9181/17/© 2017 Published by Elsevier Inc.

surgpath.theclinics.com

haematopoietic, and jaw tumors). There is considerable morphologic overlap between the different entities in these subgroups and the use of additional immunohistochemistry, and molecular diagnostics to aid in their distinction are discussed. At the molecular level, recent advances have been made in understanding the molecular background as well as in the identification of molecular targets for therapy in chordoma and Ewing sarcoma. Moreover, the group of rare round cell sarcomas other than classic *EWSR1*- or *FUS*-rearranged Ewing sarcoma was rapidly delineated with the advent of next-generation sequencing, and their workup using immunohistochemistry and molecular testing in daily practice is discussed. Several reactive and nonneoplastic processes can present primarily in bone in such a way that they pose diagnostic difficulties for the pathologist and can be mistaken for a primary bone neoplasm. In addition, articles are devoted to soft tissue sarcomas that very rarely present as a primary bone tumor, sometimes with specific histologic features (eg, myoepithelial tumors, pseudomyogenic hemangioendothelioma), and, when unaware, the pathologist can make a wrong diagnosis. Finally, with the advent of next-generation sequencing resulting in the detection of somatic but also possible germline variants, and with the recent elucidation that about half of the sarcoma patients have putatively pathogenic monogenic and polygenic variations in known and novel cancer genes in their germline,[7] it is imperative that pathologists are aware of this and that this information is included in multidisciplinary decision making. Thus, this issue of *Surgical Pathology Clinics* is meant to provide pathologists with state-of-the-art morphologic, immunohistochemical, and molecular tools to increase their diagnostic accuracy of bone tumor diagnosis.

Judith V.M.G. Bovée, MD, PhD
Professor
Department of Pathology
Leiden University Medical Center
PO Box 9600, L1-Q 2300 RC
Leiden, The Netherlands

E-mail address:
j.v.m.g.bovee@lumc.nl

REFERENCES

1. Pansuriya TC, van Eijk R, d'Adamo P, et al. Somatic mosaic IDH1 and IDH2 mutations are associated with enchondroma and spindle cell hemangioma in Ollier disease and Maffucci syndrome. Nat Genet 2011;43(12):1256–61.
2. Amary MF, Damato S, Halai D, et al. Ollier disease and Maffucci syndrome are caused by somatic mosaic mutations of IDH1 and IDH2. Nat Genet 2011;43:1262–5.
3. Behjati S, Tarpey PS, Presneau N, et al. Distinct H3F3A and H3F3B driver mutations define chondroblastoma and giant cell tumor of bone. Nat Genet 2013;45(12):1479–82.
4. Fang D, Gan H, Lee JH, et al. The histone H3.3K36M mutation reprograms the epigenome of chondroblastomas. Science 2016;352(6291):1344–8.
5. Amary MF, Berisha F, Mozela R, et al. The H3F3 K36M mutant antibody is a sensitive and specific marker for the diagnosis of chondroblastoma. Histopathology 2016;69(1):121–7.
6. Luke J, von Baer A, Schreiber J, et al. H3F3A mutation in giant cell tumour of the bone is detected by immunohistochemistry using a monoclonal antibody against the G34W mutated site of the histone H3.3 variant. Histopathology 2017;71(1):125–33.
7. Ballinger ML, Goode DL, Ray-Coquard I, et al. Monogenic and polygenic determinants of sarcoma risk: an international genetic study. Lancet Oncol 2016;17(9):1261–71.

Bone-Forming Tumors

Yaxia Zhang, MD, PhD[a], Andrew E. Rosenberg, MD[b],*

KEYWORDS

- Bone • Neoplasm • Osteoid osteoma • Osteoblastoma • Fibrous dysplasia • Osteosarcoma

---

Key points

1. Bone-forming tumors have a broad spectrum of biological behavior and morphology and their accurate diagnosis requires correlation of their clinical, pathologic, and radiological findings.

2. Benign bone-forming tumors are usually slow growing, well demarcated, and composed of cytologically benign cells that deposit neoplastic trabeculae of woven bone. These tumors have the potential to locally recur and are usually ablated or removed surgically by curettage or en bloc resection.

3. Malignant bone-forming tumors (ie, osteosarcomas) are usually rapidly growing, large, destructive neoplasms composed of malignant cells that at least focally deposit recognizable tumor bone. High-grade tumors are aggressive and need to be treated with systemic therapy, wide resection, and radiotherapy when indicated.

ABSTRACT

Bone-forming tumors are defined by neoplastic cells that differentiate along the lines of osteoblasts that deposit neoplastic bone. The morphology and biological spectrum of bone-forming tumors is broad, and their accurate diagnosis requires the careful correlation of their clinical, morphologic, and radiologic characteristics. Immunohistochemical and molecular analyses have an important role in select instances. At present, the identification of neoplastic bone largely depends on histologic analysis, which can be subjective. The major types of osteosarcoma are defined according to their morphology, origin within or on the surface of the bone, and their histologic grade.

OVERVIEW

Bone-forming tumors are defined as benign or malignant neoplasms in which the proliferating cells have an osteoblastic phenotype and manufacture and secrete the organic components of bone, which may or may not mineralize.[1] These tumors are heterogeneous and have a broad spectrum of biological behavior ranging from indolent to very aggressive with a rapidly fatal outcome. Their accurate diagnosis is critical to patient care and incorporates careful assessment of the clinical, radiological, and pathologic features; an incorrect diagnosis can result in significant mismanagement of the patient. At present, the identification of osteoblastic phenotype in surgical pathology is based on histologic analysis. Important lineage-specific molecules related to osteoblasts such as runt-related transcription factor 2 (RUNX2), Osterix, and special AT-rich sequence-binding protein 2 (SATB2) have been identified. Although these molecules are sensitive markers of osteoblastic differentiation, they are also expressed in nonosteoblastic neoplasms, therefore the immunohistochemical expression of these markers in neoplasms should be carefully assessed in the context of the morphology of the tumor.[2–4] Molecular analysis can be useful in select situations and requires tissue to be fixed and decalcified in a manner that does not degrade nucleic acids.

OSTEOID OSTEOMA

Osteoid osteoma is a benign, usually solitary, bone-forming tumor that by definition is 2 cm or less in diameter (Table 1). The neoplastic nature

---

Disclosures: The authors have no financial disclosures.
[a] Department of Pathology, Lerner College of Medicine, Robert J. Tomsich Pathology and Laboratory Medicine Institute, Cleveland Clinic, 9500 Euclid Avenue L25, Cleveland, OH 44195, USA; [b] Department of Pathology, Miller School of Medicine, University of Miami, 1400 Northwest 12th Avenue, Miami, FL 33136, USA
* Corresponding author.
E-mail address: Arosenberg@med.miami.edu

Surgical Pathology 10 (2017) 513–535
http://dx.doi.org/10.1016/j.path.2017.04.006
1875-9181/17/© 2017 Elsevier Inc. All rights reserved.

surgpath.theclinics.com

Table 1
Key points of osteoid osteoma and osteoblastoma

Osteoid Osteoma	Osteoblastoma
• Incidence: accounts for 13% of all primary benign bone tumors	• Uncommon; accounts for 1% of primary bone tumors
• Small size; <2 cm	• Larger tumor; >2 cm
• Limited growth potential	• Locally aggressive
• Severe localized pain often worse at night, relieved by aspirin or other nonsteroidal antiinflammatory medication	• Constant achy pain
• Imaging: well-defined, round, lucent tumor surrounded by zone of sclerosis	• Expansile, well-defined, oval, mixed lytic and blastic mass
• Radiofrequency ablation is treatment of choice	• Curettage or en bloc excision

of osteoid osteoma has been questioned because of its limited growth potential; however, cytogenetic studies have shown aberration of chromosome 22q, which supports the concept that the lesion is neoplastic.[5]

Osteoid osteoma accounts for approximately 10% to 12% of benign bone tumors and 3% of all primary bone tumors.[6] It most commonly develops in individuals 5 to 25 years of age, has a peak incidence in the second decade of life, and there is a male predominance of 2:1 to 3:1. Osteoid osteoma can arise in any bone in the body, but most commonly develops in the long bones of the lower extremities, with the femoral neck being the single most frequent anatomic site.

Clinically, patients typically complain of severe localized pain that is often worse at night and that is relieved by aspirin or other nonsteroidal antiinflammatory medications. Patients with lesions located close to or within joints can present with joint pain, swelling, and effusions, mimicking a primary intra-articular process. Tumors located in the vertebral column can cause painful scoliosis secondary to paravertebral muscle spasm, whereas lesions of the small bones of the hands and feet may produce soft tissue swelling, mimicking infection.

On roentgenograms the lesion is usually round to oval, 1 to 2 cm in diameter, and has a targetoid appearance. The tumor shows avid uptake of technetium and computed tomography (CT) shows a well-circumscribed, lucent mass with central mineralization that is usually surrounded by a zone of sclerosis (Fig. 1). Significant surrounding bone marrow edema can be seen on fluid-sensitive MRI sequences. Technetium bone scan, CT, and MRI studies are very important in localizing intra-articular tumors and those obscured by abundant reactive bone.[7]

Grossly, osteoid osteomas are small, round to oval, sharply demarcated, gritty, and dark red

with central tan-white speckled areas (Fig. 2). On histology, the well-circumscribed tumor is composed of haphazard, interanastomosing trabeculae and sheetlike aggregates of woven bone that are rimmed prominently by plump, metabolically active osteoblasts (Fig. 3). The stroma filling the intertrabecular spaces is composed of richly vascularized loose connective tissue containing fibroblasts and thin-walled, congested blood vessels. Osteoclasts are frequently scattered along the bony surfaces. Juxta-articular or intra-articular osteoid osteomas may be associated with a periosteal reaction and chronic synovitis that contains lymphoid follicles resembling rheumatoid arthritis.[8] The proliferating osteoblasts in osteoid osteoma show strong nuclear staining for Runx2 and Osterix.[2]

In the past, osteoid osteoma was frequently removed by curettage or en bloc resection; however, radiofrequency ablation is now the treatment of choice except for tumors that are in close proximity to crucial structures such as the spinal cord or articular cartilage. Minimally invasive techniques such as CT-guided core drill excision, cryoablation, and laser photocoagulation are other forms of effective therapy. The cure rate for osteoid osteoma varies according to technique but ranges from 80% to 90%.

OSTEOBLASTOMA

Osteoblastoma is histologically similar to osteoid osteoma but has greater growth potential and is more locally aggressive (see Table 1). The tumor is larger than 2 cm and commonly originates in the posterior elements of the spine, sacrum, mandible, and the metadiaphyseal region of the long tubular bones. Few cytogenetic abnormalities have been identified but they include a unique 3-way translocation involving

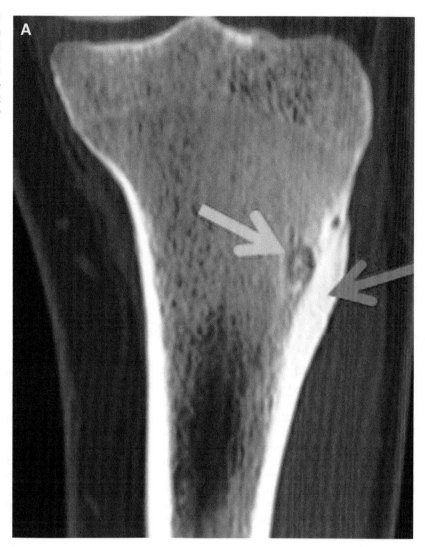

Fig. 1. (*A*) Coronal and (*B*) axial CT of the left tibia shows the small, round osteoid osteoma, which is lucent with central mineralization (*orange arrow*) with adjacent cortical thickening (*blue arrow*).

chromosomes 1, 2, and 14; a balanced translocation involving chromosomes 4,7, and 14; rearrangement of 1q42; and homozygous deletions of chromosome band 22q12.[9–11]

Osteoblastoma is uncommon and accounts for 1% of primary bone tumors. It affects young adults in the second to fourth decade of life, and occurs in men approximately twice as frequently as in women. Progressive pain is the most common symptom, and unlike osteoid osteoma the pain is constant, and insensitive to aspirin and related analgesics. Tumors in the spine can cause back pain, neurologic dysfunction, and scoliosis, whereas tumors in the craniofacial bones can lead to headache, tooth impaction, and epistaxis.

Radiographically, osteoblastoma often presents as a well-defined, mixed lytic and blastic mass with sclerotic margins, and may cause bone expansion (**Fig. 4**A). The tumor shows avid uptake on technetium scans and CT and MRI imaging reveals a well-circumscribed heterogeneous mass that may have cystic components and is surrounded by edema and reactive bone (see **Fig. 4**B). Some tumors are large and have more poorly defined margins, causing them to mimic more aggressive neoplasms.

Grossly, osteoblastoma is dark red, tan-white, and gritty. In most cases, the tumor ranges from 2 to 5 cm in diameter but some tumors are larger than 10 cm. Cystic changes (aneurysmal bone cyst–like) are present in approximately 10% of tumors. Microscopically, osteoblastoma is composed of haphazardly deposited trabeculae or sheets of woven bone rimmed by osteoblasts and scattered osteoclasts that are enmeshed in a richly vascular stroma (**Fig. 5**). The osteoblasts

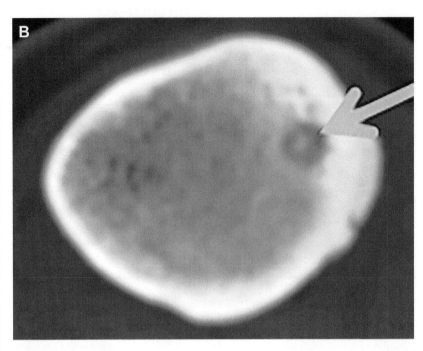

Fig. 1. (*continued*).

in conventional tumors are ovoid or round with eccentric nuclei and moderate amounts of eosinophilic or amphophilic cytoplasm. Mitoses may be present but are of normal structure and necrosis is usually absent, unless there has been pathologic fracture. Large expansile lesions usually have secondary aneurysmal bone cyst–like changes with multiple cystic blood-filled cavities. Rarely, hyaline cartilage is a component of the matrix and its presence is a diagnostic pitfall for osteosarcoma. Epithelioid osteoblastoma, previously known as aggressive osteoblastoma, is characterized by large epithelioid osteoblasts that have abundant eosinophilic cytoplasm and nuclei that are vesicular and contain prominent nucleoli (**Fig. 6**). A minority of epithelioid osteoblastomas are multinodular, consisting of a group of separate aggregates of tumor, and this configuration may simulate the infiltrative growth pattern present in osteosarcoma.[12] Rarely, osteoblastoma contains cells with enlarged hyperchromatic nuclei that are hypothesized to be degenerative and this

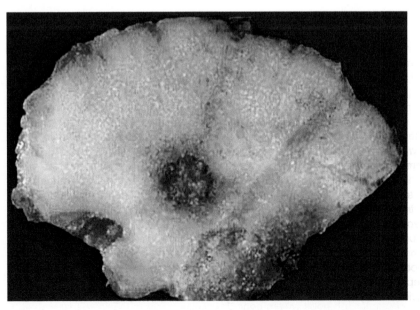

Fig. 2. Osteoid osteoma. A small, round, red-tan osteoid osteoma is centered in the outer cortex. Note the abundant adjacent reactive bone that thickens the involved cortex and partially fills the medullary cavity.

Fig. 3. (*A*, *B*) Resected osteoid osteoma shows a well-demarcated small round tumor surrounded by reactive bone. The tumor is composed of haphazardly interconnecting trabeculae of woven bone lined by plump osteoblasts.

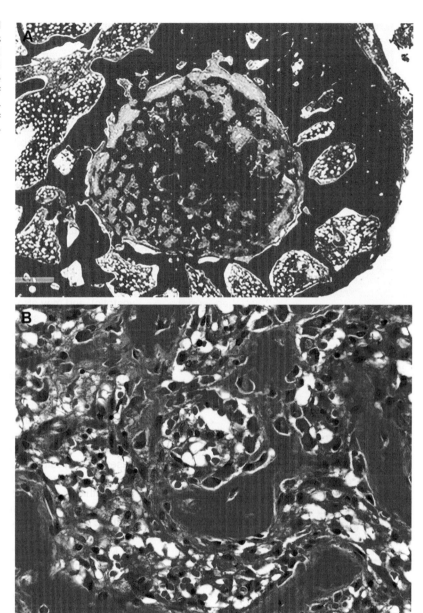

variant is known as pseudomalignant osteoblastoma. This finding has no clinical significance except that it may cause histologic confusion with osteosarcoma. High beta-catenin protein expression has been detected in osteoblastoma, which is not specific.

The treatment of osteoblastoma is either aggressive curettage with adjuvants or en bloc resection and the strategy depends on the size and location of the mass. The prognosis is based on completeness of the resection; curettage is associated with a local recurrence rate of approximately 20%. Factors reported to be associated with aggressive behavior include secondary aneurysmal bone cyst–like changes and incomplete removal. Malignant transformation of osteoblastoma to osteosarcoma is exceptionally rare.

FIBROUS DYSPLASIA

Fibrous dysplasia is a benign tumor composed of fibroblastlike spindle cells associated with scattered trabeculae of curvilinear woven bone that lacks conspicuous osteoblastic rimming. Fibrous dysplasia is caused by a missense mutation in the GNAS gene located on chromosome 20q13, which contains the genetic code for the guanine nucleotide-binding protein (G protein). In bone,

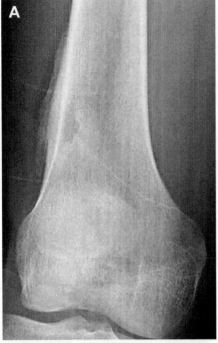

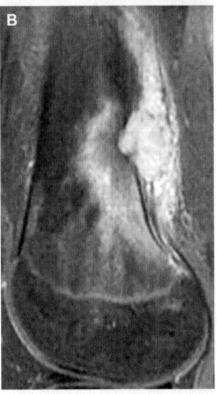

Fig. 4. (A) Radiograph of osteoblastoma manifesting as a well-circumscribed irregular lytic tumor associated with a periosteal reaction and sclerotic margin. (B) Sagittal T1 fat-saturated postcontrast image shows the oval bright tumor surrounded by edema and reactive changes.

this abnormality causes proliferation of osteoprogenitor cells and inhibits their differentiation, which results in an overproduction of fibro-osseous tissue and the bone is usually woven in architecture. Other cytogenetic structural alterations involving chromosomes 3, 8, 10, and 15 have been documented as well, and this suggests that fibrous dysplasia is neoplastic with a predisposition to somatic mutations of bone-forming mesenchymal tissue.[13,14]

The precise incidence of fibrous dysplasia is difficult to establish with certainty because many lesions are asymptomatic; however, it is estimated that it accounts for 5% to 7% of benign bone tumors. The tumors typically develop during childhood but are often not recognized until early adulthood or midadulthood and infrequently in the elderly. Fibrous dysplasia may involve a single bone (monostotic), or several or many bones (polyostotic), and may also be associated with abnormalities of the skin and endocrine glands. Monostotic solitary bone lesions are the most common clinical expression, and account for 70% to 80% of cases. In monostotic disease the tumor involves the craniofacial bones, ribs, femur, tibia, and humerus in decreasing order of frequency. Polyostotic lesions may be monomelic or polymelic in distribution. Polyostotic fibrous dysplasia without endocrine dysfunction accounts for 20% to 30% of all cases. About 2% to 3% of cases of polyostotic fibrous dysplasia is associated with café-au-lait skin pigmentation and endocrinopathies, a triad known as the McCune-Albright syndrome. A minority of patients with polyostotic disease develop multiple soft tissue myxomas; this combination of abnormalities is known as Mazabraud syndrome and is also more common in women.

Radiographically, fibrous dysplasia has a classic ground-glass appearance but can be radiolucent or radiodense, depending on the amount of bone present and its degree of mineralization. In the appendicular skeleton, the margins of the lesion are usually well defined and surrounded by a rim of sclerotic bone (Fig. 7). Fibrous dysplasia of the craniofacial skeleton seems to be less well defined and blends with the surrounding bone (Fig. 8). Extensive involvement causes bony expansion and sometimes severe deformity of the affected bone.

Grossly, fibrous dysplasia is well circumscribed, tan-white, and has a gritty and leatherlike consistency. Occasionally, it contains cystic areas, which may occupy a small or large portion of the lesion. In a minority of instances nodules of pearly white cartilage are present. Microscopically, fibrous dysplasia is composed of cellular fibrous tissue

Fig. 5. (*A, B*) Osteoblastoma has well-demarcated margins and is surrounded by preexisting and reactive bone. The tumor is composed of interconnecting trabeculae of woven bone rimmed by prominent plump osteoblasts. The intertrabecular space is filled with loose fibrovascular tissue.

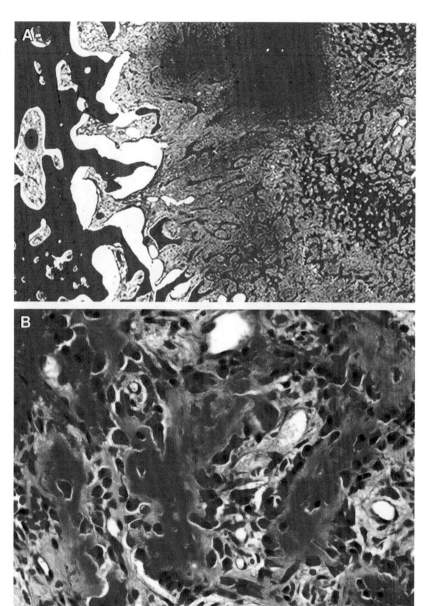

surrounding irregular, curvilinear bony trabeculae (**Fig. 9**A). The trabeculae are discontinuous and formed directly from the adjacent spindle cells because there is minimal osteoblastic rimming; however, osteoclasts may be numerous. In some tumors the bone is abundant and interconnecting, and in craniofacial tumors the lesional bone tends to fuse with the surrounding host cancellous bone, explaining the lack of demarcation radiographically. The fibrous tissue is composed of cytologically banal, plump spindle cells that lack atypia and show few mitotic figures. The spindle cells are associated with collagen fibers and are usually arranged in a storiform pattern, especially in areas devoid of bone. Some tumors have regions with very little bone; others cases have stroma that is focally myxoid in appearance and still others have collections of foamy histiocytes, thus mimicking a xanthoma or a fibroxanthoma. The collagen fibers in the stroma (Sharpey-like fibers) frequently merge with the collagen framework of the lesional trabecular bone (see **Fig. 9**B). Cellular nodules of hyaline cartilage that can resemble growth plate cartilage are present in approximately 20% of cases. Matrix resembling cementum may be found in lesions of the

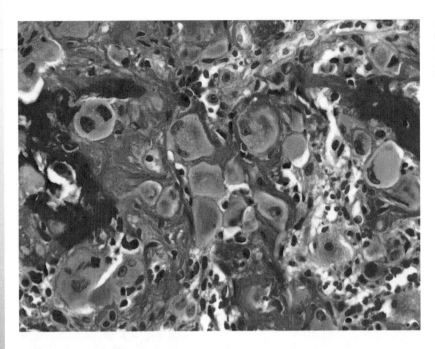

Fig. 6. Epithelioid (so-called aggressive) osteoblastoma is characterized by large epithelioid osteoblasts.

craniofacial skeleton and less frequently in the bones of the extremities. Aneurysmal bone cyst–like changes are occasionally encountered, and may be prominent.

The treatment of fibrous dysplasia depends on the extent and severity of the disease and the problems caused by individual lesions. Therapy ranges from observation to surgical removal. Medical treatment with drugs such as bisphosphonates can be helpful.

The differential diagnosis of fibrous dysplasia includes desmoplastic fibroma, osteofibrous dysplasia, and well-differentiated intramedullary osteosarcoma (Table 2).

OSTEOSARCOMA

Osteosarcoma is defined as a sarcoma that arises within or on the surface of bone in which the neoplastic cells have an osteoblastic phenotype and deposit neoplastic bone. It represents a group of heterogeneous lesions that have a wide spectrum of morphology and clinical behavior. High-grade osteosarcoma shows numerous complex genetic alterations that are a result of chromothripsis and kataegis.[15] However, cytogenetic aberrations have proved to be of little importance in understanding the molecular pathogenesis of these tumors and predicting their prognosis.[16,17] In contrast, low-grade surface and central osteosarcomas have a simple genetic profile with

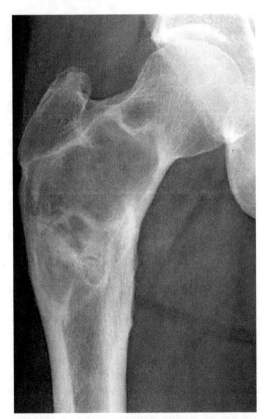

Fig. 7. Fibrous dysplasia of the proximal femur presents as a well-circumscribed tumor with sclerotic margins. The tumor has a ground glass–like appearance with areas of increased radiodensity.

Fig. 8. Coronal CT scan of polyostotic fibrous dysplasia involving the craniofacial skeleton showing multiple expansile ground-glass lesions that merge with the adjacent bone.

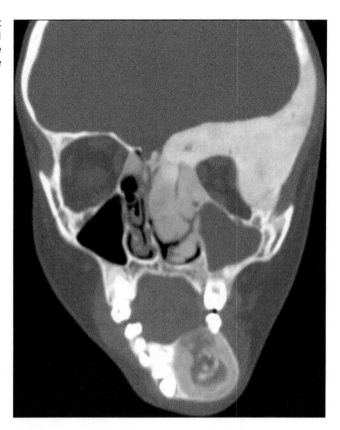

supernumerary ring chromosomes involving chromosome 12q13 to 12q15, resulting in gain or amplification of *MDM2* and *CDK4* genes so this finding is useful for diagnostic purposes.[18–20]

Osteosarcoma accounts for approximately 20% of all primary malignant bone tumors, with 1000 to 1500 new cases diagnosed annually in the United States. The age distribution is bimodal, with the first peak occurring in 10-year-old to 14-year-old age group and the second peak developing during midadulthood to late adulthood. Men are affected more frequently than women at a ratio of 1.3:1 to 1.6:1, with equal distribution among races. Any bone of the body can be affected but almost all originate in the long bones of the appendicular skeleton, especially in the distal femur, followed by the proximal tibia and proximal humerus; these sites contain the most proliferative growth plates. In the long bones, the tumor is most frequently centered in the metaphysis (90%), infrequently in the diaphysis (9%), and rarely in the epiphysis.

Osteosarcoma is classified according to a variety of characteristics, including its histologic features, biological potential (grade), relationship to the bone of origin (surface or intramedullary), multiplicity (solitary and multifocal), and the state of the underlying bone (primary or secondary). Most osteosarcomas can be categorized into 3 major groups (**Table 3**): (1) conventional intramedullary osteosarcoma and its histologic subtypes; (2) intramedullary well-differentiated osteosarcoma; and (3) surface osteosarcomas (parosteal, periosteal, and high-grade surface osteosarcoma).

CONVENTIONAL OSTEOSARCOMA AND ITS HISTOLOGIC SUBTYPES

Conventional or garden variety osteosarcoma is solitary, arises in the medullary cavity of an otherwise normal bone, is high grade, and produces neoplastic bone with or without cartilaginous or fibroblastic components. Approximately 75% to 80% of osteosarcomas are of the conventional type. It typically manifests as a progressively enlarging, painful mass. The pain is deep seated, boring in nature, frequently noted months before diagnosis, and usually increases in intensity over time, eventually producing unremitting discomfort. The overlying skin may be warm, erythematous, edematous, and cartographed by prominent engorged veins. Large tumors restrict range of motion; decrease musculoskeletal function; produce

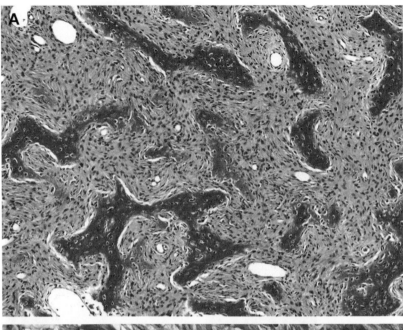

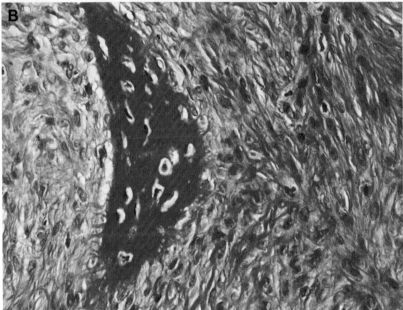

Fig. 9. (A, B) Curvilinear trabeculae of woven bone surrounded by spindle cells characterize fibrous dysplasia. The woven bone has inconspicuous osteoblastic rimming with collagen fibers of the stroma merging into the bone matrix.

joint effusions; and, in far advanced cases, result in weight loss and cachexia. In 5% to 10% of cases, the heralding event is a sudden, devastating, pathologic fracture through the destructive mass.

On plain films, conventional tumors present as large, destructive, poorly defined, mixed lytic and blastic masses that transgress the cortex and form large soft tissue masses that may be circumferential (Fig. 10). In some cases, the tumor is entirely lytic, which is often seen in the telangiectatic variant; in others it is diffusely mineralized, producing a densely sclerotic mass. The periphery of the lesion is usually the least mineralized, and soft tissue components may have a fine cloudlike pattern of radiodensity. Osteosarcoma is frequently situated eccentrically within the medullary cavity and its largest dimension parallels the long axis of the underlying bone. As the enlarging

Table 2 Differential diagnosis of fibrous dysplasia	
Fibrous Dysplasia vs	**Helpful Distinguishing Features**
Desmoplastic fibroma	1. Spindle cells are arranged in broad fascicles and not a storiform pattern 2. Bone formation is not a component
Osteofibrous dysplasia	1. Arises in the anterior cortex of the tibia and fibula rather than the medullary cavity 2. Prominent osteoblastic rimming of the lesional bone
Low-grade intramedullary osteosarcoma	1. Infiltrative growth pattern encasing preexisting trabeculae of bone 2. Amplification of MDM2, which can be detected by fluorescent in situ hybridization 3. No GNAS mutation

Table 3 Classification of osteosarcoma	
Conventional osteosarcoma and histologic subtypes	1. Conventional osteosarcoma (osteoblastic, chondroblastic, fibroblastic) 2. Telangiectatic osteosarcoma 3. Small cell osteosarcoma 4. Giant cell–rich osteosarcoma 5. Osteoblastomalike osteosarcoma
Intramedullary well-differentiated osteosarcoma	1. Intramedullary well-differentiated osteosarcoma
Surface osteosarcomas	1. Parosteal osteosarcoma (well-differentiated juxtacortical osteosarcoma) 2. Periosteal osteosarcoma (intermediate-grade, chondroblastic osteosarcoma) 3. High-grade surface osteosarcoma (high-grade osteoblastic osteosarcoma)

mass destroys and permeates the cortex, it mechanically elevates the periosteum, producing reactive bone in the form of the Codman triangle at the proximal and distal extent of the tumor, as well as a sunburst or onion skin–like pattern of periosteal bone formation along the bulk of its length. Conventional osteosarcoma is heterogeneous on CT and MRI, and these modalities provide valuable information regarding the overall dimensions of the tumor, its extent within the medullary cavity and soft tissue, and its relationship to important neighboring anatomic structures. This information is vital to planning successful limb salvage surgical resection.

Grossly, conventional osteosarcoma is a large, metaphyseal, intramedullary, hemorrhagic, tan-gray-white, and gritty mass (**Fig. 11**). Tumors containing abundant mineralized bone are diffusely tan-white and hard, and nonmineralized cartilaginous components are glistening, gray, and may be mucinous if the matrix is myxoid or rubbery if it is hyaline, and fibrous areas are pink-tan and leathery. Regions of hemorrhage and cystic change are common and, when extensive, produce a friable, bloody, and spongy mass (telangiectatic osteosarcoma) (**Fig. 12**). Intramedullary involvement is often considerable, and the tumor

usually destroys the overlying cortex and forms an eccentric or circumferential soft tissue component. The dislodged periosteum becomes a sharp interface between the mass and the bordering skeletal muscle and fat and may deposit reactive woven bone. Growth into the joint space, which in some cases may be associated with the tumor coating peripheral portions of the articular cartilage, follows pathways offering least resistance to spread: beneath the synovium via extension along the cortical surface, or through tendinous-ligamentous and joint capsule insertion sites.

Microscopically, high-grade osteosarcoma grows with a permeative pattern, replacing the marrow space, surrounding and eroding preexisting bony trabeculae, and filling and expanding haversian systems (**Fig. 13**). Soft tissue components lift and displace the periosteum, which deposits reactive woven bone in its wake. The conventional type is subclassified into osteoblastic, chondroblastic, fibroblastic, and mixed types, depending on the predominance of the neoplastic component. In osteoblastic foci, the malignant cells have an osteoblastic phenotype and are large, pleomorphic, and polyhedral or spindle-

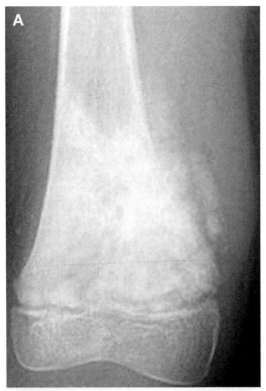

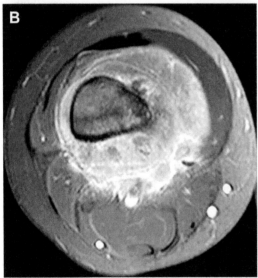

Fig. 10. (*A*) This conventional osteosarcoma manifests on radiograph as a poorly defined mixed blastic and lytic tumor centered in the distal femoral metaphysis. The tumor extends into the adjacent soft tissues and the soft tissue component has a fine cloudlike pattern of radiodensity. (*B*) In this T1-weighted fat-saturated image of osteosarcoma the tumor fills the medullary cavity and forms a large, circumferential soft tissue mass.

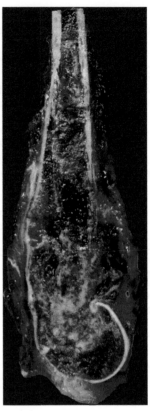

Fig. 11. Hemorrhagic red-tan osteosarcoma fills the medullary cavity, destroys areas of the cortex, and extends into the soft tissues.

shaped (**Fig. 14**). The nuclei are hyperchromatic, central or eccentric in position, and may contain prominent nucleoli. The cytoplasm is eosinophilic with a volume that correlates with cell size. The tumor cells are intimately related to the surfaces of the neoplastic bone, and, as the matrix surrounds and imprisons them, they become smaller and appear less atypical; this phenomenon is known as normalization. The neoplastic bone is woven in architecture; varies in quantity; and is deposited as primitive, disorganized trabeculae that produce a coarse, lacelike pattern or large, broad sheets fashioned by coalescing trabeculae, as seen in the sclerosing variant. Depending on its state of mineralization, the bone is eosinophilic or basophilic and may have a pagetoid appearance caused by haphazardly deposited cement lines. Neoplastic cartilage, when present, is usually hyaline but may be predominately myxoid, particularly in tumors arising in jaw bones. The malignant chondrocytes show severe cytologic atypia and reside in lacunar spaces in hyaline matrix, or float singly or in cords in myxoid matrix (**Fig. 15**). Fibroblastic foci manifest as cytologically malignant

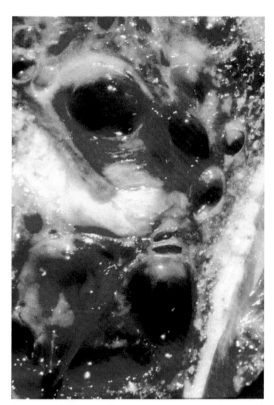

Fig. 12. Telangiectatic osteosarcoma contains multiple cystic spaces that are often filled with blood.

spindle cells arranged in herringbone or storiform patterns. The degree of atypia is variable, but is frequently severe. Mitoses are numerous and structurally abnormal forms are common.

Fig. 13. Osteosarcoma permeates the medullary cavity and cortex and extends into the soft tissues.

Telangiectatic osteosarcoma is a high-grade tumor that is lytic on radiographs and contains numerous blood-filled cystic spaces that comprise greater than 75% of the tumor. The cyst walls contain and are lined by malignant cells that produce variable amounts of neoplastic matrix (**Fig. 16**). Telangiectatic osteosarcoma is more sensitive to neoadjuvant chemotherapy and as a result may have a better prognosis, with patients having survival rates of 60% at 10 years.[21]

Small cell osteosarcoma is a microscopic variant of high-grade osteosarcoma characterized by a monotonous proliferation of malignant small cells that deposit bone matrix. The clinical and radiographic features are similar to those of conventional osteosarcoma. Microscopically, the tumor cells are round to oval with fine to coarse chromatin. Lacelike osteoid production is always present. Immunohistochemically the tumor cells may be positive for CD99 but often lack FLI-1 immunoreactivity, a marker that is useful in distinguishing the tumor from Ewing sarcoma.[22] Unlike Ewing sarcoma, small cell osteosarcoma expresses SATB2 and does not have translocation of EWSR1 or other genes associated with Ewing sarcoma.[23]

Giant cell–rich osteosarcoma accounts for approximately 3% of all osteosarcoma. As the name implies, the hallmark of this variant is numerous nonneoplastic, osteoclast-type giant cells scattered throughout the tumor (**Fig. 17**). Their presence can cause confusion with giant cell tumor of bone and other osteoclast-rich neoplasms. Mutation analysis of the H3F3A gene

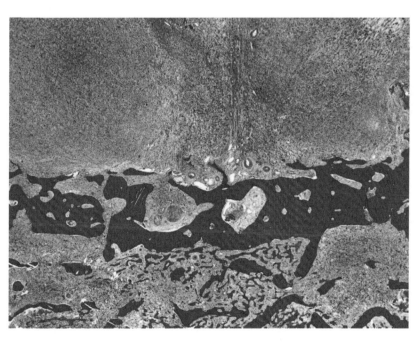

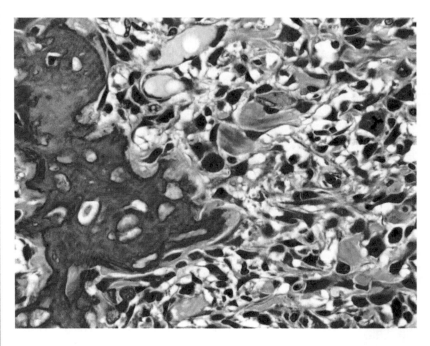

Fig. 14. Osteoblastic osteosarcoma is characterized by malignant cells intimately associated with coarse lacelike neoplastic bone.

can be used as a diagnostic tool because giant cell osteosarcoma does not have a mutation in this gene that is present in giant cell tumor of bone.[24]

Osteoblastomalike osteosarcoma is rare and histologically the tumor cells may be deceptively banal and rim the neoplastic bony trabeculae in a fashion that mimics osteoblastoma. Features that permit its distinction from osteoblastoma are the permeative growth pattern and solid cellular intertrabecular tissue that are found in osteosarcoma.

INTRAMEDULLARY WELL-DIFFERENTIATED OSTEOSARCOMA

Intramedullary well-differentiated osteosarcoma is a distinct form of osteosarcoma characterized by its comparatively indolent course, deceptively benign cytologic features, and the presence of well-formed tumor bone. It is uncommon and represents only 1% of all osteosarcomas. Most develop during the second to fifth decades of

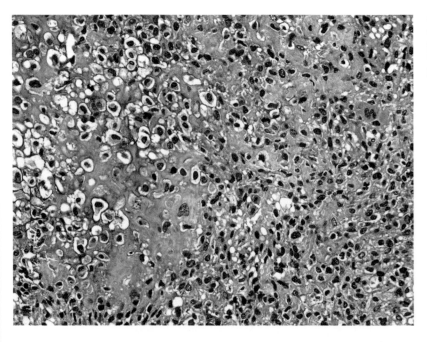

Fig. 15. Chondroblastic osteosarcoma shows high-grade malignant cartilage that merges with eosinophilic neoplastic bone.

Fig. 16. Cyst wall of telangiectatic osteosarcoma contains malignant tumor cells associated with neoplastic matrix.

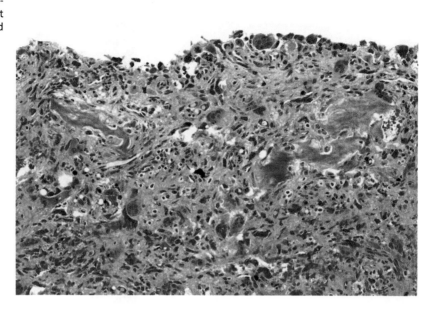

life, and almost 50% of affected individuals are in their 20s at the time of diagnosis.[25,26] Patients usually present with localized pain of variable duration, or a palpable mass. Intramedullary, well-differentiated osteosarcomas have heterogeneous radiographic findings, and are variably lytic or radiodense. The tumors usually have poorly demarcated margins, and may expand the underlying bone with little periosteal reaction (**Fig. 18**). Soft tissue extension may be present and is usually small in relation to the extent of intramedullary involvement. Intramedullary well-differentiated osteosarcoma usually arises in the metaphyseal-diaphyseal region and is centered in the medullary cavity. The tumor is hard, gritty, and tan-white, and has poorly defined margins

Fig. 17. The presence of numerous multinucleated osteoclast-type giant cells characterizes the giant cell–rich variant of osteosarcoma.

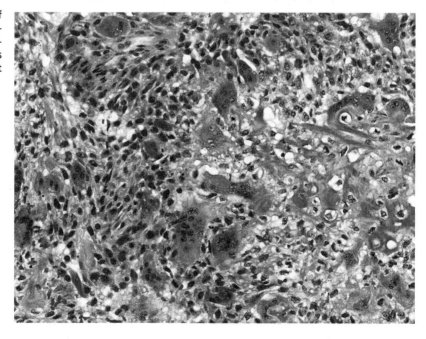

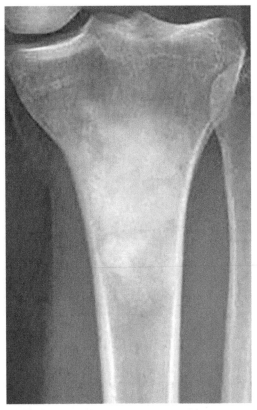

Fig. 18. Well-differentiated intramedullary osteosarcoma of the proximal tibia appears as an irregular radiodense mass within the medullary cavity.

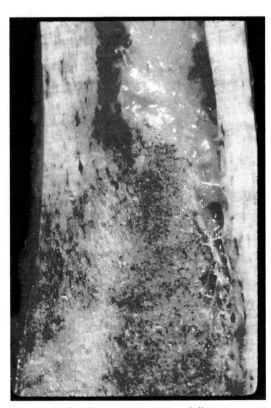

Fig. 19. Well-differentiated intramedullary osteosarcoma is hard, tan-white, and infiltrates the cortex and medullary cavity.

(Fig. 19). Microscopically, it is composed of a mild to moderately cellular cytologically bland spindle cells that are intimately associated with long trabeculae or round islands of woven bone, which may have a pagetoid appearance (Fig. 20). Unlike fibrous dysplasia, which it may resemble, the tumor grows with an infiltrative pattern, replacing the marrow space and surrounding preexisting bony trabeculae that serve as scaffolding for the deposition of tumor bone (see Fig. 20). Immunohistochemistry for the detection of MDM2 and CDK4 and fluorescence in situ hybridization for amplification of MDM2 can help distinguish it from other benign fibro-osseous tumors. The treatment of choice is wide excision. The prognosis is very good and approaches 90%. High-grade transformation or dedifferentiation occurs in 10% to 26% of cases and it is this phenomenon that is responsible for most cases that develop metastases.

SURFACE OSTEOSARCOMAS

Surface osteosarcomas originate and grow predominantly on the surface of bone and are divided into 2 main categories: well-differentiated juxtacortical osteosarcoma (parosteal) and biologically high-grade juxtacortical osteosarcomas (periosteal and high-grade surface). Occasionally, parosteal osteosarcoma dedifferentiates into a high-grade tumor.

Parosteal osteosarcoma usually arises during the third decade of life, whereas juxtacortical, intermediate-grade, chondroblastic osteosarcoma (periosteal osteosarcoma) and high-grade, osteoblastic osteosarcoma (high-grade surface osteosarcoma) commonly develop in the second decade of life. Parosteal and periosteal osteosarcomas have a predilection for women, whereas high-grade surface osteosarcomas more frequently affect men. Parosteal osteosarcoma is most commonly based on the posterior femoral cortex in the metaphyseal-diaphyseal area of the popliteal region, followed by the metaphyseal-diaphyseal zone of the proximal tibia (Fig. 21). Periosteal osteosarcoma originates from the cortex of the diaphysis or metaphysis of the tibia, followed in frequency by the femur. High-grade surface osteosarcoma arises on the metaphyseal surface of long bones in a distribution similar to conventional

Fig. 20. (*A, B*) Well-differentiated intramedullary osteosarcoma permeates the cortex and medullary cavity. The tumor is composed of trabeculae of woven bone surrounded by fascicles of minimally atypical spindle cells.

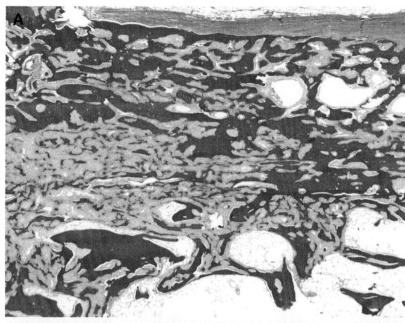

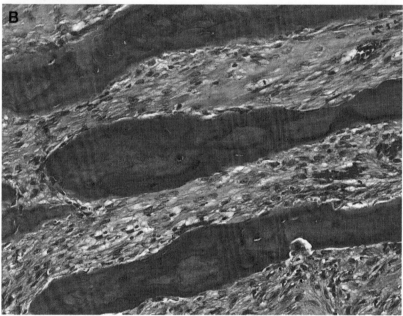

osteosarcoma and most frequently involves the distal femur and proximal humerus.

Clinically, surface osteosarcoma may or may not be associated with pain but usually presents as an enlarging, fixed, firm mass. The low-grade variant is slow growing, may be painless, and is frequently of long duration. The authors have seen some cases in which the neoplasm is discovered incidentally. Surface osteosarcomas have a broad base of attachment to the underlying cortex.

Parosteal tumors may be circumferential or mushroom shaped and are usually densely mineralized. They may have radiolucent areas or a lobular contour with little or no periosteal reaction. A radiolucent line separating the base of the tumor from the adjacent cortex is sometimes present. Periosteal osteosarcomas are fusiform, predominately lucent, and frequently associated with a periosteal reaction in the form of a Codman triangle and perpendicular linear striae that radiate from the

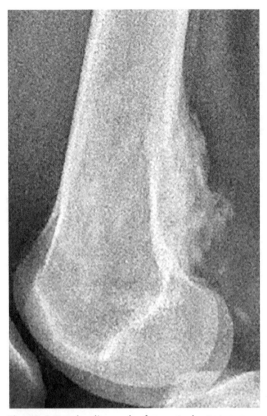

Fig. 21. Lateral radiograph of parosteal osteosarcoma showing an irregular elongate radiodense mass on the posterior cortex of the distal femur.

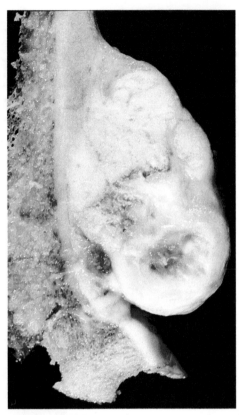

Fig. 22. Resected parosteal osteosarcoma from the distal femur appears as a hard, solid, tan-white mass.

underlying bone. High-grade surface osteosarcoma is similar in appearance to periosteal osteosarcoma but, in addition, tends to have fine, cloudlike areas of radiopacity. CT is helpful in assessing invasion of the cortex and medullary canal. MRI facilitates the identification of cartilage, which may be in the form of a peripheral cap in parosteal osteosarcoma or scattered throughout the mass in cases of periosteal or high-grade surface osteosarcoma.

Grossly, surface osteosarcomas are broad based, rigidly attached to the underlying cortex, and usually well demarcated from the neighboring soft tissues. Well-differentiated juxtacortical tumors are solid, tan-white, hard, and gritty and may have a gray, firm, glistening, hyaline cartilage cap or areas that are softer and fish flesh–like, representing fibrosarcomatous elements (**Fig. 22**). High-grade juxtacortical osteosarcomas (periosteal and high-grade surface) may be dominated by cartilaginous tissue or composed of hard, tan-white areas admixed with fish flesh–like regions. Destruction of the underlying cortex and invasion into the medullary canal is usually absent and,

when present, is often limited. If medullary cavity invasion is extensive, it is difficult, and sometime impossible, to distinguish an intramedullary tumor with an eccentric soft tissue component from a surface neoplasm with extensive invasion of the medullary canal.

Microscopically, parosteal osteosarcoma is distinguished by the presence of well-formed, long, linear trabeculae of woven bone, surrounded by a mildly to moderately cellular spindle cell proliferation enmeshed in a collagenous stroma (**Fig. 23**). The spindle cells have elongate nuclei with pointed ends and show limited degrees of cytologic atypia. In the deceptively bland-appearing cases, the nuclei have finely stippled chromatin, small nucleoli, poorly defined eosinophilic cytoplasm, and few mitoses, thus resembling fibromatosis. The spindle cells are often oriented in fascicles that parallel the direction of the neoplastic trabeculae (**Fig. 24**); in areas in which bone is not present the spindle cells may be arranged in a herringbone pattern. Malignant cartilage is sometimes a component of parosteal osteosarcoma and, when present,

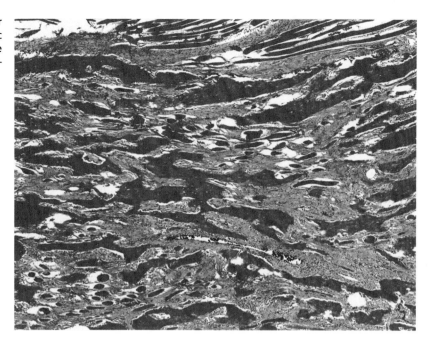

Fig. 23. Long linear trabeculae of neoplastic woven bone are commonly found in parosteal osteosarcoma.

has a hyaline matrix, contains mildly to moderately atypical chondrocytes, and grows as a cap covering the periphery of the tumor (**Fig. 25**). The cartilage can undergo enchondral ossification and this configuration can cause confusion with osteochondroma. Rarely, parosteal osteosarcoma contains foci of pleomorphic spindle cell sarcoma or even high-grade osteosarcoma. In this instance, the term dedifferentiated parosteal osteosarcoma is used to denote these lesions. Cytogenetics and immunohistochemistry for MDM2 and CDK4 cytogenetics and immunoreactivity are often helpful to differentiate parosteal osteosarcoma from other fibro-osseous lesions.[20,27]

Periosteal osteosarcoma is a grade 2 or 3 chondroblastic osteosarcoma. Therefore, lobules of neoplastic cartilage, frequently hyaline,

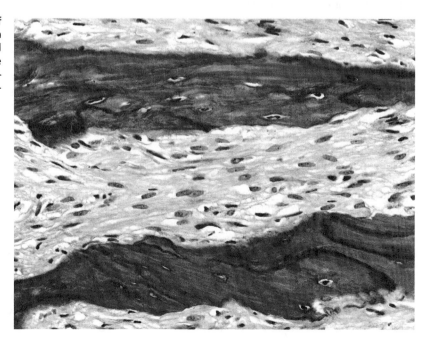

Fig. 24. Spindle cells of parosteal osteosarcoma grow in fascicles parallel to the long axis of the neoplastic bone trabeculae and show mild cytologic atypia.

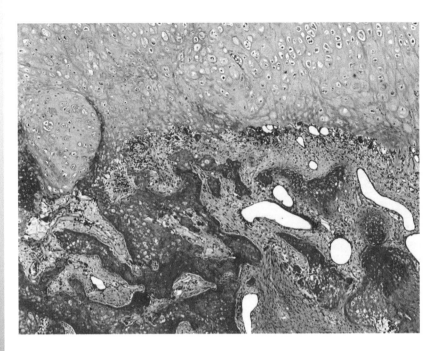

Fig. *25.* Cartilaginous cap of parosteal osteosarcoma with underlying tumor bone.

predominate, with the chondrocytes showing moderate to severe cytologic atypia as well as mitotic activity (**Fig. 26**). The neoplastic bone usually has a coarse, lacelike pattern and either merges with or is surrounded by the cartilage, or arises in the background of significantly atypical proliferating spindle-shaped or polyhedral tumor cells.

High-grade surface osteosarcoma is essentially a high-grade osteoblastic osteosarcoma that arises on the external surface of the cortex. The tumor cells show pronounced cytologic atypia, mitotic activity, and areas of necrosis. As in all high-grade osteosarcomas, neoplastic cartilage and fibroblastic components may be present.

The treatment of osteosarcoma is tailored to the age of the patient and the location, size, grade, and stage of the tumor. The goal of therapy is eradication of the primary tumor and the elimination of any metastases. Local therapy is usually limb salvage, wide surgical resection with negative margins for appendicular tumors, and surgical excision in combination with radiation for tumors that are not resectable in their entirety (as can be the case for neoplasms involving the axial skeleton). Adjuvant chemotherapy (methotrexate, cisplatin, doxorubicin, ifosfamide) is usually used in the preoperative setting for all high-grade intramedullary and surface osteosarcomas, and continues after the surgical resection has been completed and

wound healing has begun. The integration of aggressive polychemotherapy into treatment protocols for high-grade osteosarcomas has had a dramatic impact on an otherwise fatal disease. Low-grade central osteosarcoma and parosteal osteosarcomas are usually treated by surgery alone, because they are associated with a low risk of dissemination.

The histologic response of the tumor to preoperative chemotherapy is thought to be one of the most important prognostic features for localized high-grade osteosarcoma of the extremities (almost all of the tumors): a good response is considered to be 90% or greater necrosis (**Fig. 27**); poor response is less than 90% necrosis. The histologic assessment of tumor necrosis requires extensive sampling and evaluation of the treated neoplasm. A recent study has shown that the quantitation of the extent of residual viable tumor may be a better parameter than the percentage of necrosis.[28] Of conventional osteosarcoma subtypes, the chondroblastic variant has been shown to be associated with a poor preoperative chemotherapy response and, in some studies, has a worse prognosis than other variants.[28,29] Relapse-free survival rates for patients with localized conventional high-grade osteosarcoma of the extremity have been reported to vary from 50% to 80%. Actuarial 10-year survival rates for patients with axial tumors are approximately 27% for patients presenting with metastatic disease, 53% for

Fig. 26. (*A, B*) Periosteal osteosarcoma with neoplastic lobules of cartilage and bone, showing the underlying cortex. The tumor consists of malignant intermediate-grade hyaline cartilage that merges with foci of neoplastic bone.

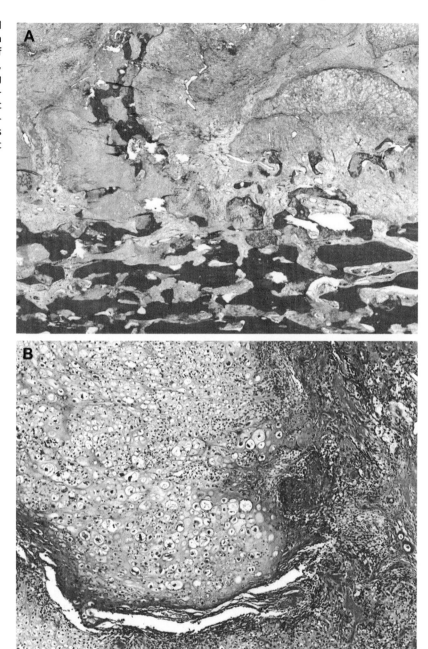

patients with large tumors (more than one-third the length of involved bone), 47% for patients with tumors with a poor response, and 73% for patients with tumors with a good response. Parosteal osteosarcoma and intramedullary well-differentiated osteosarcoma have an excellent prognosis and at least 90% of patients are long-term survivors. Periosteal osteosarcoma has a survival rate of approximately 75%, although a recent study using chemotherapy achieved a 10-year metastasis-free survival rate of 100%. High-grade surface osteosarcoma has a prognosis similar to conventional intramedullary osteosarcoma. Neoadjuvant chemotherapy improves outcome in osteosarcoma; however, failure to improve survival over the last 20 years emphasizes the importance of developing new treatments for this disease.[30]

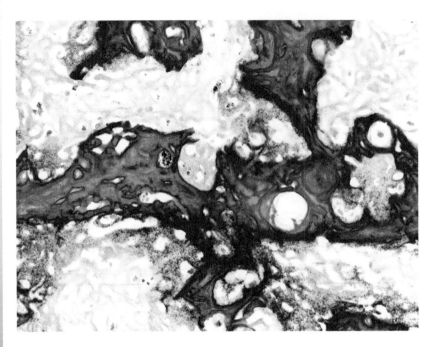

Fig. 27. Treated osteosarcoma with residual neoplastic bone without viable tumor cells.

REFERENCES

1. Fletcher CDM, Bridge JA, Hogendoorn PCW, et al. WHO classification of tumours of soft tissue and bone. Lyon (France): IARC; 2013.

2. Dancer JY, Henry SP, Bondaruk J, et al. Expression of master regulatory genes controlling skeletal development in benign cartilage and bone forming tumors. Hum Pathol 2010;41(12):1788–93.

3. Conner JR, Hornick JL. SATB2 is a novel marker of osteoblastic differentiation in bone and soft tissue tumours. Histopathology 2013;63(1):36–49.

4. Davis JL, Horvai AE. Special AT-rich sequence-binding protein 2 (SATB2) expression is sensitive but may not be specific for osteosarcoma as compared with other high-grade primary bone sarcomas. Histopathology 2016;69(1):84–90.

5. Baruffi MR, Volpon JB, Neto JB, et al. Osteoid osteomas with chromosome alterations involving 22q. Cancer Genet Cytogenet 2001;124(2):127–31.

6. Unni KK, Inwards CY. Dahlin's bone tumors: general aspects and data on 10,165 cases. 6th edition. Philadelphia: Lippincott Williams & Wilkins; 2010.

7. Allen SD, Saifuddin A. Imaging of intra-articular osteoid osteoma. Clin Radiol 2003;58(11):845–52.

8. Bauer TW, Zehr RJ, Belhobek GH, et al. Juxta-articular osteoid osteoma. Am J Surg Pathol 1991;15(4):381–7.

9. Giannico G, Holt GE, Homlar KC, et al. Osteoblastoma characterized by a three-way translocation: report of a case and review of the literature. Cancer Genet Cytogenet 2009;195(2):168–71.

10. Baker AC, Rezeanu L, Klein MJ, et al. Aggressive osteoblastoma: a case report involving a unique chromosomal aberration. Int J Surg Pathol 2010;18(3):219–24.

11. Nord KH, Nilsson J, Arbajian E, et al. Recurrent chromosome 22 deletions in osteoblastoma affect inhibitors of the Wnt/beta-catenin signaling pathway. PLoS One 2013;8(11):e80725.

12. Zon Filippi R, Swee RG, Krishnan Unni K. Epithelioid multinodular osteoblastoma: a clinicopathologic analysis of 26 cases. Am J Surg Pathol 2007;31(8):1265–8.

13. Garcia RA, Inwards CY, Unni KK. Benign bone tumors–recent developments. Semin Diagn Pathol 2011;28(1):73–85.

14. Dorfman HD. New knowledge of fibro-osseous lesions of bone. Int J Surg Pathol 2010;18(3 Suppl):62s–5s.

15. Kuijjer ML, Hogendoorn PC, Cleton-Jansen AM. Genome-wide analyses on high-grade osteosarcoma: making sense of a genomically most unstable tumor. Int J Cancer 2013;133(11):2512–21.

16. Ragland BD, Bell WC, Lopez RR, et al. Cytogenetics and molecular biology of osteosarcoma. Lab Invest 2002;82(4):365–73.

17. Sadikovic B, Park PC, Selvarajah S, et al. Array comparative genomic hybridization in osteosarcoma. Methods Mol Biol 2013;973:227–47.

18. Gisselsson D, Palsson E, Hoglund M, et al. Differentially amplified chromosome 12 sequences in low- and high-grade osteosarcoma. Genes Chromosomes Cancer 2002;33(2):133–40.

19. Tarkkanen M, Bohling T, Gamberi G, et al. Comparative genomic hybridization of low-grade central osteosarcoma. Mod Pathol 1998;11(5):421–6.

20. Dujardin F, Binh MB, Bouvier C, et al. MDM2 and CDK4 immunohistochemistry is a valuable tool in the differential diagnosis of low-grade osteosarcomas and other primary fibro-osseous lesions of the bone. Mod Pathol 2011;24(5):624–37.

21. Angelini A, Mavrogenis AF, Trovarelli G, et al. Telangiectatic osteosarcoma: a review of 87 cases. J Cancer Res Clin Oncol 2016;142(10):2197–207.

22. Lee AF, Hayes MM, Lebrun D, et al. FLI-1 distinguishes Ewing sarcoma from small cell osteosarcoma and mesenchymal chondrosarcoma. Appl Immunohistochem Mol Morphol 2011;19(3):233–8.

23. Righi A, Gambarotti M, Longo S, et al. Small cell osteosarcoma: clinicopathologic, immunohistochemical, and molecular analysis of 36 cases. Am J Surg Pathol 2015;39(5):691–9.

24. Cleven AH, Hocker S, Briaire-de Bruijn I, et al. Mutation analysis of H3F3A and H3F3B as a diagnostic tool for giant cell tumor of bone and chondroblastoma. Am J Surg Pathol 2015;39(11):1576–83.

25. Choong PF, Pritchard DJ, Rock MG, et al. Low grade central osteogenic sarcoma. A long-term followup of 20 patients. Clin Orthop Relat Res 1996;(322):198–206.

26. Bertoni F, Bacchini P, Fabbri N, et al. Osteosarcoma. Low-grade intraosseous-type osteosarcoma, histologically resembling parosteal osteosarcoma, fibrous dysplasia, and desmoplastic fibroma. Cancer 1993;71(2):338–45.

27. Mejia-Guerrero S, Quejada M, Gokgoz N, et al. Characterization of the 12q15 MDM2 and 12q13-14 CDK4 amplicons and clinical correlations in osteosarcoma. Genes Chromosomes Cancer 2010;49(6):518–25.

28. Chui MH, Kandel RA, Wong M, et al. Histopathologic features of prognostic significance in high-grade osteosarcoma. Arch Pathol Lab Med 2016;140:1231–42.

29. Bacci G, Longhi A, Versari M, et al. Prognostic factors for osteosarcoma of the extremity treated with neoadjuvant chemotherapy: 15-year experience in 789 patients treated at a single institution. Cancer 2006;106(5):1154–61.

30. Whelan JS, Jinks RC, McTiernan A, et al. Survival from high-grade localised extremity osteosarcoma: combined results and prognostic factors from three European Osteosarcoma Intergroup randomised controlled trials. Ann Oncol 2012;23(6):1607–16.

Integrating Morphology and Genetics in the Diagnosis of Cartilage Tumors

Carlos E. de Andrea, MD, PhD[a], Mikel San-Julian, MD, PhD[b],
Judith V.M.G. Bovée, MD, PhD[c],*

KEYWORDS

- Cartilaginous tumors • Enchondroma • Osteochondroma • Chondrosarcoma • IDH mutations
- HEY1-NCOA2 fusion

Key points

- Cartilaginous tumors of bone form a histologic spectrum ranging from benign (enchondroma, osteochondroma) to intermediate (atypical cartilaginous tumor/chondrosarcoma grade 1) to malignant (grade 2 and grade 3 chondrosarcoma, dedifferentiated chondrosarcoma).
- The diagnosis of a cartilage tumor can be made only in a multidisciplinary team.
- Criteria to distinguish between benign and malignant are different depending on age, the presence of multiple lesions, and the location of the tumor.
- Molecular alterations that can be used for diagnosis include *IDH1* (R132C; R132H) or *IDH2* (R172S) mutations in enchondromas, atypical cartilaginous tumor/grade 1 central chondrosarcoma, grade 2/3 central chondrosarcoma, and dedifferentiated chondrosarcoma; and HEY-NCOA2 fusion genes in mesenchymal chondrosarcoma.

ABSTRACT

Cartilage-forming tumors of bone are a heterogeneous group of tumors with different molecular mechanisms involved. Enchondromas are benign hyaline cartilage–forming tumors of medullary bone caused by mutations in *IDH1* or *IDH2*. Osteochondromas are benign cartilage-capped bony projections at the surface of bone. *IDH* mutations are also found in dedifferentiated and periosteal chondrosarcoma. A recurrent *HEY1-NCOA2* fusion characterizes mesenchymal chondrosarcoma. Molecular changes are increasingly used to improve diagnostic accuracy in chondrosarcomas. Detection of *IDH* mutations or *HEY1-NCOA2* fusions has already proved their immense value, especially on small biopsy specimens or in case of unusual presentation.

OVERVIEW

Cartilaginous tumors are the most common primary bone neoplasms, characterized by the production of a cartilaginous matrix. They are classified based on their clinical and histologic features and location within bone. A multidisciplinary approach is imperative for appropriate diagnosis and management. Conventional radiography is the cornerstone of the diagnosis of cartilage tumors. The presence of matrix mineralization in the form of "popcorn" calcifications in the tumor is characteristic. Cartilaginous tumors are

---

Disclosure Statement: The authors have no conflict of interest to declare.
[a] Department of Histology and Pathology, University of Navarra, Irunlarrea 1, Navarra, Pamplona 31008, Spain; [b] Department of Orthopaedic Surgery and Traumatology, University Clinic of Navarra, Irunlarrea 1, Navarra, Pamplona 31008, Spain; [c] Department of Pathology, Leiden University Medical Center, PO Box 9600, L1-Q, 2300 RC Leiden, The Netherlands
* Corresponding author.
E-mail address: J.V.M.G.Bovee@lumc.nl

clinically divided according to their behavior into benign, intermediate, and malignant. The most common benign lesions are enchondromas and osteochondromas, which together constitute more than 60% of benign bone tumors. They can be the precursor lesions of central and peripheral chondrosarcoma, respectively, accounting for 10% to 20% of malignant bone tumors.

Histologically, enchondromas and osteochondromas are formed by chondrocytes embedded in a cartilaginous extracellular matrix (ECM). The ECM is a rich network of cartilage-specific collagens (predominantly type II collagen) and proteoglycans (including heparan sulfate proteoglycans). Its function goes beyond providing physical support for chondrocytes and cartilage integrity and elasticity: it is a dynamic structure that is constantly remodeled to control tissue development and homeostasis.[1]

Cartilaginous tumors are complex diseases and different molecular mechanisms are involved in the different subtypes. Point mutation(s) in a single gene underlies the formation of enchondromas and osteochondromas. They may occur early during development, resulting in a somatic mosaicism causing nonhereditary enchondromatosis or can be present in the germline causing hereditary multiple osteochondromas syndrome. Additional secondary mutations drive multistep malignant progression forward. On the other hand, in mesenchymal chondrosarcoma a recurrent translocation is found.[2]

Here, we summarize the morphology as well as the molecular and genetic mechanisms involved in enchondromas, osteochondromas, and different subtypes of chondrosarcomas.

ENDOCHONDRAL BONE FORMATION

Most of the skeleton develops by endochondral ossification, a process in which the skeletal elements are preformed in a cartilage model. Cartilage tumors arise mainly in those parts of the skeleton formed by endochondral ossification. The face and skull are therefore rarely affected. Endochondral ossification is a stepwise physiologic process in which chondrocytes undergo a coordinated process of cell proliferation, differentiation, and programmed cell death within the normal growth plate. Cartilaginous matrix surrounding apoptotic chondrocytes mineralizes and blood vessels bring in osteoblasts replacing hyaline cartilage by bone.[3]

Endochondral ossification is coordinated by various growth factors, signaling molecules and cytokines.[4,5] Some of these molecules function in a gradient fashion, generating short- and long

ranges of signaling activity.[6,7] Proteoglycans (eg, heparan sulfate proteoglycans) are involved in signaling gradients formation.[8–10] Prehypertrophic chondrocytes secrete the growth factor Indian Hedgehog (IHH). IHH diffuses away from its site of synthesis, and signals to the proliferating chondrocytes to increase their proliferation rate.[3,4] IHH also acts as a long-range signaling molecule stimulating perichondral cells to secrete parathyroid hormonelike hormone (PTHLH; also known as parathyroid hormone–related protein). PTHLH inhibits both chondrocyte differentiation and the expression of IHH, keeping chondrocytes in a proliferating state. When the PTHLH levels decrease below a certain threshold, chondrocytes stop proliferating and begin hypertrophic differentiation and ossification.[3,5] Deregulation of signaling pathways that coordinate endochondral ossification (eg, IHH signaling pathway) are associated with the formation of enchondromas, osteochondromas, and chondrosarcomas (**Table 1**).[2,11]

The ECM in cartilage is mainly composed of type II collagen. Mutations in several different types of collagen I, II, IX, X, and XI genes are related to cartilage abnormalities in humans.[12] Mutations in the COL2A1 gene have been found in many forms of chondrodysplasias, cartilage tumors, and in cartilage degeneration. COL2A1 gene mutations alter the formation of the triple helical assembly of collagen in cartilage. Several studies in humans have shown that the severity of the clinical phenotype corresponds to the number of altered collagen fragments left unfolded and to their altered mobility.[13]

BENIGN CARTILAGE TUMORS

Chondromas are relatively frequent, and most are located centrally within the medulla of bone (enchondroma), whereas a minority are classified as periosteal (juxtacortical) chondromas. The incidence of these benign tumors cannot reliably be assessed, as they often go unnoticed and are detected by coincidence, with a radiological examination that was requested for other reasons. Occasionally there is a pathologic fracture.

ENCHONDROMA

Enchondromas are benign hyaline cartilage–forming tumors of medullary bone. They are located in the metaphyses and diaphysis of short and long tubular bones of limbs, especially hands and feet.[14] Enchondromas usually appear as single lesions (solitary enchondromas) (**Fig. 1**). Multiple lesions are seen in the setting of nonhereditary

Table 1
The distinctive histologic and molecular features of cartilaginous tumors

	Histology	Genetic Alterations
Central tumors		
Enchondroma	Encasement; low cellularity; no atypia.	PTHR1 (~8%); **IDH1 (R132C; R132H) or IDH2 (R172S) (~40% in solitary lesions, ~90% in multiple lesions).**
Atypical cartilaginous tumor (ACT)	Host bone entrapment; small, densely stained nuclei; chondroid or myxoid matrix.	**IDH1 or IDH2 (~60%);** COL2A1 (~40%); TP53 (~20%); RB1 pathway (~30%); Indian Hedgehog (IHH) signaling (~20%); NRAS (~20%).
Chondrosarcoma grade 1 (skull base lesion)	Same as ACT.	
Chondrosarcoma grade 2/3	Moderate/high cellularity; myxoid changes; mitosis; spindle cells at the edge of lobules.	
Peripheral tumors		
Osteochondroma	Cartilage-capped bony projections containing a marrow cavity that is continuous with that of the underlying bone.	EXT1 (~65%); EXT2 (~35%); No mutation (~10%).
ACT	Evidence of a preexisting osteochondroma; low cellularity; lobular growth pattern; chondroid or myxoid matrix.	RB1 pathway; CDKN2A (p16INK4a); TP53.
Chondrosarcoma grade 1 Tumors located in pelvis	Same as ACT.	
Chondrosarcoma grade 2/3	Evidence of a preexisting osteochondroma; high cellularity; mitosis; lobular growth pattern; chondroid or myxoid matrix.	
Rare chondrosarcoma subtypes		
Clear cell chondrosarcoma	Low-grade variant; bland clear cells (resembling growth plate hypertrophic chondrocytes); hyaline cartilage.	H3F3B (K36M; ~7%); Loss of p16 protein expression with no identifiable p16 mutation.
Mesenchymal chondrosarcoma	Biphasic pattern: small cells and islands of atypical cartilage.	**HEY1-NCOA2 fusion (~90%)** IRF2BP2-CDX1 fusion
Periosteal chondrosarcoma	Moderately cellular matrix; mucoid-myxoid changes; intramedullary extension; host bone entrapment.	IDH1 (R132C; ~15%); loss of p16 protein expression with no identifiable CDK4, TP53, or MDM2 mutations.
Dedifferentiated chondrosarcoma	A well-differentiated cartilaginous tumor, juxtaposed to a high-grade noncartilaginous sarcoma, with a sharp interface.	**IDH1 or IDH2 (~50%).**

In bold: molecular alterations that can be used for diagnosis.

enchondromatosis including Ollier disease (multiple enchondromas with a unilateral predominance) and Maffucci syndrome (multiple enchondromas combined with [spindle cell] hemangiomas).[15]

The potential for malignant progression is greater when multiple lesions are present, and is reported to be up to 35% in Ollier disease and greater than 50% in Maffucci syndrome,

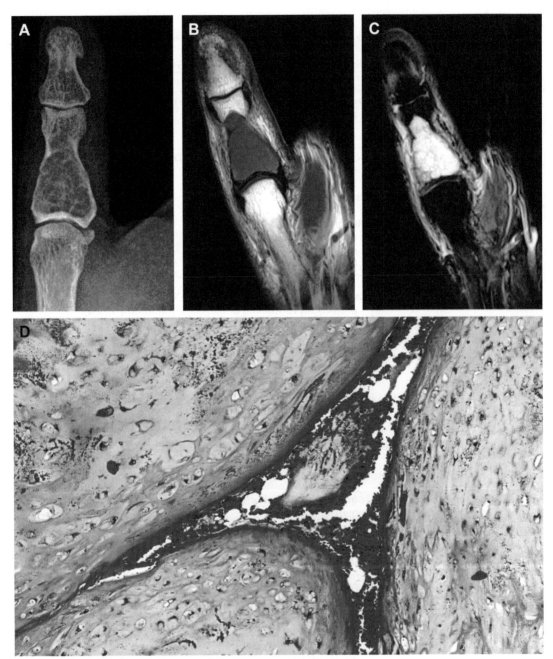

Fig. 1. Enchondroma. (*A*) A lytic expansile lesion, with thinning of the cortex but is still intact. (*B, C*) The lesion shows high signal intensity at T2-weighted MRI. (*C, D*) Poorly cellular proliferation of small tumor cells, embedded in abundant hyaline cartilaginous matrix.

depending on the location of the tumors.[16] The risk of developing chondrosarcoma is increased when enchondromas are located in the pelvis.[17]

Histologically, enchondromas are lobular, relatively cell-poor hyaline cartilage, often separated by a zone of reactive bone formation (encasement) (see **Fig. 1**). Chondrocytes have nuclei with condensed chromatin and are evenly dispersed.

Binucleated cells are rarely seen and mitoses are absent. Degenerative features, such as ischemic necrosis or calcifications, can be prominent.

Enchondromas in the phalanges display more myxoid features, and the lesion may have increased cellularity. At this location, the main characteristics of malignancy are the presence of mitoses, cortical breakthrough, and soft tissue involvement.[18] Malignant progression toward secondary central chondrosarcoma is documented for approximately 1% of solitary enchondromas (although areas of preexisting enchondroma are frequently seen in central chondrosarcoma) and up to approximately 50% in patients with multiple enchondromas.[17]

Enchondromas are caused by somatic mutations in the *isocitrate dehydrogenase* genes *IDH1* and *IDH2* (see Table 1). In 87% of syndromic enchondromas and in 52% of sporadic enchondromas, *IDH1* or *IDH2* mutations are found, indicating that these are an early, driving event for enchondroma formation[19,20] (Fig. 2). Similarly,

chondrosarcomas arising in these enchondromas contain *IDH* mutations in approximately 86%. In primary central chondrosarcomas, the frequency is 38% to 70%.[19,20] Hot spot mutations are exclusively found at the *IDH1* R132 and the *IDH2* R172 positions. Interestingly, within the tumor, chondrocytes with and without *IDH1* mutation are found, indicating intraneoplastic mosaicism.[20]

In patients with nonhereditary Ollier disease or Maffucci syndrome, also some cells in the surrounding normal tissue contain the mutation (somatic mosaicism), supporting the hypothesis that *IDH1* or *IDH2* mutations in Ollier disease or Maffucci syndrome occur early during embryonic

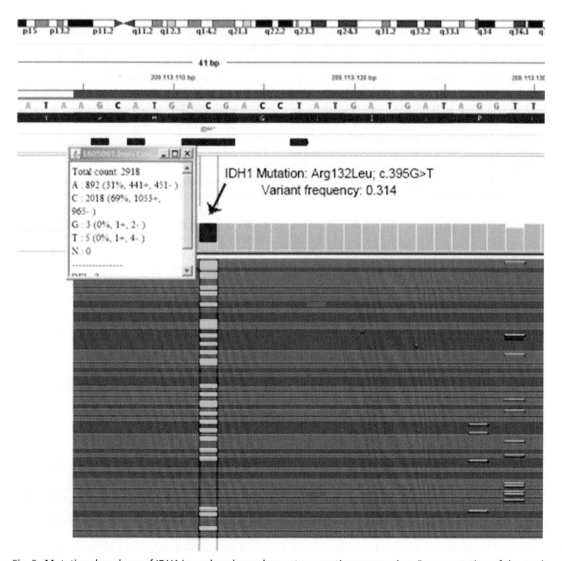

Fig. 2. Mutational analyses of IDH1 in enchondroma by next-generation sequencing. Representation of the reads aligned to the reference genome (Integrative Genomics Viewer software—IGV v 2.1, Broad Institute, Cambridge, Massachusetts, United States) for an IDH1 mutation p.R132L (c.395G>T) in exon 4 in an enchondroma.

development in the mesoderm (from which the skeleton is formed) after gastrulation. A small percentage of *IDH1* or *IDH2* mutated mesenchymal stem cells in the body may initiate the development of enchondromas at different locations in the skeleton, with a unilateral predominance. Other enchondromatosis subtypes, distinct from Ollier disease and Maffucci syndrome, are extremely rare and caused by mutations in different genes.[20]

The *IDH* genes encode isocitrate dehydrogenase, an enzyme involved in the conversion of isocitrate to α-ketoglutarate in the tricarboxylic acid cycle. Three isoforms of IDH are known. IDH1 is localized in the cytoplasm, whereas IDH2 and IDH3 act in the mitochondria. Gain-of-function mutations are exclusively found on the arginine residues R132 in *IDH1* and R140 and R172 in *IDH2*, which give the mutant enzyme the activity to convert α-ketoglutarate into D-2-hydroxyglutarate (D-2-HG). Increased levels of D-2-HG have been found in cartilage tumors with an *IDH1* or *IDH2* mutation.[19] In addition, elevated intracellular and extracellular levels of D-2-HG have been identified in cell lines with endogenous mutations in *IDH1* or *IDH2*.[21] Increased levels of the oncometabolite D-2-HG are found to cause DNA hypermethylation at CpG sites in enchondromas, causing a CpG island methylator phenotype (CIMP), similar to the CIMP phenotype described in colon carcinoma and glioblastoma.[20,22]

OSTEOCHONDROMA

Osteochondromas, previously called (osteocartilaginous) exostoses, are benign cartilage-capped bony projections containing a marrow cavity that is continuous with that of the underlying bone[23,24] (Fig. 3). They arise as sporadic (nonfamilial/solitary) or multiple (hereditary) lesions on the external surface of bone near the epiphyseal growth plate of long bones, ribs, and vertebrae. Sporadic occurrence is approximately 6 times more common.

Osteochondromas develop while the epiphyseal growth plate is active, and cease to increase in size when the growth plate closes at puberty.[7,25] Thus, osteochondromas behave like a displaced growth-plate cartilage growing at an angle from the normal bone.[16]

Histologically, 3 distinct layers are seen in an osteochondroma: perichondrium, cartilage cap, and bone (see **Fig. 3**). The size of an osteochondroma is given by the cap thickness.[26] Chondrocytes embedded in a cartilaginous matrix form the osteochondroma cap. Endochondral ossification is seen at the cartilage bone interface. Cellularity is variable, depending on the age of the patient. Binucleated cells, calcification, necrosis, nodularity, and cystic changes can be seen. The organization is, however, less organized as compared with the normal growth plate. A reliable histologic diagnosis cannot be made without adequate radiographic correlation, emphasizing the importance of multidisciplinary team meetings in establishing a final diagnosis.[27]

Multiple osteochondroma (MO) is an autosomal dominant disease and has an estimated incidence of 1 in 50,000. Patients with MO often display a wide phenotypic and genetic variation. The severity of the disease varies from patient to patient and even within family members. It makes clinical presentation and treatment of MO often unique to each patient. Treatment may vary according to the severity of symptoms, the number

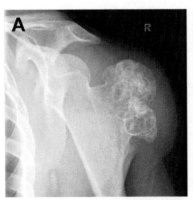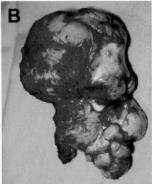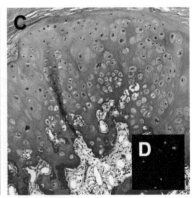

Fig. 3. Osteochondroma. (*A*) The medullary cavity of the lesion is continuous with the medullary cavity of the underlying bone. (*B*) Gross specimen of osteochondroma showing a lobular cartilaginous cap. (*C*) The lesion consists of 3 layers: perichondrium, cartilage, and bone. The organization of the cells within the cartilaginous cap resembles the growth plate with resting, proliferating, and hypertrophic chondrocytes. (*D*) The lack of the *EXT1* locus (*red*) probes with retained centromere-8 (*green*) probes indicates a homozygous loss of *EXT1* in osteochondroma.

of osteochondromas, and their locations. Patients may be treated with observation, or marginal excision.[28-30]

Osteochondroma formation requires a stochastic loss of heterozygosity for either *EXT* allele in cartilage[31,32] (see **Table 1**). *EXT1* or *EXT2* loss of function results in significantly shorter heparan sulfate chains, causing a loss and/or an uneven distribution of heparan sulfates at the cell surface and in the cartilaginous ECM.[10,33] Loss of *EXT* function results in altered gradient distribution of proteoglycans in human osteochondroma cells, which will result in abnormal diffusion and signaling of IHH, causing increased proliferation and delayed differentiation.[34-37] The abnormal diffusion of IHh ligands in the cartilaginous extracellular matrix environment results in a larger area in which IHH can diffuse, potentially leading to loss of polar organization allowing growth-plate chondrocytes located immediately adjacent to the perichondrium to grow at an angle from the normal bone.[38]

During osteochondroma formation, wild-type chondrocytes are integrated into the cartilaginous cap. Mixed populations of chondrocytes bearing homozygous loss of the *EXT1* gene and chondrocytes bearing functional copies of the *EXT1* gene can be found.[37,39] *EXT* wild-type chondrocytes may create an environment conducive for chondrocytes bearing homozygous loss of either *EXT* genes to proliferate and grow, probably providing

a certain threshold level and an even distribution of heparan sulfate throughout the osteochondroma cap.[10]

MALIGNANT CARTILAGE TUMORS

Chondrosarcomas are a heterogeneous group of malignant bone tumors. Chondrosarcomas are divided mainly into 5 distinct subtypes, including conventional (80%–85%), dedifferentiated (6%–10%), periosteal (2%), mesenchymal (2%), and clear cell chondrosarcoma (1%). Conventional chondrosarcomas are divided into 2 groups depending on their location in bone: central chondrosarcomas (85%–90%) and peripheral chondrosarcomas (10%–15%).[23]

HISTOLOGIC GRADING

Conventional chondrosarcomas are histologically graded according to Evans and colleagues[40] (grade 1, 2, and 3 tumors) (**Fig. 4**). Grading is so far the most important prognostic predictor for metastasis. In grade 2 chondrosarcomas, the cellularity and nuclear atypia are increased, and mitoses, although scarce, can be seen. The matrix becomes more mucomyxoid. In grade 3 chondrosarcomas, the cellularity is high, with nuclear atypia, and mitoses are even more easily identified. At the periphery of the lobules, spindle

Fig. 4. Spectrum of histologic features observed in cartilaginous tumors. Criteria to distinguish benign from malignant are depending on context as shown. EC, enchondroma; ACT, atypical cartilaginous tumor; CS1, grade 1 chondrosarcoma; CS2, grade 2 chondrosarcoma; CS3, grade 3 chondrosarcoma.

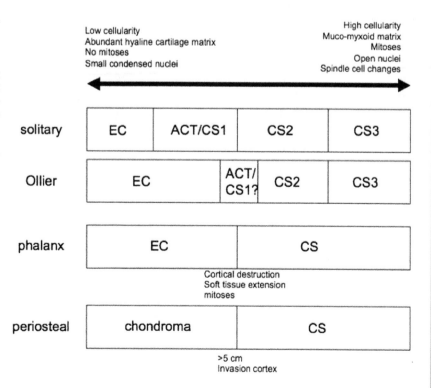

cell change may occur. Histologic grading was not proven useful for conventional chondrosarcomas located in the phalanx and the larynx.[18,41] The risk of developing metastasis increases with increasing tumor grade.[23] In central chondrosarcoma, metastasis of grade 1 chondrosarcomas is extremely rare, whereas 10% to 33% of grade 2 and approximately 70% of grade 3 metastasize.[40]

Metastases of grade 1 chondrosarcoma occurs predominantly after local recurrence with progression to grade 2 chondrosarcoma. The term "atypical cartilaginous tumor" (ACT) was therefore introduced in the World Health Organization 2013 classification to replace chondrosarcoma grade 1, to account for the locally aggressive, rarely metastasizing behavior of most chondrosarcomas grade 1[23] (see Fig. 4). Similar to the use of different terminology for histologically identical lipomatous tumors depending on their location (atypical lipomatous tumor in the extremities and well-differentiated liposarcoma in the retroperitoneum, reflecting different clinical behavior),[23] one could consider a similar approach in chondrosarcoma. Future studies should reveal whether it is justified to use the term "atypical cartilaginous tumor" in the long bones, and chondrosarcoma grade 1 for similar lesions located in the skull base, and perhaps for axial tumors. Also, for large lesions arising in pelvic osteochondromas (secondary peripheral ACT/CS1) that are difficult to operate, a similar approach could be considered.

CONVENTIONAL CENTRAL CHONDROSARCOMA

Histologically, the distinction between enchondroma and atypical cartilaginous tumor/chondrosarcoma grade 1 (ACT/CS1) is often difficult and highly observer dependent[42–44] (Fig. 5). Immunohistochemistry or molecular approaches cannot help in this differential diagnosis. ACT/CS1 is often more cellular when compared with enchondroma; the cells are irregularly arranged, and binucleated cells are frequently seen. Mucomyxoid matrix degeneration (>20%), entrapment of preexisting host bone, and the absence of encasement favor the diagnosis of ACT/CS1 over enchondroma[43] (see Fig. 5). Phalangeal enchondromas, however, may display high cellularity with a high number of binucleated cells with open chromatin, without this leading to an increased risk of recurrence or metastasis. Here, cortical destruction and/or the presence of mitoses lead to a diagnosis of chondrosarcoma. Similarly, this different "threshold" to diagnose ACT/CS1 is also obvious for tumors in the context of enchondromatosis, and for tumors in patients before puberty (before growth-plate fusion). In addition, an extraosseous cartilage tumor (periosteal/juxta-cortical) is much less aggressive when compared with a histologically similar tumor in the long bones.[45] This effect is even stronger in case of synovial chondromatosis; malignant subtypes of these lesions are extremely rare.[46–48] In daily practice, this means that a pathologist cannot sign out cartilage tumors

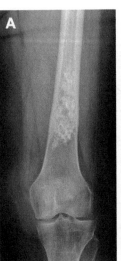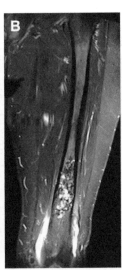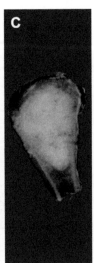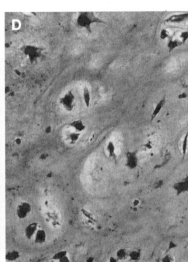

Fig. 5. Atypical cartilaginous tumor/central conventional chondrosarcoma grade 1. (A) Conventional radiograph demonstrating the typical popcornlike calcifications strongly suggesting a cartilaginous tumor. (B) MRI showing high signal intensity, endosteal scalloping, and cortical thinning. (C) Gross specimen of chondrosarcoma of the fibula head. The tumor occupies much of the medulla. (D) The cellularity is increased and myxoid change of the matrix can be seen.

without being aware of the exact location of the tumor, the patient age, and the absence or presence of enchondromatosis.

Genetically, mutations in *IDH1* or *IDH2* genes are found in 86% of secondary central chondrosarcomas[19,20] (see **Table 1**). Progression of enchondroma toward chondrosarcoma is characterized by aneuploidy and complex karyotypes with increasing histologic grade, with aberrations in the p53 and Rb pathways. Mutations in *COL2A1* gene, comprising insertions, deletions, and rearrangements, have been found in approximately 45% of secondary central chondrosarcomas[2,49] (see **Table 1**). *COL2A1* gene encodes the alpha chain of type II collagen fibers, the major collagen constituent of articular cartilage. Mutations in *YEATS2*, involved in histone H3 repression of transcription of target genes, were found in 12.3% of chondrosarcomas, were more frequent in high-grade tumors, and were mutually exclusive with *COL2A1*.[49] The functional roles of COL2A1 and YEATS2 mutations in chondrosarcoma are still unresolved. *NRAS* (Q61K and Q61H) mutations have been identified in a subset of conventional central chondrosarcomas (6/50, 12%).[50] This activating *NRAS* mutation may be related with conventional central chondrosarcoma initiation, maintenance, or progression. In addition, mutations in *TP53* (20%), the RB1 pathway (33%), and IHH signaling (18%) have been identified[2,49] (see **Table 1**).

As *IDH1* or *IDH2* mutations are early events, already present in enchondroma, they cannot be used to distinguish enchondromas from ACT/CS1. *IDH* mutation analysis can be helpful on biopsy specimens to confirm the diagnosis of chondrosarcoma over chordoma, over fibrous dysplasia with extensive cartilaginous metaplasia, or over chondroblastic osteosarcoma.[51,52]

Treatment may vary according to the severity of the symptoms, the size of the lesion, and its location. Patients with ACT/CS1 are usually treated by curettage with local adjuvants, whereas grade 2 and grade 3 chondrosarcomas should be treated with en bloc resection.[29,30]

SECONDARY PERIPHERAL CHONDROSARCOMA

Secondary peripheral chondrosarcoma arises in a preexisting osteochondroma. Approximately 1% of patients with solitary osteochondromas and 1% to 5% of patients with MOs at the age of 30 to 60 years will eventually develop a secondary peripheral chondrosarcoma.[23]

Imaging studies and gross macroscopic documentation of the cartilaginous cap size are the most reliable methods for diagnosis of ACT/CS1 arising in an osteochondroma, as it was shown that size of the cap was most predictive[27] (**Fig. 6**). A cap exceeding 1.5 to 2.0 cm in adults is suggestive of malignancy.[23]

Histologically, secondary peripheral chondrosarcomas are often low-grade, cartilaginous matrix-producing lesions that grow in a lobular pattern.[27] Evidence of a preexisting osteochondroma can often be identified. In high-grade secondary peripheral chondrosarcomas, the cellularity and nuclear atypia are increased, and mitoses are often easily seen (see **Fig. 6**). At the periphery of the neoplastic cartilaginous lobules, spindle cell changes may occur.

Malignant transformation of an osteochondroma is associated with increased expression of type X collagen and increased vascularization.[53] Mouse study of peripheral chondrosarcoma genesis has shown that loss of the tumor suppressor regulators Cdkn2a or Trp53 weakens cell-cycle checkpoint regulation and promotes chondrocyte proliferation[54] (see **Table 1**). In this model, deficient primary ciliogenesis has been identified. Primary cilia are organelles that function in sensory and signaling pathways and in cell polarity processes. Loss of polarity in the setting of deficient ciliogenesis may provide selective pressure, favoring the growth of clones of chondrocytes that have lost cell-cycle regulatory genes.[54] These clones of proliferating, deciliated chondrocytes, unable to transduce the polarity signal, may cause the irregular, bulky surface of the secondary chondrosarcoma cap consisting of lobules of cartilage separated from the main mass and invading soft tissue.[24]

Even though in osteochondromas *EXT* is inactivated in most tumor cells, in the cartilaginous cap of secondary peripheral chondrosarcoma, most cells have at least one functional copy of the *EXT1* and *EXT2* genes (see **Table 1**). This indicates that other (genetic) events, different from *EXT1* or *EXT2* mutations, take place in the *EXT1* or *EXT2* wild-type cells to promote malignant transformation.[7] Massively parallel sequencing of the whole genome of 4 low-grade secondary peripheral chondrosarcomas has shown that the proportion of *EXT1* or *EXT2* mutated alleles among all *EXT* alleles is approximately 40% (ranging from 27% to 50%), indicating that *EXT* mutant alleles and EXT wild-type alleles are coexisting in these tumors.[49] Genome profiling of chondrosarcomas arising in patients with MO typically shows chromosome instability with gains and losses and genomic diversity that increases with increasing grade of malignancy.[55,56] Frequent loss of heterozygosity for the chromosomal bands bearing the *RB1* and *CDKN2A* (*p16INK4a*) tumor suppressor genes

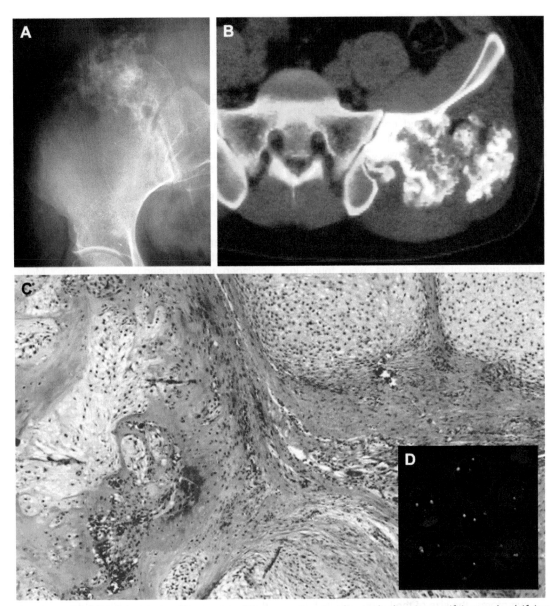

Fig. 6. Secondary peripheral chondrosarcoma. (*A*) Conventional radiograph showing ossifying and calcifying mass in close relation to the surface of the bone. (*B*) Often the stalk of the original osteochondroma is seen (computed tomography image). (*C*) Lobules of tumor cartilage separated by fibrous tissue are seen invading soft tissue. (*D*) Most cells retained *EXT1* (*red; centromere-8 in green*), suggesting functional *EXT1* gene in secondary peripheral chondrosarcoma.

has been described[55] (see **Table 1**). Inactivation of the CDKN2A locus at chromosome 9p21 is one of the most common genetic alterations in human cancers.[57] *CDKN2A* inactivation in secondary peripheral chondrosarcomas may occur by mutations[55] or less frequently by homozygous deletions.[2] Mutations in the *COL2A1* gene have not been identified in secondary peripheral chondrosarcomas.[2]

Treatment may vary according to the severity of the symptoms, the size of the lesion, and its location. Patients may be treated with en bloc resection, including removal of the pseudo-capsule.[29,30] The most common location for malignant transformation of an osteochondroma is the pelvis, where large lesions can be difficult to excise completely. Local recurrences can occur and, generally, are related to incomplete excision. Metastasis is very rare. Patients with secondary peripheral chondrosarcomas may die of recurrent tumors in the trunk that become inoperable.[58]

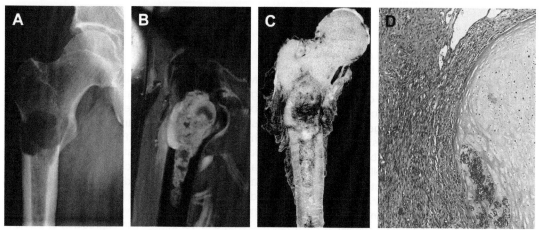

Fig. 7. Dedifferentiated chondrosarcoma. (A) Conventional radiograph showing an aggressive lytic lesion with destructive growth pattern. Distal from this lesion there are popcornlike calcifications suggesting juxtaposition to a low-grade cartilaginous lesion characteristic of dedifferentiated chondrosarcoma. (B) Corresponding T2-weighted MRI. (C) Corresponding gross specimen indicating the presence of a conventional cartilaginous lesion with lobular appearance in the distal part of the lesion, adjacent to an aggressive tumor with fish-flesh appearance, hemorrhage, and necrosis. (D) Abrupt transition between the conventional low-grade cartilaginous component (right) and the high-grade spindle cell sarcoma (left).

DEDIFFERENTIATED CHONDROSARCOMA

Dedifferentiated chondrosarcoma is a highly malignant variant of chondrosarcoma (~10% of all chondrosarcomas). It is characterized by the occurrence of 2 clearly defined components: a well-differentiated cartilage tumor (enchondroma, ACT, or grade 2 chondrosarcoma), juxtaposed to a high-grade noncartilaginous sarcoma with a sharp interface[23] (Fig. 7). The high-grade anaplastic component often resembles undifferentiated

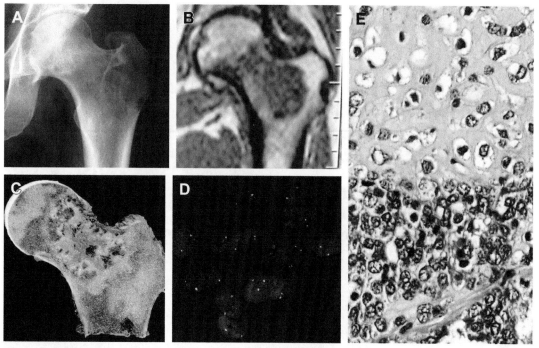

Fig. 8. Mesenchymal chondrosarcoma. (A) Conventional radiograph showing a calcified, eccentric, osteolytic lesion. (B) MRI showing a well-demarcated lesion composed of calcified and noncalcified areas. (C) Gross specimen of mesenchymal chondrosarcoma, the cartilaginous nature is not grossly evident. (D) Fluorescence in situ hybridization using probes for NCOA2 (red) and HEY1 (green) demonstrating the fusion (yellow dot) of HEY1 and NCOA2 caused by the inversion on chromosome 8 (Courtesy of D. de Jong and K Szuhai). (E) Areas with more or less differentiated hyaline cartilage admixed with cellular areas containing undifferentiated small round cells with scant or no cytoplasm.

pleomorphic sarcoma, but also can show various levels of differentiation resulting in the appearance of osteosarcoma, leiomyosarcoma, or even angiosarcoma, which can be a cause of misdiagnosis at small needle biopsies. Both components have been shown to share identical genetic aberrations with additional genetic changes in the anaplastic component, suggesting that both components share a common precursor cell.[59,60] Genetically, approximately 50% of dedifferentiated chondrosarcomas carry mutations in *IDH1* or *IDH2* in both components[19,60] (see **Table 1**). The mutation in *IDH* can therefore be very useful diagnostically in case of small biopsy specimens demonstrating only the anaplastic sarcoma and lacking the conventional chondrosarcoma part (see **Table 1**).

MESENCHYMAL CHONDROSARCOMA

Mesenchymal chondrosarcoma is a rare high-grade malignant neoplasm characterized by a biphasic pattern composed of poorly differentiated small round cells and islands of well-differentiated hyaline cartilage[23] (**Fig. 8**). The small cells often lack any cytoplasm, and staghorn vessels are characteristic. In biopsy specimens, the cartilaginous areas can be absent, rendering a broad differential diagnosis of a small blue round cell tumor. Immunohistochemistry will reveal positivity for CD99, SOX9, and bcl-2.[61–63] The expression of SOX9 is, however, not specific, as it is also found in other cartilaginous and noncartilaginous tumors, including synovial sarcoma.[64] Occasionally,

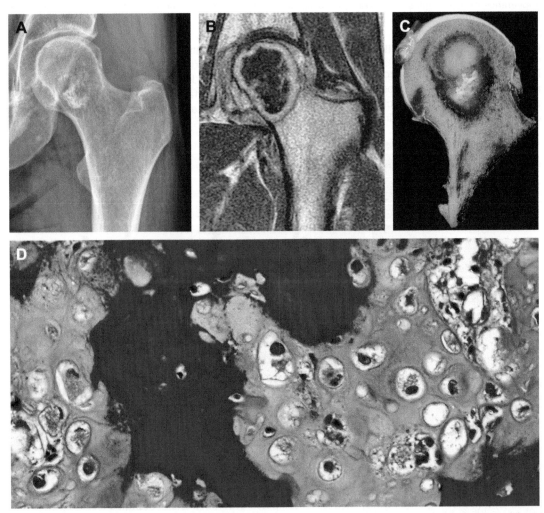

Fig. 9. Clear cell chondrosarcoma. (*A*) Conventional radiograph showing a lytic lesion with calcifications. (*B*) MRI T1 with gadolinium displays a lesion with relatively homogeneous low to intermediate signal intensity. (*C*) Gross specimen of clear cell chondrosarcoma showing a lobulated mixed soft and solid lesion. (*D*) Well-defined cellular margins and abundant clear or pale eosinophilic cytoplasm. Nuclei with prominent central nucleoli and soft chromatin are typical. Small regular deposits of osteoid, which may be calcified, are characteristic.

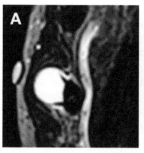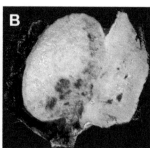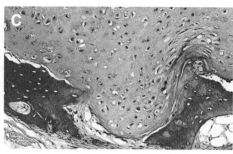

Fig. 10. Periosteal chondrosarcoma. (*A*) T2-weighted MRI reveals a sharply delineated mass with high signal intensity arising from the periosteum of the fourth rib. (*B*) Corresponding gross specimen in which the periosteal localization is evident; the lesion starts to invade the underlying cortex. (*C*) A cellular hyaline cartilaginous tumor invades the preexisting bone.

aberrant expression of desmin (35%) and epithelial membrane antigen (50%) can be found, whereas smooth muscle actin, myogenin, MyoD1, glial fibrillary acidic protein, and keratins are negative.[65] A recurrent *HEY1-NCOA2* fusion has been identified in approximately 90% of mesenchymal chondrosarcomas,[66] which can be used in the differential diagnosis with other small blue round cell sarcomas, including small cell osteosarcoma (see **Table 1**). An *IRF2BP2-CDX1* fusion has been reported in a *HEY1-NCOA2* negative case.[67]

Additionally, downregulation of Rb pathways has been reported.[60] IDH mutations are absent in this tumor.[19]

CLEAR CELL CHONDROSARCOMA

Clear cell chondrosarcoma is a rare, low-grade variant of chondrosarcoma characterized histologically by bland clear cells, resembling the hypertrophic cells in the growth plate, in addition to hyaline cartilage[23] (**Fig. 9**). The cells have typical round nuclei with fine chromatin and a prominent nucleolus. There is a regular deposition of osteoid, and small osteoclastic giant cells can be seen. *IDH* mutations are absent.[19] Although complete loss of p16 protein expression has been reported in most clear cell chondrosarcomas, no p16 point mutations have been identified[60] (see **Table 1**). Additionally, a recurrent loss or rearrangements of chromosome arm 9p are found.[68] One of 15 clear cell sarcomas harbored a *H3F3B* p.Lys36Met mutation, which is identical to the mutation that is found in almost 100% of chondroblastomas.[69,70] Chondroblastoma and clear cell chondrosarcoma both have the epiphysis of the bone as their preferential location, and therefore often enter the same radiological differential diagnosis. Histologically, however, they are distinct, as chondroblastoma is characterized by sheets of uniform small chondroblastlike cells, large osteoclast-type giant cells, and an amorphous eosinophilic matrix.

PERIOSTEAL CHONDROSARCOMA

Periosteal chondrosarcoma is a rare malignant cartilaginous tumor arising from the external surface of bone. It is characterized by a moderately to highly cellular lobulated cartilage mass, with low to moderate nuclear pleomorphism (**Fig. 10**). Mucoid-myxoid matrix changes are often seen. In most tumors, neocortex formation, the formation of a layer of compact mature bone surrounding the tumor, is found. Occasional intramedullary extension and subsequent host bone entrapment is also identified.[71] Histologic grading was not shown to be predictive of clinical behavior in periosteal chondrosarcoma. Periosteal chondrosarcoma is distinguished from periosteal chondroma by the presence of cortical invasion, and size larger than 5 cm.[71,72]

Genetically, only a small subset (~15%) of the periosteal chondrosarcomas showed *IDH1* mutation. Loss of p16 protein expression is found in approximately 50% of the cases, whereas no genetic alterations were found in *CDK4*, *TP53*, or *MDM2* genes[71] (see **Table 1**).

SUMMARY

Although great progress has been made toward understanding the genetic and molecular mechanisms of enchondromas, osteochondromas, and chondrosarcomas, many questions remain unanswered. Powerful techniques, such as massively parallel sequencing, are already providing valuable information about molecular genetics of cartilage tumors. These techniques allow screening of thousands of loci for cancer-causing mutations or structural rearrangements that may be very useful in the diagnostic setting, as well as identifying novel therapeutic targets. Even though the classical morphology remains at the cornerstone of bone tumor diagnosis, the additional detection of *IDH* mutations or *HEY1-NCOA2* fusions have already proven their immense value in improving diagnostic accuracy on small biopsy specimens or in case of unusual presentation.

Pitfalls

! Criteria to distinguish between benign and malignant depend on age, the presence of multiple lesions, and the location of the tumor and therefore the pathologist will inevitably make mistakes when evaluating cartilaginous tumours without this information.

! The immunohistochemical marker for mutant IDH1 that is commonly used in neuropathology detects only ~ 30% of all *IDH1* mutations in chondrosarcoma; negativity does not rule out the presence of an *IDH1* mutation.

! Histological grade does not predict outcome in phalangeal, laryngeal and periosteal chondrosarcoma.

REFERENCES

1. Bonnans C, Chou J, Werb Z. Remodelling the extracellular matrix in development and disease. Nat Rev Mol Cell Biol 2014;15(12):786–801.
2. Tarpey PS, Behjati S, Cooke SL, et al. Frequent mutation of the major cartilage collagen gene COL2A1 in chondrosarcoma. Nat Genet 2013;45(8):923–6.
3. Kronenberg HM. Developmental regulation of the growth plate. Nature 2003;423(6937):332–6.
4. Jochmann K, Bachvarova V, Vortkamp A. Heparan sulfate as a regulator of endochondral ossification and osteochondroma development. Matrix Biol 2014;34:55–63.
5. Lanske B, Karaplis AC, Lee K, et al. PTH/PTHrP receptor in early development and Indian hedgehog-regulated bone growth. Science 1996;273(5275):663–6.
6. Vortkamp A, Lee K, Lanske B, et al. Regulation of rate of cartilage differentiation by Indian hedgehog and PTH-related protein. Science 1996;273(5275):613–22.
7. de Andrea CE, Hogendoorn PC. Epiphyseal growth plate and secondary peripheral chondrosarcoma: the neighbours matter. J Pathol 2012;226(2):219–28.
8. Cortes M, Baria AT, Schwartz NB. Sulfation of chondroitin sulfate proteoglycans is necessary for proper Indian hedgehog signaling in the developing growth plate. Development 2009;136(10):1697–706.
9. Yan D, Lin X. Shaping morphogen gradients by proteoglycans. Cold Spring Harb Perspect Biol 2009;1(3):a002493.
10. de Andrea CE, Prins FA, Wiweger MI, et al. Growth plate regulation and osteochondroma formation: insights from tracing proteoglycans in zebrafish models and human cartilage. J Pathol 2011;224(2):160–8.
11. Tiet TD, Hopyan S, Nadesan P, et al. Constitutive hedgehog signaling in chondrosarcoma up-regulates tumor cell proliferation. Am J Pathol 2006;168(1):321–30.
12. Warman ML, Cormier-Daire V, Hall C, et al. Nosology and classification of genetic skeletal disorders: 2010 revision. Am J Med Genet A 2011;155A(5):943–68.
13. Donahue LR, Chang B, Mohan S, et al. A missense mutation in the mouse Col2a1 gene causes spondyloepiphyseal dysplasia congenita, hearing loss, and retinoschisis. J Bone Miner Res 2003;18(9):1612–21.
14. Pansuriya TC, Kroon HM, Bovee JV. Enchondromatosis: insights on the different subtypes. Int J Clin Exp Pathol 2010;3(6):557–69.
15. Gnoli M, Ponti F, Sangiorgi L. Tumor syndromes that include bone tumours; an update. Surg Pathol Clin 2017.
16. Bovee JV, Hogendoorn PC, Wunder JS, et al. Cartilage tumours and bone development: molecular pathology and possible therapeutic targets. Nat Rev Cancer 2010;10(7):481–8.
17. Verdegaal SH, Bovee JV, Pansuriya TC, et al. Incidence, predictive factors, and prognosis of chondrosarcoma in patients with Ollier disease and Maffucci syndrome: an international multicenter study of 161 patients. Oncologist 2011;16(12):1771–9.
18. Bovee JV, van der Heul RO, Taminiau AH, et al. Chondrosarcoma of the phalanx: a locally aggressive lesion with minimal metastatic potential: a report of 35 cases and a review of the literature. Cancer 1999;86(9):1724–32.
19. Amary MF, Bacsi K, Maggiani F, et al. IDH1 and IDH2 mutations are frequent events in central chondrosarcoma and central and periosteal chondromas but not in other mesenchymal tumours. J Pathol 2011;224(3):334–43.
20. Pansuriya TC, van Eijk R, d'Adamo P, et al. Somatic mosaic IDH1 and IDH2 mutations are associated with enchondroma and spindle cell hemangioma in Ollier disease and Maffucci syndrome. Nat Genet 2011;43(12):1256–61.
21. Suijker J, Oosting J, Koornneef A, et al. Inhibition of mutant IDH1 decreases D-2-HG levels without affecting tumorigenic properties of chondrosarcoma cell lines. Oncotarget 2015;6(14):12505–19.

22. Hughes LA, Melotte V, de Schrijver J, et al. The CpG island methylator phenotype: what's in a name? Cancer Res 2013;73(19):5858–68.

23. Fletcher CDM, Centre international de recherche sur le cancer. WHO classification of tumours of soft tissue and bone. 4th edition. Lyon (France): International Agency for Research on Cancer; 2013.

24. de Andrea CE, Hogendoorn PC, Bovee JVMG. Molecular genetics of multiple osteochondromas. eLS. Chichester (England): John Wiley & Sons Ltd; 2016. Available at: http://www.els.net.

25. Passanise AM, Mehlman CT, Wall EJ, et al. Radiographic evidence of regression of a solitary osteochondroma: a report of 4 cases and a literature review. J Pediatr Orthop 2011;31(3):312–6.

26. Sternberg SS, Mills SE, Carter D, Ovid Technologies Inc. Sternberg's diagnostic surgical pathology. 5th edition. Philadelphia: Wolters Kluwer/Lippincott Williams & Wilkins; 2010.

27. de Andrea CE, Kroon HM, Wolterbeek R, et al. Interobserver reliability in the histopathological diagnosis of cartilaginous tumors in patients with multiple osteochondromas. Mod Pathol 2012;25(9):1275–83.

28. Stieber JR, Dormans JP. Manifestations of hereditary multiple exostoses. J Am Acad Orthop Surg 2005; 13(2):110–20.

29. Gelderblom H, Hogendoorn PC, Dijkstra SD, et al. The clinical approach towards chondrosarcoma. Oncologist 2008;13(3):320–9.

30. van Maldegem AM, Bovee JV, Gelderblom H. Comprehensive analysis of published studies involving systemic treatment for chondrosarcoma of bone between 2000 and 2013. Clin Sarcoma Res 2014;4:11.

31. Hameetman L, Szuhai K, Yavas A, et al. The role of EXT1 in nonhereditary osteochondroma: identification of homozygous deletions. J Natl Cancer Inst 2007;99(5):396–406.

32. Reijnders CM, Waaijer CJ, Hamilton A, et al. No haploinsufficiency but loss of heterozygosity for EXT in multiple osteochondromas. Am J Pathol 2010; 177(4):1946–57.

33. Busse M, Feta A, Presto J, et al. Contribution of EXT1, EXT2, and EXTL3 to heparan sulfate chain elongation. J Biol Chem 2007;282(45):32802–10.

34. Bellaiche Y, The I, Perrimon N. Tout-velu is a Drosophila homologue of the putative tumour suppressor EXT-1 and is needed for Hh diffusion. Nature 1998;394(6688):85–8.

35. The I, Bellaiche Y, Perrimon N. Hedgehog movement is regulated through tout velu-dependent synthesis of a heparan sulfate proteoglycan. Mol Cell 1999; 4(4):633–9.

36. Benoist-Lasselin C, de Margerie E, Gibbs L, et al. Defective chondrocyte proliferation and differentiation in osteochondromas of MHE patients. Bone 2006;39(1):17–26.

37. Hilton MJ, Gutierrez L, Martinez DA, et al. EXT1 regulates chondrocyte proliferation and differentiation during endochondral bone development. Bone 2005;36(3):379–86.

38. de Andrea CE, Wiweger M, Prins F, et al. Primary cilia organization reflects polarity in the growth plate and implies loss of polarity and mosaicism in osteochondroma. Lab Invest 2010;90(7):1091–101.

39. de Andrea CE, Reijnders CM, Kroon HM, et al. Secondary peripheral chondrosarcoma evolving from osteochondroma as a result of outgrowth of cells with functional EXT. Oncogene 2012;31(9): 1095–104.

40. Evans HL, Ayala AG, Romsdahl MM. Prognostic factors in chondrosarcoma of bone: a clinicopathologic analysis with emphasis on histologic grading. Cancer 1977;40(2):818–31.

41. Chin OY, Dubal PM, Sheikh AB, et al. Laryngeal chondrosarcoma: a systematic review of 592 cases. Laryngoscope 2017;127(2):430–9.

42. Mirra JM, Gold R, Downs J, et al. A new histologic approach to the differentiation of enchondroma and chondrosarcoma of the bones. A clinicopathologic analysis of 51 cases. Clin Orthop Relat Res 1985;(201):214–37.

43. Eefting D, Schrage YM, Geirnaerdt MJ, et al. Assessment of interobserver variability and histologic parameters to improve reliability in classification and grading of central cartilaginous tumors. Am J Surg Pathol 2009;33(1):50–7.

44. Skeletal Lesions Interobserver Correlation among Expert Diagnosticians Study Group. Reliability of histopathologic and radiologic grading of cartilaginous neoplasms in long bones. J Bone Joint Surg Am 2007;89(10):2113–23.

45. Boriani S, Bacchini P, Bertoni F, et al. Periosteal chondroma. A review of twenty cases. J Bone Joint Surg Am 1983;65(2):205–12.

46. McCarthy C, Anderson WJ, Vlychou M, et al. Primary synovial chondromatosis: a reassessment of malignant potential in 155 cases. Skeletal Radiol 2016; 45(6):755–62.

47. Bertoni F, Unni KK, Beabout JW, et al. Chondrosarcomas of the synovium. Cancer 1991;67(1):155–62.

48. Davis RI, Hamilton A, Biggart JD. Primary synovial chondromatosis: a clinicopathologic review and assessment of malignant potential. Hum Pathol 1998;29(7):683–8.

49. Totoki Y, Yoshida A, Hosoda F, et al. Unique mutation portraits and frequent COL2A1 gene alteration in chondrosarcoma. Genome Res 2014;24(9): 1411–20.

50. Zhang YX, van Oosterwijk JG, Sicinska E, et al. Functional profiling of receptor tyrosine kinases and downstream signaling in human chondrosarcomas identifies pathways for rational targeted therapy. Clin Cancer Res 2013;19(14):3796–807.

51. Arai M, Nobusawa S, Ikota H, et al. Frequent IDH1/2 mutations in intracranial chondrosarcoma: a possible diagnostic clue for its differentiation from chordoma. Brain Tumor Pathol 2012;29(4):201–6.

52. Kerr DA, Lopez HU, Deshpande V, et al. Molecular distinction of chondrosarcoma from chondroblastic osteosarcoma through IDH1/2 mutations. Am J Surg Pathol 2013;37(6):787–95.

53. de Andrea CE, Wiweger MI, Bovee JV, et al. Peripheral chondrosarcoma progression is associated with increased type X collagen and vascularisation. Virchows Arch 2012;460(1):95–102.

54. de Andrea CE, Zhu JF, Jin H, et al. Cell cycle deregulation and mosaic loss of Ext1 drive peripheral chondrosarcomagenesis in the mouse and reveal an intrinsic cilia deficiency. J Pathol 2015;236(2): 210–8.

55. Bovee JV, Cleton-Jansen AM, Kuipers-Dijkshoorn NJ, et al. Loss of heterozygosity and DNA ploidy point to a diverging genetic mechanism in the origin of peripheral and central chondrosarcoma. Genes Chromosomes Cancer 1999;26(3):237–46.

56. Hallor KH, Staaf J, Bovee JV, et al. Genomic profiling of chondrosarcoma: chromosomal patterns in central and peripheral tumors. Clin Cancer Res 2009; 15(8):2685–94.

57. Kamb A, Gruis NA, Weaver-Feldhaus J, et al. A cell cycle regulator potentially involved in genesis of many tumor types. Science 1994;264(5157):436–40.

58. Ahmed AR, Tan TS, Unni KK, et al. Secondary chondrosarcoma in osteochondroma: report of 107 patients. Clin Orthop Relat Res 2003;(411):193–206.

59. Bovee JV, Cleton-Jansen AM, Rosenberg C, et al. Molecular genetic characterization of both components of a dedifferentiated chondrosarcoma, with implications for its histogenesis. J Pathol 1999; 189(4):454–62.

60. Meijer D, de Jong D, Pansuriya TC, et al. Genetic characterization of mesenchymal, clear cell, and dedifferentiated chondrosarcoma. Genes Chromosomes Cancer 2012;51(10):899–909.

61. van Oosterwijk JG, Meijer D, van Ruler MA, et al. Screening for potential targets for therapy in mesenchymal, clear cell, and dedifferentiated chondrosarcoma reveals Bcl-2 family members and TGFbeta as potential targets. Am J Pathol 2013;182(4): 1347–56.

62. Wehrli BM, Huang W, De Crombrugghe B, et al. Sox9, a master regulator of chondrogenesis, distinguishes mesenchymal chondrosarcoma from other small blue round cell tumors. Hum Pathol 2003;34(3):263–9.

63. de Jong Y, van Maldegem AM, Marino-Enriquez A, et al. Inhibition of Bcl-2 family members sensitizes mesenchymal chondrosarcoma to conventional chemotherapy: report on a novel mesenchymal chondrosarcoma cell line. Lab Invest 2016;96(10): 1128–37.

64. Cajaiba MM, Jianhua L, Goodman MA, et al. Sox9 expression is not limited to chondroid neoplasms: variable occurrence in other soft tissue and bone tumors with frequent expression by synovial sarcomas. Int J Surg Pathol 2010;18(5):319–23.

65. Fanburg-Smith JC, Auerbach A, Marwaha JS, et al. Immunoprofile of mesenchymal chondrosarcoma: aberrant desmin and EMA expression, retention of INI1, and negative estrogen receptor in 22 female-predominant central nervous system and musculoskeletal cases. Ann Diagn Pathol 2010; 14(1):8–14.

66. Wang L, Motoi T, Khanin R, et al. Identification of a novel, recurrent HEY1-NCOA2 fusion in mesenchymal chondrosarcoma based on a genome-wide screen of exon-level expression data. Genes Chromosomes Cancer 2012;51(2):127–39.

67. Nyquist KB, Panagopoulos I, Thorsen J, et al. Whole-transcriptome sequencing identifies novel IRF2BP2-CDX1 fusion gene brought about by translocation t(1;5)(q42;q32) in mesenchymal chondrosarcoma. PLoS One 2012;7(11):e49705.

68. Nishio J, Reith JD, Ogose A, et al. Cytogenetic findings in clear cell chondrosarcoma. Cancer Genet Cytogenet 2005;162(1):74–7.

69. Behjati S, Tarpey PS, Presneau N, et al. Distinct H3F3A and H3F3B driver mutations define chondroblastoma and giant cell tumor of bone. Nat Genet 2013;45(12):1479–82.

70. Cleven AH, Hocker S, Briaire-de Bruijn I, et al. Mutation analysis of H3F3A and H3F3B as a diagnostic tool for giant cell tumor of bone and chondroblastoma. Am J Surg Pathol 2015;39(11): 1576–83.

71. Cleven AH, Zwartkruis E, Hogendoorn PC, et al. Periosteal chondrosarcoma: a histopathological and molecular analysis of a rare chondrosarcoma subtype. Histopathology 2015;67(4):483–90.

72. Huvos AG. Malignant surface lesions of bone. Curr Diagn Pathol 2001;7:247–50.

Giant Cell–Containing Tumors of Bone

Zsolt Orosz, MD, PhD, Nicholas A. Athanasou, MD, PhD, MRCP, FRCPath*

KEYWORDS

• Giant cell tumors • Bone • Osteoclast

Key points

- Histologic appearances of different giant cell–containing lesions, especially in biopsy samples, can be significantly overlapping. For correct diagnosis, it is essential to take into consideration the age of the patient, location of the lesion, radiologic findings, comorbidities, and laboratory results.

- The distribution of the giant cells, appearance of mononuclear cells, presence or absence of mitotic activity, presence or absence of atypical mitoses, and the quality of the stroma are important cornerstones to the correct diagnosis.

- Immunohistochemical analysis of giant cell tumors (GCTs) led to the discovery of the receptor activator for nuclear factor κB (RANK) and to the development of targeted therapy for GCT of bone by denosumab.

- Molecular profiling of histone H3.3 variant resulted in the diagnostically useful K36M antibody for chondroblastoma identification.

ABSTRACT

Giant cell–containing tumors of bone are characterized morphologically by the presence of numerous osteoclastic giant cells. Correlation of clinical, radiologic, and laboratory findings is required for accurate histopathologic diagnosis and treatment of a giant cell–containing tumor of bone. In differential diagnosis, it is particularly important to note the age of the patient and the skeletal location of the lesion. This article considers the range of neoplastic and nonneoplastic lesions, which histologically contain numerous osteoclastic giant cells, and focuses on several lesions that frequently enter into the differential diagnosis.

OVERVIEW

Giant cell–containing tumors of bone (GCTs) represent a large category of tumors and tumor-like lesions, which are characterized morphologically by the presence of numerous osteoclasts or osteoclast-like giant cells. Osteoclasts are formed by the fusion of mononuclear phagocyte (macrophage) precursors, which express receptor activator for nuclear activator κB (RANK).[1] In the presence of macrophage-colony stimulating factor, these cells interact with osteoblasts that express RANK ligand (RANKL) and differentiate into multinucleated osteoclasts. There is a decoy receptor for RANKL, termed osteoprotegerin, which inhibits osteoclast formation/activity. Numerous cytokines and growth factors, including tumor necrosis factor α and interleukin 6, promote RANKL-induced osteoclast formation/activity. Mononuclear stromal cells in giant cell tumor of bone (GCTB) and other GCTs express RANKL.[2–4]

Several discrete neoplastic and non-neoplastic lesions of bone enter into the differential diagnosis of a GCT (Box 1). For this reason, correlation of histology with clinical, radiologic, and laboratory findings is essential for diagnosis. It is particularly

Disclosure Statement: There are no commercial or financial conflicts of interest. No funding has been received for this work.
Nuffield Department of Orthopaedics, Rheumatology and Musculoskeletal and Sciences, Nuffield Orthopaedic Centre, Windmill Road, University of Oxford, Oxford OX3 7HE, UK
* Corresponding author.
E-mail address: nick.athanasou@ndorms.ox.ac.uk

surgpath.theclinics.com

Box 1
Bone lesions containing numerous osteoclasts/osteoclast-like giant cells

GCTB

Chondroblastoma

CMF

ABC

LCH

NOF

Giant cell reparative granuloma (jaw/small bones)

FD

Giant cell–rich osteosarcoma

Telangiectatic osteosarcoma

Simple bone cyst (with fracture)

Other bone tumors (eg, osteoblastoma) associated with excessive bone remodeling activity

Paget disease

Fracture

Hyperparathyroidism (brown tumor)

important to note patient age because certain GCTs occur more commonly in skeletally mature or immature patients (Table 1). GCTs present with pain and/or swelling but a few can present with a pathologic fracture. Laboratory investigations, such as serum calcium and phosphate, are often useful to exclude a metabolic disorder, such as hyperparathyroidism.

The precise location of a GCT within bone provides important diagnostic information (see Table 1). GCTB and chondroblastoma typically involve the epiphysis of a long bone and it is always important to exclude these lesions when dealing with an epiphyseal GCT. Other radiologic features useful to note include whether the growth plate is open or closed, whether the bone containing the lesion is normal or abnormal, and whether the zone of transition, that is, the interface between the lesion and the surrounding bone, is well or poorly defined. A sclerotic rim is present around a very slow growing tumor whereas a non-sclerotic margin is usually found around a more rapidly growing lytic lesion. It may be possible to radiologically identify specific matrix components, such as bone and cartilage, or calcification within the lesion. Rapidly growing malignant lesions are evidenced by destruction of the host bone by

Table 1
Age groups and involved sites of giant cell tumors

	Most Commonly Involved Age Group	Most Commonly Involved Sites
GCTB	Third and fourth decades	Epiphysis of femur, tibia, humerus
Chondroblastoma	Skeletally immature patients	Epiphysis of femur, tibia, and humerus
ABC	Most common but not exclusive in skeletally immature patients	Metaphysis of long bones Lumbar and cervical vertebrae
Giant cell lesion of the small bones	Children, adolescents, and young adults	Hands and feet
Brown tumor of hyperparathyroidism	Skeletally mature patients	Hands, facial bones, pelvis, ribs, femur
NOF	Children, adolescents, young adults	Metaphysis of femur, tibia, fibula, humerus
LCH	First decade of life	Skull, jaws, ribs, vertebrae, proximal long bones
CMF	Adolescent, young adults	Metaphysis of long bones, proximal tibia, bones of the feet
FD	First 3 decades	Skull, facial bones, jaw, rib, pelvis, metaphysis of femur and tibia
Telangiectatic osteosarcoma	Second decade	Distal femoral metaphysis, proximal tibia, proximal humerus

infiltrating tumor. The extent of intraosseous and extraosseous tumor involvement is generally more accurately assessed using CT or MRI. Bone scintigraphy is particularly useful in conditions where multiple lesions are suspected.

GIANT CELL TUMOR OF BONE (GCTB)

GCTB is a common primary tumor of bone that arises in the epiphysis of a long bone. GCTB accounts for approximately 5% of all primary bone tumors.[5,6] GCTB usually presents with bone pain and swelling in a skeletally mature patient. GCTB most often arises in the distal femur and proximal tibia but the end of any tubular bone may be involved. It may also arise in flat bones, principally the pelvis, vertebral body, and sacrum.

RADIOGRAPHIC FEATURES

GCTBs are usually well-defined lytic lesions that lie eccentrically in the epiphysis of a long bone or in an apophysis. The tumor often extends up to the articular surface and may involve the metaphysis (Fig. 1). Where the tumor extends into soft tissue, it usually maintains a well-defined rounded border and evokes little periosteal reaction.

GROSS FEATURES

A GCTB is usually well defined, red-brown, and fleshy; it may contain areas of hemorrhage and cystic change.

MICROSCOPIC FEATURES

GCTB is characterized by the presence of very large numbers of osteoclast-like giant cells, which appear uniformly scattered among numerous round or spindle-shaped mononuclear cells (Fig. 2A). The (RANKL+) mononuclear stromal cells are often elongated and have spindle-shaped or ovoid nuclei in which mitotic activity and nuclear hyperchromasia can be seen. Macrophage-like mononuclear cells and giant cells contain vesicular nuclei with prominent nucleoli. Many of the giant cells are larger than normal osteoclasts and may contain more than 20 nuclei. The giant cells in GCTB, like normal osteoclasts, are distinguished immunohistochemically from macrophages and macrophage polykaryons by the expression of CD51 and a restricted range of macrophage-associated antigens (eg, CD68+, CD11/18−, CD14−, and HLA-DR−).[7] The tumor stroma is often well vascularized and may contain prominent cellular or collagenous fibrous tissue, areas of recent hemorrhage, hemosiderin deposition, and collections of foamy macrophages. Most GCTBs

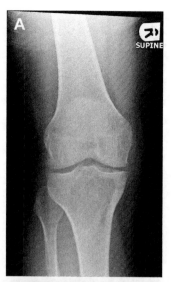

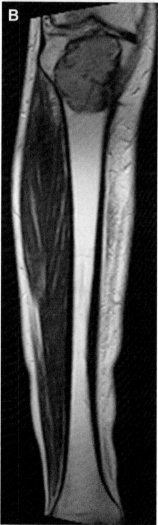

Fig. 1. (A) Radiograph and (B) MRI of GCTB of proximal tibia showing epiphyseal location. The lesion is well-defined and extends up to the articular surface.

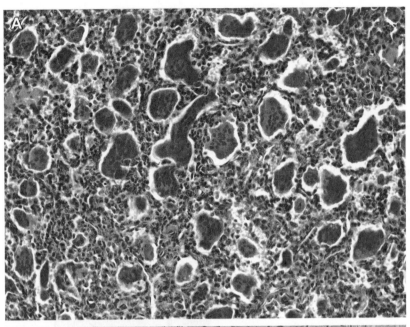

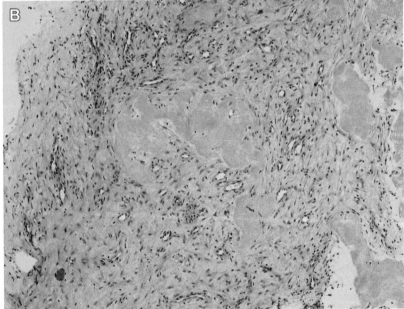

Fig. 2. (*A*) GCTB showing numerous osteoclastic giant cells and mononuclear cells (hematoxylin-eosin, original magnification ×400). (*B*) GCTB post-denosumab therapy showing absence of osteoclasts and formation of fibrous tissue and bone (hematoxylin-eosin, original magnification ×250).

show p63 and smooth muscle actin positivity, but their differential diagnostic or prognostic role is limited. A fibrous histiocytoma-like storiform pattern and secondary aneurysmal bone cyst (ABC)–like change may be noted. An organized host woven bone reaction is commonly present at the edge of the tumor. Focally, some mononuclear stromal cells within the lesion may be associated with osteoid and woven bone formation.

Intravascular extension of GCTB may occur. Grading the histologic features of GCT has not been shown to have prognostic significance in terms of predicting recurrence or metastasis.

MOLECULAR GENETIC FEATURES

The replication-independent histone H3.3 is involved in S-phase independent regulation of chromatin template processes, including transcription, and mutation of this gene has been associated with several childhood and young adult tumors. H3.3 is encoded by 2 genes, H3F3A on chromosome 1 and H3F3B on chromosome 17. These genes have different DNA sequences but both encode histone H3.3 of identical amino acid sequence. The percentage of detected histone H3.3 driver mutations of H3F3A in GCTBs depends on the sensitivity of the technique used, ranging from 69% in case of Sanger sequencing to 96% when targeted next generation sequencing is used.[8,9] Mutation analysis of H3F3A can be used to distinguish GCTB from other GCTs.[9,10] H3.3 mutations have also been identified rarely in chondrosarcoma, including clear cell chondrosarcoma, and osteosarcoma. GCTB does not show other driver mutations, including IDH1, IDH2, and TP53 or USP6 translocation.[8,10]

PROGNOSIS AND TREATMENT

GCTB should be regarded as a locally aggressive and rarely metastasizing lesion. Lung metastases of GCTB are usually single, develop within a few years of surgical treatment of the primary tumor, and frequently show focal osteoid or bone formation but otherwise histologically resemble the primary tumor, often remaining unchanged in size for many years. In most cases, these lung lesions are thought to represent tumor implants rather than metastases from a primary malignant tumor. Sarcomatous transformation, mostly to an undifferentiated pleomorphic sarcoma or osteosarcoma, may rarely occur in an otherwise typical GCTB (malignant GCTB).

GCTB is generally treated by curettage but recurrence occurs in up to one-third of cases. En bloc excision of the lesion is curative but not always possible. Intraoperative implantation of tumor in soft tissues may lead to recurrence outside the bone. The discovery of RANKL has led to the use of a fully human anti-RANKL monoclonal antibody, denosumab, to control GCTB growth of recurrent or surgically unsalvageable tumors and preoperatively to facilitate surgical resection of aggressive GCTBs. Treatment with denosumab usually results in disappearance of osteoclasts and an increase in cellular and collagenous fibrous tissue with focal osteoid and woven bone formation[11] (see Fig. 2B).

CHONDROBLASTOMA

Chondroblastoma (Codman tumor) is a rare cartilaginous tumor that arises in the epiphysis and contains immature cartilage cells (chondroblasts).

It accounts for less than 1% of all bone tumors.[6,12] Chondroblastoma has been reported over a wide age range but most commonly presents in children, adolescents, and young adults. It almost always involves the epiphysis and occurs mainly around the knee joint and proximal humerus. There is usually a long history of pain, local tenderness, swelling, joint effusion, or limited joint movement.

RADIOLOGIC FEATURES

Chondroblastoma is usually a well-demarcated radiolucent lesion lying within the epiphysis and occasionally extending into the metaphysis (Fig. 3). The tumor may also arise in an apophysis. Fine matrix calcification may be present within the lesion. Most tumors have a sclerotic border and occupy less than one-half of the diameter of the epiphysis.

GROSS FEATURES

The tumor is well-defined white, yellow, or brown and composed mainly of cartilage with focal areas of calcification.

MICROSCOPIC FEATURES

The lesion is composed largely of small uniform chondroblasts (S100+), which have a well-defined cell membrane, clear cytoplasm, and a hyperchromatic round nucleus that frequently contains a longitudinal groove. There is often a variable amount of amorphous chondroid, or chondrosteoid matrix and delicate lacy, or chicken wire, calcification around individual tumor cells (Fig. 4). Mitotic figures are present but are not usually numerous and never atypical. There are scattered osteoclastic giant cells (occasionally very large), particularly around areas of chondroid matrix or calcified cartilage. Akpalo and colleagues[13] reported strong positive membranous DOG1 expression in chondroblastomas parallel with negative reaction in chondromyxoid fibromas (CMFs) and GCTBs, suggesting diagnostic usefulness of DOG1. Cleven and colleagues,[14] however, found the DOG1 expression only focal and less sensitive in chondroblastomas; therefore, especially on core biopsy samples, the results should be interpreted with caution.[14]

MOLECULAR GENETIC FEATURES

Driver mutations, mostly on the H3F3B gene, are present in more than 90% of chondroblastomas.[8,9] This results in the production of an aberrant K36M protein, which inhibits at least 2

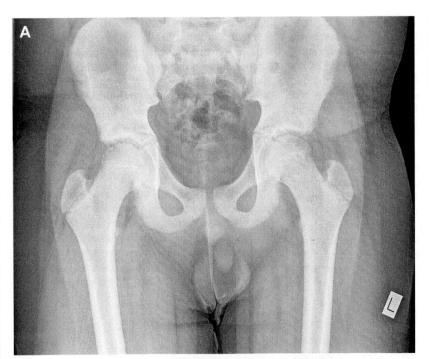

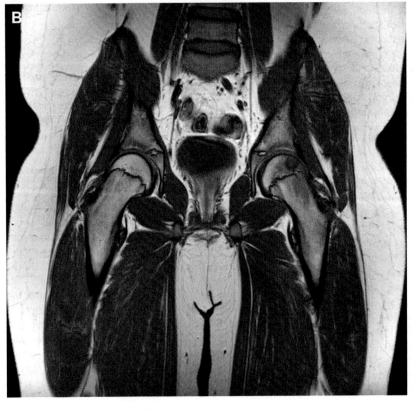

Fig. 3. (*A*) Radiograph and (*B*) MRI of chondroblastoma of the proximal femur showing a small, lytic, well-defined lesion in the epiphysis.

Fig. 4. Chondroblastoma showing chicken wire calcification within chondroid matrix and surrounding chondroblasts and osteoclast-like giant cells (hematoxylin-eosin, original magnification ×250).

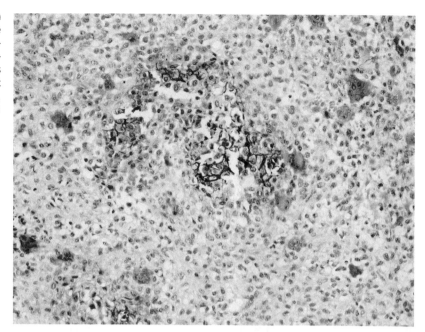

methyltransferases MMSET and SETD2, leading to altered expression of several genes involved in tumor formation and progression.[15] Mutation analysis by polymerase chain reaction and the H3F3 K36M mutant antibody are useful tools in the diagnosis of chondroblastoma.[8,16] H3.3 mutations have not been seen in CMF. Other driver mutations, including IDH1 and IDH2, are absent in chondroblastoma.

PROGNOSIS AND TREATMENT

The tumor is of intermediate malignancy, rarely metastasizing and usually cured by curettage. Local recurrence occurs in 5% to 10% of cases and may follow incomplete removal. Implantation of tumor in soft tissue after curettage can result in local recurrence. Benign pulmonary metastasis, similar to GCTB, can rarely occur with chondroblastomas and usually follows surgical intervention.

ANEURYSMAL BONE CYST (ABC)

ABC is an uncommon benign, rapidly expanding, and locally destructive multicystic lesion of bone, which is characterized by the presence of numerous blood-filled spaces.[6,17] It may occur as a primary bone lesion (primary ABC) or be associated with a preexisting bone lesion (secondary ABC). Primary ABC accounts for approximately 2.5% of all primary bone tumors and may occur at any age, although most lesions develop between the ages of 5 years and 20 years. The

proximal and distal femur, proximal tibia and proximal humerus, and lumbar and cervical vertebrae are most frequently affected but ABC may arise in any bone. Most patients complain of pain and swelling of variable duration.

RADIOLOGIC FEATURES

The lesion is osteolytic and commonly multiloculated and results in eccentric expansion of the affected bone. In long bones, ABC is often centered on the metaphysis. The intramedullary component usually has a well-circumscribed margin. If the cortex is disrupted, the lesion balloons into soft tissue and is covered by a shell of reactive new bone. In the spine, ABC typically involves the posterior elements. CT and MRI are particularly useful in establishing the multicystic nature of the lesion and in identifying fluid within the cyst (**Fig. 5**).

GROSS FEATURES

Grossly, ABC is often large and red-brown and composed of cystic spaces filled with blood or brown fluid.

MICROSCOPIC FEATURES

An ABC contains numerous cystic blood-filled spaces that are separated by cellular fibrous tissue lined in part by osteoclastic giant cells and macrophages (**Fig. 6**). Within the cyst wall there are also scattered giant cells and macrophages, many of which contain hemosiderin. Fibrous septa

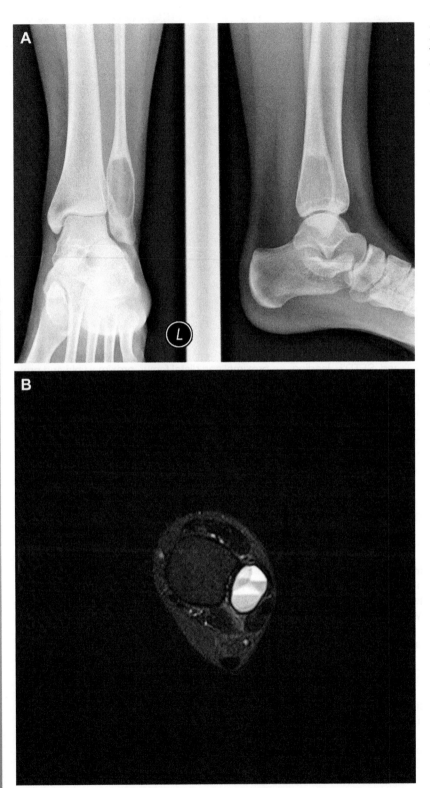

Fig. 5. (*A*) Radiographs and (*B*) MRI of ABC of the distal fibula showing expansion of bone by a metaphyseal lytic well-defined tumor. MRI shows characteristic fluid-fluid levels.

Fig. 6. ABC showing cyst wall containing macrophages, scattered osteoclasts and thin woven bone trabeculae (hematoxylin-eosin, original magnification ×250).

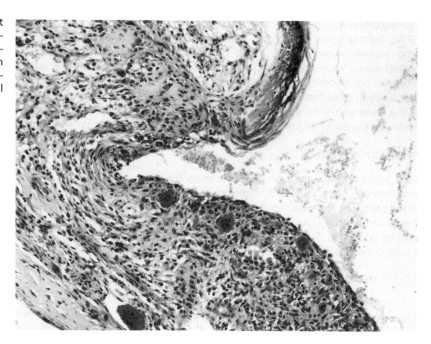

separating cystic spaces may contain focal areas of hemorrhage, myxoid degeneration, or thin woven bone trabeculae or strands of osteoid, some of which may be partly mineralized. There are mitotic figures but there is no significant pleomorphism. The external surface is usually covered by periosteal fibrous tissue beneath which there is reactive new bone formation.

The solid variant of ABC is composed mainly of cellular fibrous tissue containing numerous macrophages, osteoclast-like giant cells, and areas of (benign) osteoid and woven bone formation. Spindle-shaped fibroblasts may show increased mitotic activity but there is no cytologic atypia. Typically, the bone appears more mature and organized toward the periphery. These solid lesions also usually contain small focal areas of typical cystic change.

MOLECULAR GENETIC FEATURES

In primary ABC, cytogenetic rearrangement of the USP6 gene at chromosome 17p13 has been noted in 70% of cases[18–20]; this rearrangement, which is not seen in secondary ABC or other forms of GCT, is useful in the diagnosis of ABC. The USP6 rearrangement, however, may be difficult to detect, because the ratio of abnormal cells can vary from 8% to 82%.[19]

PROGNOSIS

Primary ABC is usually treated by curettage and bone grafting. The recurrence rate is high and most recurrences are within 2 years of treatment; recurrence is more common in patients younger than 20 years of age. ABC stromal cells express RANKL and treatment with denosumab has proved effective in a few cases.[3,21]

Giant cell lesion of small bones is a rare benign giant cell–rich lesion, which arises in the bones of the hands and feet.[22] Genetic studies have identified a UPS6 gene rearrangement in this lesion indicating that it is a true ABC.[23] The lesion has been reported over a wide age range but occurs most often in children, adolescents, and young adults. It usually arises in the phalanges but may develop in the metacarpals or metatarsals and rarely in carpal and tarsal bones. Radiologically, the lesion is expansile and radiolucent and may occupy the entire length of a phalanx. Histologically, the lesion resembles a solid ABC and contains numerous scattered giant cells, which lie in a prominent fibrous stroma. Reactive osteoid or bone formation and evidence of recent or past hemorrhage may be seen in the fibrous stroma. The differential diagnosis includes GCTB, hyperparathyroidism, and GCT of tendon sheath eroding bone. The lesion usually requires curettage and bone grafting but not uncommonly recurs.

CHONDROMYXOID FIBROMA (CMF)

CMF is a rare tumor in which there are lobules of chondromyxoid or fibromyxoid matrix containing spindle-shaped or stellate cells.[6,24] It accounts for less than 1% of all bone tumors.

Up-regulation of the glutamate receptor gene GRM1 through gene fusion and promoter swapping has been noted in CMF.[25] CMF has been reported over a wide age range but develops most often in adolescents and young adults, more frequently in male than in female patients. Bones of the lower extremity are most often affected, in particular the proximal tibia and bones of the feet.

RADIOLOGIC FEATURES

CMF arises in the metaphysis and is an eccentric, well-defined, often lobulated, radiolucent lesion, which produces expansion of the overlying cortex. The lesion typically has a sclerotic border, which may be scalloped. Rarely, the tumor may arise in a subperiosteal location.

GROSS FEATURES

CMF is a well-defined, firm, gray-white, and lobulated lesion. The periosteum around eccentrically located lesion is intact.

MICROSCOPIC FEATURES

Histologically, the tumor contains lobules of spindle-shaped or stellate cells, which lie within a myxoid or chondroid matrix (**Fig. 7**). The lobules are separated by bands of cellular fibrous tissue, containing fibroblasts and a few osteoclast-like giant cells. Tumor cells within the myxoid stroma have an indistinct cell border and abundant, often vacuolated cytoplasm, with degenerate, occasionally hyperchromatic nuclei. Mitotic activity is unusual. Cystic degeneration, ABC change, more mature cartilaginous differentiation, and matrix calcification may uncommonly be noted. Immunohistochemistry shows staining of cells for S100 with focal expression of smooth muscle actin and muscle specific actin and matrix staining for SOX9 and collagen II.[24]

PROGNOSIS AND TREATMENT

CMF is a locally aggressive tumor of intermediate malignancy. The curettage may be followed by local recurrence and, if multiple recurrences occur, en bloc resection may be the treatment of choice.

NON-OSSIFYING FIBROMA (NOF)

NOF is a common benign fibrohistiocytic lesion, which occurs most often in the metaphysis of the long bone.[6,26] Smaller lesions of similar morphology are termed, metaphyseal fibrous defect or fibrous cortical defect. This condition does not seem to be neoplastic and is thought to be a developmental abnormality of bone modeling, which occurs as a consequence of increased subperiosteal osteoclastic resorption at sites of ligament or tendon insertion into bone. Trauma or stress injury to the bone may play a role. Most metaphyseal fibrous defects are

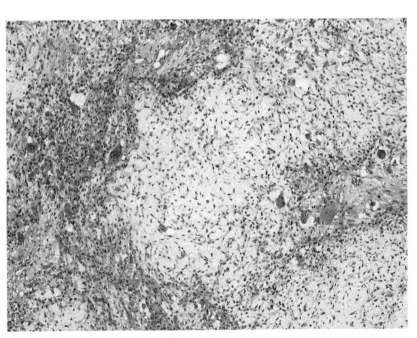

Fig. 7. CMF showing areas of cellular fibrous tissue and osteoclastic giant cells around fibromyxoid and chondromyxoid tissue (hematoxylin-eosin, original magnification ×100).

asymptomatic and usually noted as an incidental finding on radiographs. NOF is rarely encountered beyond the second decade and is also uncommon in children under 5 years. Male and female patients are equally affected. Large lesions are symptomatic and patients usually complain of pain. Bones most often affected are the femur, tibia, fibula, and humerus.

RADIOLOGIC FEATURES

A metaphyseal fibrous defect is a well-defined lytic lesion that lies against the cortex and has a sclerotic, often scalloped border. The lesion may migrate toward the diaphysis and may gradually disappear over time. NOFs are large lytic lesions that occupy a significant portion of the metaphysis and frequently extend into the diaphysis. They are eccentrically located and usually do not occupy more than one-half of the width of the bone.

GROSS FEATURES

NOF is a cortically based lesion, composed of firm yellow, white, or brown tissue. The cortical bone can be significantly thinned. Cystic change or hemorrhage may be present.

MICROSCOPIC FEATURES

NOF is composed of fibroblasts and macrophages that are arranged in a prominent whorled or storiform pattern (Fig. 8). There is a variable amount of collagen formation. Fibroblasts may be plump and have large nuclei, which show occasional typical mitotic activity. There are scattered osteoclast-like giant cells and often focal collections of foamy macrophages or hemosiderin deposition. Secondary ABC change may be noted. Bone or osteoid formation is not seen within the lesion. Reactive new bone formation may be seen at the periphery.

PROGNOSIS AND TREATMENT

Large lesions in which there is a risk of pathologic fracture may require curettage and bone grafting. Malignant change does not occur.

Benign fibrous histiocytoma (BFH) is a rare benign tumor of bone, which is identical histologically to an NOF but arises at skeletal sites in which NOF does not occur that is, in nonmetaphyseal regions of long bones and in the pelvis.[6,26] BFH has been described most often in adults after the third decade of life. Males and females are equally affected. The lesion is asymptomatic or associated with pain.

LANGERHANS CELL HISTIOCYTOSIS (LCH)

LCH designates a group of conditions that are characterized by the presence of a mixed, polymorphic inflammatory infiltrate that includes Langerhans cells.[27] Langerhans cells are antigen-presenting cells found in the skin, lymph nodes, and other tissues. LCH occurs most commonly in

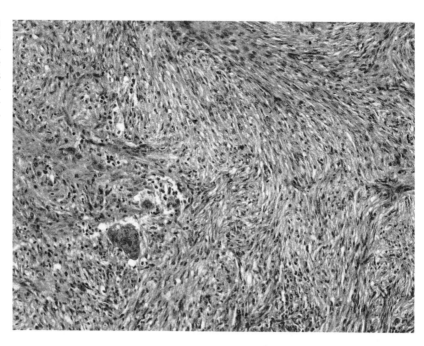

Fig. 8. NOF showing numerous spindle-shaped cells arranged in a storiform pattern. There are numerous macrophages and scattered osteoclast-like giant cells (hematoxylin-eosin, original magnification ×250).

the first decade of life and is uncommon after 30 years of age. Patients may be asymptomatic or present with bone pain, local tenderness, or pathologic fracture. Solitary lesions (eosinophilic granuloma) are encountered much more commonly than multiple lesions, which usually present within the first 3 years of life. Lesions may arise in any bone but the skull, jaw, ribs, vertebral bodies, and proximal long bones are most often affected.

RADIOLOGIC FEATURES

Bone lesions in LCH are usually located in the metaphysis or diaphysis and show a wide range of radiographic features. Lesions lie in the medulla and are well-defined, round or ovoid, and osteolytic and show little or no surrounding sclerosis. Lesions may grow to a large size and result in cortical erosion and soft tissue involvement. A periosteal reaction may or may not be present. In some cases, the lesion is poorly defined and there is a permeative or moth-eaten pattern of bone destruction and a prominent periosteal reaction. This appearance is most commonly seen in young children and can mimic other benign (eg, osteomyelitis) and malignant (eg, Ewing sarcoma) conditions. In the spine, lesions are usually found in the vertebral body, where they may cause collapse and flattening (*vertebra plana*).

MACROSCOPIC FEATURES

Grossly, the lesions are often well-defined and red-gray and contain flecks of yellow material.

MICROSCOPIC FEATURES

LCH contains a variable mixture of inflammatory cells, including identifiable Langerhans cells and macrophages, eosinophils, lymphocytes, plasma cells, and scattered giant cells (Fig. 9A). Langerhans cells may be scanty or numerous within the infiltrate and are identified as large ovoid cells with abundant cytoplasm and variably shaped indented or lobulated nuclei, which have a longitudinal groove; nuclear chromatin is either delicately dispersed or condensed along the prominent nuclear membrane. Eosinophil polymorphs may be numerous and occasionally form large aggregates (eosinophil abscesses). Langerhans cells are characterized ultrastructurally by intracytoplasmic tennis racquet–shaped inclusion bodies called Birbeck granules. Langerhans cells are positive for leukocyte common antigen, CD68, HLA-DR, S100 protein, CD1a, and Langerin (CD207) (see Fig. 9B).

MOLECULAR GENETIC FEATURES

BRAFV600E mutation has been identified in 50% to 65% of LCH cases. This mutation leads to activation of RAS/RAF/MEK/ERK signaling pathway, which is also involved in other malignant diseases (including malignant melanoma and colorectal carcinoma). The activated RAS/RAF/MEK/ERK pathway has been observed also in BRAF wild-type cases and subsequently, in a significant proportion of these cases, activating mutations of MAP2K1 and ARAF genes have been identified.[28,29]

PROGNOSIS AND TREATMENT

Solitary bone lesions in LCH tend to stabilize or regress spontaneously but can be treated by simple curettage or injection of steroids.

LCH is discussed in more detail in this issue (See Arjen H.G. Cleven and Pancras C.W. Hogendoorn's article, "Haematopoietic Tumors Primarily Presenting in Bone," in this issue).[30]

FIBROUS DYSPLASIA (FD)

FD is a common benign bone lesion composed of cellular fibrous tissue and irregular woven bone trabeculae.[6,31] FD accounts for approximately 8% of all bone tumors. Most cases involve only a single bone (monostotic). In 20% of cases, the condition is polyostotic and more than 1 bone is involved. Monostotic FD may present over a wide age range but is most often diagnosed in the first 3 decades of life. Male and female patients are affected equally. Most patients present with swelling, deformity, and bone pain, which may be of long duration. Most monostotic lesions cease to enlarge after skeletal growth has ended. Pregnancy may reactivate the growth of some lesions. Any bone may be affected in monostotic or polyostotic FD, but those most often involved are the skull, facial bones, jaw, rib, pelvis, and long tubular bones, especially the femur and tibia.

RADIOLOGIC FEATURES

Lesions are usually well defined and radiolucent and have a ground-glass appearance. There is often a sclerotic rim around the lesion. There may be endosteal scalloping of the cortex and expansion of the bone. In long bones, the metaphysis and diaphysis are most often affected;

Fig. 9. (*A*) LCH with multi-nucleated giant cells (hematoxylin-eosin, original magnification ×400). (*B*) LCH with abundant eosinophils. Langerhans cells contain grooved nuclei. (*Insert*)   CD1a-positive Langerhans cells (hematoxylin-eosin,   original magnification ×400).

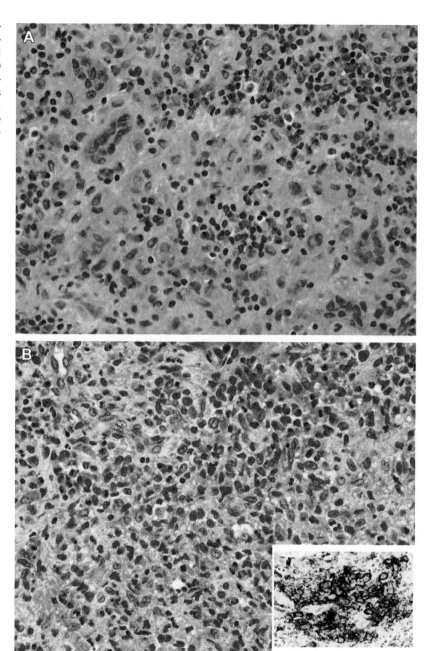

epiphyseal involvement is unusual. There may be associated bony deformity (eg, shepherd's crook deformity of the proximal femur).

MACROSCOPIC FEATURES

FD consists of a well-defined mass of firm, white, gritty, fibrous tissue, which fills the medulla and extends into the cortex. Cystic change and nodules of cartilage may be noted.

MICROSCOPIC FEATURES

FD is composed of small irregular trabeculae of woven bone that lie in a cellular fibrous stroma. Woven bone trabeculae are thin and irregular in

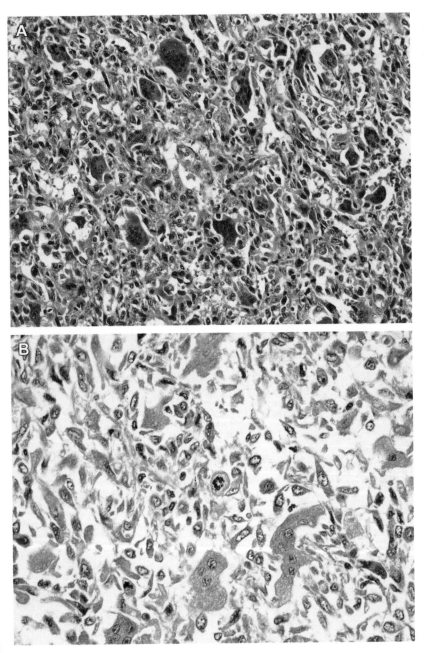

Fig. 10. (*A*) Giant cell–rich osteosarcoma. Even distribution of giant cells in this field mimics GCTB (hematoxylin-eosin, original magnification ×200). (*B*) Giant cell–rich osteosarcoma. On higher magnification pleomorphic mononuclear cells and abnormal mitotic figures are evident (hematoxylin-eosin, original magnification ×400).

shape and are not covered by plump osteoblasts. Bone trabeculae appear to be formed by fibro-osseous metaplasia and contain prominent cement lines. The fibrous stroma contains numerous spindle-shaped fibroblasts, which do not show mitotic activity or pleomorphism and are separated by abundant cellular or collagenous fibrous tissue. The fibrous stroma may exhibit a prominent storiform pattern or contain few fibroblasts and abundant collagen. Foci of calcification, which resembles cementum or psammoma bodies, and areas of myxoid and cystic change may be noted and there may be collections of lipid-laden foamy macrophages and multinucleated osteoclast-like giant cells, particularly around areas of hemorrhage. Small and large nodules of cartilage may be present.

MOLECULAR GENETICS

In FD, there is an activating mutation of the gene that codes for the G_s-α subunit (GNAS1), which stimulates the activity of adenyl cyclase and results in elevation of intracellular cyclic AMP in mesenchymal precursor cells; this leads to over-expression of the Fos protein and consequent enhancement of osteoblast differentiation. GNAS1 mutation detection can be useful in establishing a diagnosis of FD.[32,33]

PROGNOSIS AND TREATMENT

Myxoid/cystic degeneration or ABC change may result in rapid growth of the lesion and suggest sarcomatous change. Sarcomatous transformation to osteosarcoma, fibrosarcoma, or chondrosarcoma can occur but is a rare complication; it has been associated with previous radiation therapy. Treatment of symptomatic lesions is essentially surgical. Recurrence after incomplete curettage or marginal resection may occur.

OSTEOSARCOMAS CONTAINING NUMEROUS OSTEOCLASTS

Giant cell–rich osteosarcoma is a rare histologic subtype of conventional osteosarcoma in which there are numerous scattered osteoclast-like giant cells as well as features of a high-grade malignant bone-forming tumor.[6,34] This tumor enters into the differential diagnosis of GCTB (**Fig. 10**A). Giant cell–rich osteosarcoma can contain very large

numbers of evenly distributed osteoclast-like giant cells. The neoplastic osteoid formation, especially in small biopsy samples, is not always obvious. In these cases, recognition of nuclear pleomorphism and the presence of atypical mitoses leads to the correct diagnosis (see **Fig. 10**B). Telangiectatic osteosarcoma is a rare subtype of intramedullary osteosarcoma characterized by the presence of numerous blood-filled spaces separated by fibrous tissue septa containing malignant bone-forming tumor cells and scattered osteoclasts[6,35] (**Fig. 11**). Most osteosarcomas occur in the metaphysis of long bones and cause bone pain, swelling, or pathologic fracture. Telangiectatic osteosarcoma resembles an ABC, composed of multiple cystic spaces separated by fibrous tissue in which there are numerous benign osteoclast-like giant cells. In addition, in contrast to ABC, there are pleomorphic, atypical tumor cells, some of which exhibit osteoid or bone formation, lining cystic spaces and within fibrous septa. Correlation with radiologic appearances, especially when a sample is limited, is of paramount importance in the differential diagnosis GCTB, ABC, and osteosarcoma variants (**Fig. 12**).

OTHER BONE LESIONS CONTAINING NUMEROUS OSTEOCLASTS

Osteoclasts are seen whenever there is remodeling of bone and thus are commonly seen in non-neoplastic lesions, such as hyperparathyroidism, Paget disease, and fracture repair. A brown tumor

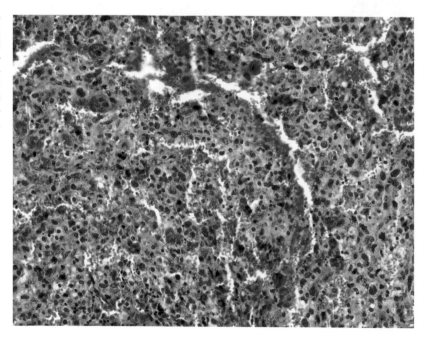

Fig. 11. Telangiectatic osteosarcoma showing irregular blood-filled spaces scattered osteoclasts and malignant tumor cells with atypical nuclei in fibrous septa (hematoxylin-eosin, original magnification ×250).

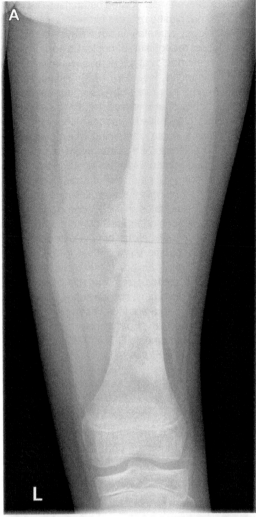

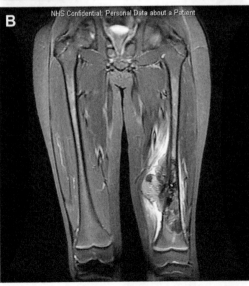

of hyperparathyroidism represents an area where much of the bone has been resorbed by osteoclasts.[6] There is abundant cellular fibrous tissue and some newly formed woven bone filling the medullary cavity that also contains areas of hemorrhage and numerous scattered osteoclasts and macrophages (Fig. 13). The surrounding bone frequently shows features of hyperparathyroidism with increased bone resorption, numerous thin bone trabeculae, and evidence of dissecting resorption and paratrabecular fibrosis. Rare giant cell–rich tumors have been reported in Paget disease, mostly in association with fracture of a pagetic bone.[36] Giant cells in bone can also be found in infective and noninfective granulomatous lesions involving bone, including the foreign body reaction to implant-derived wear particles[37] and when pigmented villonodular synovitis erodes bone.

Osteoclasts can be prominent when a simple bone cyst (unicameral bone cyst; solitary bone cyst) is complicated by fracture (Fig. 14). This lesion occurs most often in the metaphysis of a long tubular bone, in particular the proximal humerus; the cyst lies typically in the metaphysis just below the growth plate and has characteristic radiologic features. Hemorrhage into a simple bone cyst needs to be distinguished from ABC and cystic change in FD. Massive osteolysis (Gorham-Stout disease; disappearing bone disease) is a rare, massively resorptive condition that occurs most commonly in children, adolescents, and young adults characterized radiologically by extensive dissolution of cortical and cancellous bone and histologically by vascular proliferation with numerous anastomosing cavernous or capillary-size thin-walled vessels lying between bone trabeculae, which are undergoing active osteoclastic bone resorption. Osteoclasts may be prominent in clear cell chondrosarcoma, a rare, low-grade variant of chondrosarcoma that usually arises in the epiphysis of a long bone and needs to be distinguished from chondroblastoma, and in certain cases from undifferentiated high-grade pleomorphic sarcoma of bone.

Fig. 12. (*A*) Radiograph and (*B*) MRI appearances of telangiectatic osteosarcoma of the distal femur showing partly lytic partly sclerotic infiltrative tumor involving bone and soft tissues.

Fig. 13. Brown tumor of hyperparathyroidism showing cellular fibrous tissue in which there are focal areas of hemorrhage and (GCTB-like) scattered osteoclasts and macrophages (hematoxylin-eosin, original magnification ×250).

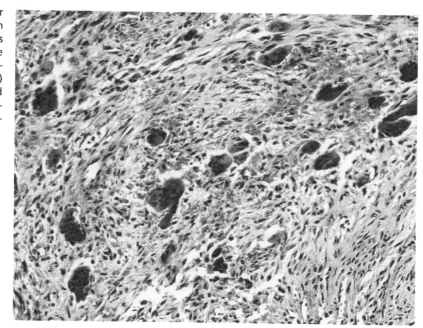

Fig. 14. Simple bone cyst of the right femur complicated by pathologic fracture.

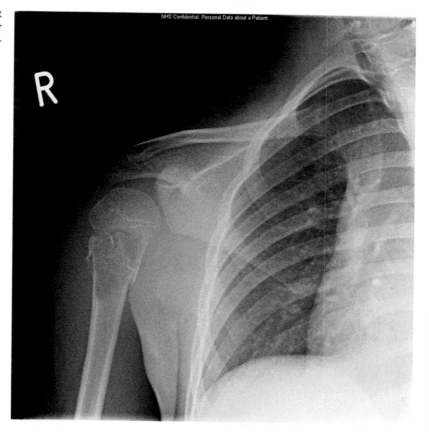

Differential Diagnosis
OF GIANT CELL–CONTAINING TUMORS OF BONE

	Helpful Distinguishing Features	Underlying Molecular Changes
GCTB	• Skeletally mature patients • Most common in distal femur and proximal tibia • Eccentric, lytic, well-defined, fleshy • Uniformly distributed osteoclast-like giant cells, round to spindle-shaped mononuclear cells • Mitotic activity can be high, but true pleomorphism and atypical mitoses are absent • Common secondary aneurysmal cyst formation, fibrohistiocytic proliferation	• Histone H3.3 driver mutation in H3F3A on chromosome 1
Chondroblastoma	• Skeletally immature patients • Chondroid matrix ± chicken wire calcification • Chondroblasts with nuclear grooves • Usually low mitotic activity without atypical forms • S100 and K36M positivity; focal DOG1 positivity	• Histone H3.3 driver mutation in H3F3B on chromosome 17
CMF	• Common metaphyseal location in 2nd and 3rd decades • Sharp, sclerotic border • Lobules of chondromyxoid matrix with stellate and spindle cells • Peripherally cellular areas • Minimal if any mitotic activity • Sparse giant cells • Chondroblastic differentiation: S100 positive • Smooth muscle actin and muscle-specific actin focally positive	• Up-regulation of GRM1 gene
ABC	• Common in skeletally immature patients • Cystic spaces lined by histiocytes, giant cells • Uneven distribution of giant cells • Uniform fibroblast-like spindle cells • Variable mitotic activity without atypical mitoses • Woven bone, osteoid formation in long strands	• UPS6 gene rearrangement in 70% of primary ABCs • No UPS6 gene rearrangement in secondary ABCs
NOF	• Skeletally immature patients, metaphyseal location, cortically based lesion • Plump fibroblasts in storiform or whorled pattern • Xanthoma cells, unevenly distributed giant cells • Strong CD68 and CD163 positivity	
Brown tumor of hyperparathyroidism	• Serum calcium increased • Serum phosphate decreased • Paratrabecular fibrosis • Dissecting bone resorption	

(continued on next page)

LCH	• Young individuals; 50% of the patients are in their first decade of life. • Craniofacial bones, vertebral bodies, ribs, pelvis, and femur are commonly involved. • Multisystem form: involvement of skin, lymph nodes, liver can occur • Two main components: Langerhans cells and eosinophilic granulocytes • Variable proportion of foamy macrophages, lymphocytes, plasma cells, and fibroblasts • Langerhans cells with nuclear groove • Langerhans cells are S100, CD1a, and Langerin positive • EM: tennis racquet–shaped Birbeck granules	• Activation of RAS/RAF/MEK/ERK pathway by • BRAFV600E mutation (50%–65%) or by • MAP2K1 mutation or by • ARAF mutation
FD	• Most common in first 3 decades of life • Wide anatomic distribution: skull, gnathic bones, pelvis, femur, tibia • Medullary lesion, radiolucent with ground-glass appearance • Fibro-osseous proliferation: whorled and storiform bland fibroblastic proliferation and irregular fish hook woven bone trabeculae • Around the bone trabeculae no osteoblast rimming is present • Osteoclast-like giant cells, xanthoma cells, hemorrhages and secondary aneurysmal cysts can occur within FD	• GNAS1 mutation
Telangiectatic osteosarcoma Giant cell–rich osteosarcoma	• Uneven distribution of giant cells • Osteoid formation • Blood-filled cystic spaces – in telangiectatic variant • Angulated or spindle cells • Marked cytologic atypia • Atypical mitoses	• No specific molecular genetic marker is known

Pitfalls
IN DIAGNOSIS OF GIANT CELL TUMORS

! Radiographic correlation is required to establish the precise anatomic location of the tumor within bone.

! Check serum calcium and phosphate to exclude hyperparathyroidism in cases of GCTB.

! Do not misdiagnose ABC for teleangiectatic osteosarcoma (or vice versa); check radiology and look for evidence of nuclear atypia and osteoid formation.

! Overinterpretation of mitotic activity and necrosis in GCTB could lead to misdiagnosis of a malignant giant cell–rich sarcoma.

! Ignoring the presence of atypical mitoses could result in misdiagnosis of a benign giant cell–rich lesion.

! In CMF, cellular pleomorphism and hyperchromasia within the area of myxoid change can lead to confusion with chondrosarcoma.

REFERENCES

1. Athanasou NA. The osteoclast–what's new? Skeletal Radiol 2011;40:1137–40.
2. Lau YS, Sabokbar A, Gibbons CLMH, et al. Phenotypic and molecular studies on giant cell tumours of bone and soft tissues. Hum Pathol 2005;36:945–54.
3. Taylor R, Kashima TG, Hemingway F, et al. CD14-molecular stromal cells support CD14+ monocyte-osteoclast differentiation in aneurysmal bone cyst. Lab Invest 2012;92:600–5.
4. Huang L, Cheng YY, Chow LT, et al. Receptor activator of NF-kappa B ligand (RANKL) is expressed in chondroblastoma; possible involvement in osteoclastic giant cell recruitment. Mol Pathol 2003;56:116–20.
5. Athanasou NA, Bansal M, Forsyth R, et al. Giant cell tumour of bone. In: Fletcher CDM, Bridge JA, Hogendoorn PCW, et al, editors. WHO classification of tumours of soft tissue and bone. 4th edition. Lyon (France): International Agency for Research on Cancer; 2013. p. 321–4.
6. Unni KK, Inwards CY, Bridge JA, et al. Tumors of the Bones and Joints. AFIP Atlas of Tumor Pathology Vol. 2. Publisher: American Registry of Pathology 2006.
7. Maggiani F, Forsyth R, Hogendoorn PCW, et al. Immunophenotype of osteoclasts and macrophage polykaryons. J Clin Pathol 2011;64:701–5.
8. Cleven AH, Hocker S, Briaire-de-Bruijn I, et al. Mutation analysis of H3F3A and H3F3B as a diagnostic tool for giant cell tumour of bone and chondroblastoma. Am J Surg Pathol 2015;39:1576–83.
9. Presneau N, Baumhoer D, Behiati S, et al. Diagnostic value of H3F3A mutations in giant cell tumours of bone compared to osteoclast-rich mimics. J Pathol Clin Res 2015;1:113–23.
10. Bahjati S, Tarpey PS, Presneau N, et al. Distinct H3F3A and H3F3B driver mutations define chondroblastoma and giant cell tumour of bone. Nat Genet 2013;45:1479–82.
11. Girolami I, Mancinic I, Simoni A, et al. Denosumab treated giant cell tumour of bone: a morphological immunohistochemical and molecular analysis of a series. J Clin Pathol 2016;69:240–7.
12. Kilpatrick SE, Romeo S. Chondroblastoma. In: Fletcher CDM, Bridge JA, Hogendoorn PCW, et al, editors. WHO classification of tumours of soft tissue and bone. 4th edition. Lyon (France): International Agency for Research on Cancer; 2013. p. 262–3.
13. Akpalo H, Lange C, Zustin J. Discovered on gastrointestinal stromal tumour 1 (DOG1): a useful immunohistochemical marker for diagnosing chondroblastoma. Histopathology 2012;60:1099–106.
14. Cleven AH, Briaire-de Bruijn I, Szuhai K, et al. DOG1 expression in giant-cell-containing bone tumours. Histopathology 2016;68:942–5.
15. Fang D, Gan H, Lee JH, et al. The histone H3.3K36M mutation reprograms the epigenome of chondroblastomas. Science 2016;10(352):1344–8.
16. Amary MF, Berisha F, Mozella R, et al. The H3F3 K36M mutant antibody is a sensitive and specific marker for the diagnosis of chondroblastoma. Histopathology 2016;69:121–7.
17. Lielsen JA, Fletcher JA, Oliveira AM. Aneurysmal bone cyst. In: Fletcher CDM, Bridge JA, Hogendoorn PCW, et al, editors. WHO classification of tumours of soft tissue and bone. 4th edition. Lyon (France): International Agency for Research on Cancer; 2013. p. 348–9.
18. Oliveira AM, His BL, Weremowica S, et al. USP6 (Tre2) Fusion oncogenes in aneurysmal bone cyst. Cancer Res 2004;64:1920–6.
19. Oliveira AM, Perez-Atayde AR, Inwards CY, et al. USP6 and CDH11 oncogenes identify the neoplastic cell in primary aneurysmal bone cysts and are absent in so-called aneurysmal bone cysts. Am J Pathol 2004;165:1773–80.
20. Althof PA, Ohmori K, Zhou M, et al. Cytogenetic and molecular cytogenetic findings in 43 aneurysmal bone cysts: aberrations of 17p mapped to 17p13.2 by fluorescence in situ hybridization. Mod Pathol 2004;17:518–25.
21. Skubitz KM, Peltola JC, Santos ER, et al. Response of aneurysmal bone cysts to denosumab. Spine 2015;40:E1201–4.
22. Forsyth R, Jundt G. Giant cell lesion of the small bones. In: Fletcher CDM, Bridge JA, Hogendoorn PCW, et al, editors. WHO classification of tumours of soft tissue and bone. 4th edition. Lyon (France): International Agency for Research on Cancer; 2013. p. 320.
23. Agaram NP, LeLoarer FV, Zhang L, et al. USP6 gene rearrangements occur preferentially in giant cell reparative granulomas of the hands and feet but not in gnatic location. Hum Pathol 2014;45:1147–52.
24. Romeo S, Aigner T, Bridge JA. Chondromyxoid fibroma. In: Fletcher CDM, Bridge JA, Hogendoorn PCW, et al, editors. WHO classification of tumours of soft tissue and bone. 4th edition. Lyon (France): International Agency for Research on Cancer; 2013. p. 255–6.
25. Nord KH, Lilljeborn H, Vezzi F, et al. GRM1 is upregulated through gene fusion and promoter swapping in chondromyxoid fibroma. Nat Genet 2014;46:474–7.
26. Nielsen GP, Kyriakos M. Non-ossifying fibroma/benign fibrous histiocytoma of bone. In: Fletcher CDM, Bridge JA, Hogendoorn PCW, et al, editors. WHO classification of tumours of soft tissue and bone. 4th edition. Lyon (France): International Agency for Research on Cancer; 2013. p. 302–4.
27. De Young B, Egeler RM, Rolling BJ. Langerhans cell histiocytosis. In: Fletcher CDM, Bridge JA, Hogendoorn PCW, et al, editors. WHO classification of tumours of soft tissue and bone. 4th edition. Lyon

(France): International Agency for Research on Cancer; 2013. p. 356–7.

28. Chakraborty R, Hampton OA, Shen X, et al. Mutually exclusive recurrent somatic mutations in MAP2K1 and BRAF support a central role for ERK activation in LCH pathogenesis. Blood 2014;124:3007–15.

29. Nelson DS, Quispel W, Badalian-Very G, et al. Somatic activating mutations in Langerhans cell histiocytosis. Blood 2014;123:3152–5.

30. Cleven AHG, Hoogendoorn PCW. Haemopoietic tumours primary presenting in bone. Surg Pathol Clinic. Elsevier 2017, in press.

31. Siegal GP, Bianco P, Dai Cin P. Fibrous dysplasia. In: Fletcher CDM, Bridge JA, Hogendoorn PCW, et al, editors. WHO classification of tumours of soft tissue and bone. 4th edition. Lyon (France): International Agency for Research on Cancer; 2013. p. 351–3.

32. Idowu BD, Al-Adnani M, O'Donnell P. A sensitive mutation-specific screening technique for GNAS1 mutations in cases of fibrous dysplasia: the first report of a codon 227 mutation in bone. Histopathology 2007;50:691–704.

33. Lee SE, Lee EH, Park H, et al. The diagnostic utility of the GNAS mutation in patients with fibrous dysplasia: meta-analysis of 168 sporadic cases. Hum Pathol 2012;43:1234–42.

34. Rosenberg AM, Cleton-Jansen A, de Pinieux G, et al. Conventional osteosarcoma. In: Fletcher CDM, Bridge JA, Hogendoorn PCW, et al, editors. WHO classification of tumours of soft tissue and bone. 4th edition. Lyon (France): International Agency for Research on Cancer; 2013. p. 282–8.

35. Oliveira A, Okada K, Squire J. Telangiectatic osteosarcoma. In: Fletcher CDM, Bridge JA, Hogendoorn PCW, et al, editors. WHO classification of tumours of soft tissue and bone. 4th edition. Lyon (France): International Agency for Research on Cancer; 2013. p. 289–90.

36. Gamage NM, Kashima TG, McNally MA, et al. Giant-cell-rich pseudotumour in Paget's disease. Skeletal Radiol 2013;42:595–9.

37. Athanasou NA. The pathobiology and pathology of aseptic implant failure. Bone Joint Res 2016;5:162–8.

Ewing Sarcoma, an Update on Molecular Pathology with Therapeutic Implications

Enrique de Alava, MD, PhD

KEYWORDS

- Sarcoma • Ewing sarcoma • Small round cell sarcoma • Molecular pathology • Diagnosis

Key points

- Ewing sarcoma is a small round cell sarcoma showing pathognomonic molecular findings and varying degrees of neuroectodermal differentiation detected by light, electron microscopy, or immunohistochemistry.

- Ewing sarcoma pathogenesis is driven by pathognomonic and etiologic EWS-ETS gene fusions that encode chimeric transcription factors that are expressed in these tumors.

- Of patients with Ewing sarcoma, 85% have *EWSR1-FLI1* fusions and *EWSR1-ERG* fusions are present in 10% of cases, whereas, in 3% of cases, fusions between *EWSR1* and other members of the ETS family of transcription factors are detected. Ancillary techniques, detecting these fusions/rearrangements, help to perform an accurate differential diagnosis of Ewing sarcoma.

- The development of new therapies in Ewing sarcoma would benefit from the improvement in representative animal models, data, or sample collection, among others.

- The pathologist, within a multidisciplinary team, has an important role in the research and validation of new therapies.

ABSTRACT

Ewing sarcoma is a developmental tumor characterized by balanced chromosomal translocations and formation of new fusion genes. Despite the large amount of knowledge regarding the molecular aspects obtained in the last few years, many questions still remain. This article focuses on research on the molecular pathology and possible developments in targeted therapies in this malignancy and discusses some related bottlenecks, as well as the possible role of pathologists, the availability of samples, the lack of appropriate animal models, and the resources needed to carry out preclinical and clinical research.

EWING SARCOMA

The most recent World Health Organization classification considers Ewing sarcoma (ES) as a single entity that encompasses different clinical presentations and histologic appearances: bone and soft tissue sites, peripheral primitive neuroectodermal tumor (pPNET), skin tumors, and other less frequent examples.[1]

ES is a rare malignancy that affects mainly children and young adults. It is a small round cell

Disclosure Statement: The author has no conflicts of interest to disclose. E.de Alava is supported by Ministry of Economy and Competitiveness of Spain-FEDER grants (CIBERONC, RD12/0036/0017, PI14/01466), María García-Estrada, Mari Paz Jiménez Casado Foundation, La Sonrisa de Alex Foundation, CRIS contra el Cáncer Foundations, Pablo Ugarte Association and EU-funded projects (EEC-Euroewing and EUROSARC).
Department of Pathology, Institute of Biomedicine of Sevilla-Virgen del Rocío University Hospital, Hospital Universitario Virgen del Rocío, CSIC-University of Seville-CIBERONC, Edificio Anatomía Patológica, Avenida Manuel Siurot s/n, 41013 Seville, Spain
E-mail address: enrique.alava.sspa@juntadeandalucia.es

sarcoma showing pathognomonic molecular findings, and varying degrees of neuroectodermal differentiation detected by light, electron microscopy, or immunohistochemistry. The term PNET was classically used for ES with evidence of neuroectodermal differentiation. ES is molecularly characterized by recurrent balanced translocations that lead to the formation of novel fusion oncogenes that are the key to pathogenesis. ES pathogenesis is driven by pathognomonic and etiologic EWS-ETS gene fusions that encode chimeric transcription factors that are expressed in these tumors. EWS-ETS fusion proteins activate or repress specific sets of target genes and generate a widespread epigenomic reprograming that, in the right timing and cellular context, give rise to the transformed phenotype of ES.[2] Recent data point to either mesenchymal stem cells or neural crest-derived stem cells as the cell of origin of ES[3,4]

CLINICAL FEATURES

ES is the second most common bone or soft tissue sarcoma in the pediatric age group. It usually affects male patients 10 to 25 years old, although well-documented cases with molecular confirmation have been reported in patients older than 40 years. ES predominantly affects the bones in the distal extremity (23%), proximal extremity (22%), the thorax or abdomen (20%), or the pelvis (19%).[5] Approximately 20% of ESs are extraskeletal and usually arise (in descending order of frequency) in the thigh, pelvis, paraspinal area, and foot.[5] Approximately 25% of patients have clinically detectable metastases at the time of diagnosis, although it is likely that nearly all patients have micrometastasis at diagnosis because the cure rate using only local treatment (resection and radiation therapy) is less than 20%.[6]

HISTOPATHOLOGY

Gross examination of untreated ES specimens is now uncommon because of the standard use of neoadjuvant chemotherapy. The cut surface is gray-white and soft, frequently with areas of hemorrhage and necrosis. ES can be large; in fact, the volume of a Ewing tumor is an important prognostic factor. Resection specimens of treated tumors show reparative features, such as marked sclerosis and hemorrhage, often with no visible residual foci of viable tumor.

Histologically, conventional ES is composed of sheets of packed cells with relatively small, round nuclei, displaying a monomorphous pattern under low-power examination (Fig. 1). The chromatin is finely granular, and nucleoli are inconspicuous. A small number of darker cells are seen among more common lighter cells; electron microscopy suggests that dark cells are probably undergoing apoptosis.[7] There are usually extensive deposits of glycogen in the cytoplasm; periodic acid or Schiff stain is positive in more than half of tumors, especially in well-fixed specimens. Nevertheless, all other round cell sarcomas can show variable

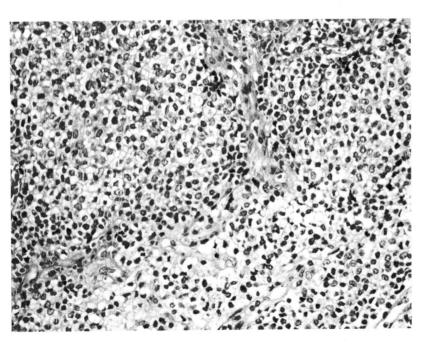

Fig. 1. ES. Conventional appearance of ES. Note the vaguely lobular pattern and clear cytoplasm secondary to abundant glycogen.

proportions of periodic acid or Schiff–positive cells. This feature is, therefore, not useful for differential diagnosis. Reticulin stains show a lack of matrix among tumor cells. A large cell, or atypical, variant has been reported[8] that shows a low-magnification appearance similar to that of conventional ES. The main differences are the larger size and the more irregular contours of the nuclei; conspicuous nucleoli can be seen, and periodic acid or Schiff stain is frequently negative (Fig. 2). The immunophenotypic and molecular features are similar to those of conventional ES and current literature reports no consistent prognostic importance to this variant. Availability of molecular diagnostics, and growing awareness by soft tissue and bone pathologists, has helped to categorize some of these cases into CIC-rearranged or BCOR-rearranged sarcomas,[9] whereas bona fide atypical ES has EWSR1-ETS fusions.

ESs showing a higher degree of neural differentiation (formerly called PNET) contain Homer-Wright rosettes, with a central fibrillary core lacking vascular lumina, similar to those seen in neuroblastoma. More frequently, tumors with a rosette-like configuration contain ill-defined groups of up to 10 cells oriented toward a central space (Fig. 3). They show a higher expression level of neuron-specific enolase and other (nonspecific) neuroectodermal markers, such as Leu-7 (CD57),

than conventional (undifferentiated) ES. No consistent prognostic differences have been found between these 2 groups.

Tumor cells show a variable degree of necrosis after induction chemotherapy, and they are replaced by loose connective tissue. Histopathologic assessment of tumor necrosis after therapy using various grading systems correlates with overall survival. Several different grading systems have been reported. Similar to osteosarcoma, the prognostically relevant cutoff in most systems is 10% residual viable tumor cells.[6]

IMMUNOHISTOCHEMISTRY

CD99 is a cell surface glycoprotein, the product of the MIC2 gene. Strong, diffuse membranous expression is seen in approximately 95% of ESs[1] (Fig. 4). MIC2 expression is unrelated to the gene products of the specific translocations found in ESs. CD99 expression is not specific for ES and has been seen in a large group of normal tissues and tumor types, including other round cell sarcomas. For example, between 71% and 93% of lymphoblastic lymphomas and leukemias express MIC2.[10] Few neoplastic cells exhibited weak, cytoplasmic staining in all 33 cases studied in a recent series of small cell osteosarcoma,[11] as well as almost all mesenchymal chondrosarcomas,[12]

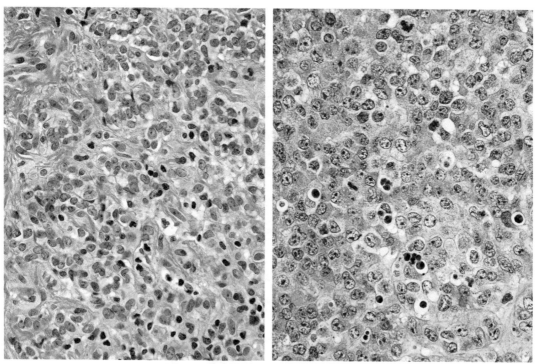

Fig. 2. ES. Large cell variant of ES (*right*), compared with conventional ES (*left*) in terms of nuclear size, nuclear irregularity, and prominent nucleoli.

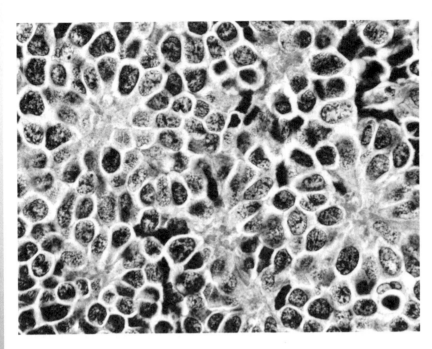

Fig. 3. ES. Well-formed pseudorosettes in an ES with extensive neural differentiation (pNET). Note the absence of nucleoli and the finely granular chromatin.

between 10% and 25% of rhabdomyosarcomas, and approximately 20% of desmoplastic small round cell tumors (DSRCTs).[13] In DSRCTs and rhabdomyosarcomas, CD99 usually shows a cytoplasmic staining pattern, in contrast to the membranous pattern typical of ES. Importantly, neuroblastomas lack CD99 immunoreactivity in all locations and age groups.[14] Clearly, CD99 is a sensitive but not a specific marker for ES.

Immunohistochemical detection of *FLI1* has proven to be more specific for ES than CD99, with a somewhat lower sensitivity. Specificity of *FLI1* is limited by its expression in lymphoblastic leukemias or lymphomas, non-Hodgkin lymphomas, and endothelial cells and derived neoplasms. Sensitivity is limited by occasionally low levels of expression of *FLI1* and by the occurrence of variant translocations that do not involve the *FLI1* gene.[15]

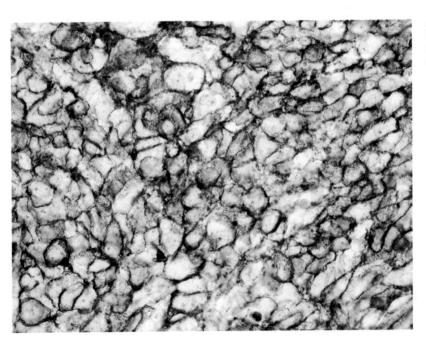

Fig. 4. CD99 in ES. Diffuse membranous immunoreactivity for CD99 is characteristic of ES.

MOLECULAR PATHOLOGY

Approximately 85% of patients with ES have *EWSR1-FLI1* fusions; *EWSR1-ERG* fusions are present in 10% of cases, whereas, in 3% of cases, fusions between *EWSR1* and other members of the ETS family of transcription factors are detected, such as *FEV1*.[1] ESs may show occasionally fusions between *EWSR1* and non-ETS gene family members (*PATZ1, SP3, NFATc2, SMARCA5*); these tumors may have some atypical morphology (scattered enlarged cells, more prominent nucleoli) or present at older ages but show a significant pathologic overlap with conventional ES with ETS-including fusions. Finally, a small group of ESs shows *FUS* gene instead of *EWSR1* rearranged with an ERG or *FEV* gene partner; *FUS* positive tumors seem to be morphologically and immunohistochemically similar to *EWSR1*-positive ES.[16] *FUS* gene rearrangements should be studied in cases of small round cell sarcomas with morphology concordant with ES and strong CD99 expression but lacking *EWSR1* rearrangements.[17]

All these rearrangements are characteristic of this tumor type because polymerase chain reaction (PCR) and Fluorescent in situ hybridization (FISH) studies of other small round cell tumors that would enter into the differential diagnosis, such as neuroblastoma, rhabdomyosarcoma, adamantinoma, or giant cell tumor of bone, are negative for these particular fusion genes. A reference laboratory for small round cell tumor diagnosis may have either FISH or reverse transcription (RT)-PCR or, preferably, both methods available. The introduction of next-generation sequencing is highly advisable in this setting. The choice of technique depends on the specific experience of the laboratory,[18] although RT-PCR is suitable when frozen tissue is available, whereas FISH is a good choice when only formalin-fixed, paraffin-embedded tissue is available. There are several commercial sources for *EWSR1* break-apart probes. Importantly, however, assays using *EWSR1* break-apart probes do not detect *EWSR1-FLI1* fusions *per se* but only *EWSR1* gene rearrangements, which should not be a problem in most cases. The impact of technologies such as massively parallel sequencing technologies and associated computational algorithms (next-generation sequencing) in ES diagnosis will likely be the generation of a relevant amount of new information, some of which could be used to identify and validate targetable molecular alterations in ES.[19] Next-generation sequencing application to ES has shown, in fact, the potential pitfall of relying only on FISH-based assays to detect *EWSR1*-containing fusions.[17] For a list of tumors showing *EWSR1* gene rearrangements, see **Table 1**.

HOW TO USE ANCILLARY STUDIES FOR DIFFERENTIAL DIAGNOSIS

A basic immunohistochemical panel for small round cell tumors, such as that shown in **Table 2**, in the appropriate clinical and histologic context, should be sufficient to allow a confident diagnosis of ES and, in particular, to exclude nonsarcomatous entities. Moreover, FISH or RT-PCR analysis is helpful to confirm the diagnosis in difficult cases, as previously discussed.

In the author's experience, the 2 major differential diagnostic considerations for (extraskeletal) ES within the round cell sarcoma category are poorly differentiated synovial sarcoma and alveolar rhabdomyosarcoma.

ES can have an infiltrative pattern (sometimes referred to in the literature as a filigree pattern), with irregular strands of tumor cells in a fibrous

Table 1
Most prevalent gene fusions of diagnostic utility in Ewing sarcoma, useful for differential diagnosis with other small round cell morphologic features

Entity	Gene Fusion
ES	• *EWSR1* with any of the following: *FLI1, ERG, PATZ1, SP3, NFATc2, SMARCA5* • *FUS* with *ERG* or *FEV*
Alveolar rhabdomyosarcoma	*PAX3-FOXO1A* *PAX7-FOXO1A*
Embryonal rhabdomyosarcoma	None
DSRCT	*EWSR1-WT1*
Poorly differentiated synovial sarcoma	*SYT-SSX1* *SYT-SSX2*
Round cell or myxoid liposarcoma	*FUS-CHOP* *EWSR1-CHOP*
Mesenchymal chondrosarcoma	*HEY1-NCOA2*
CIC-rearranged sarcoma[a]	*CIC-DUX4/DUX4L* *CIC-FOXO4*
BCOR-rearranged sarcoma[a]	*BCOR-CCNB3* *BCOR-MAML3* *ZC3H7B-BCOR*

[a] There are cases with CIC or BCOR rearrangements with still unknown partners.

Table 2
Expected immunophenotype of Ewing sarcoma and other small round cell tumors

	Epithelial Membrane Antigen or Keratins	S-100 Protein	Lymphoid Markers[a]	Desmin	Myogenin	FLI1	WT1	CD99
ES	+	–	–	–	–	++	–	++
Rhabdomyosarcoma	–	–	–	++	++[b]	–	–	+
DSRCT	++	–	–	++	–	–	++[c]	+
Poorly differentiated synovial sarcoma	++	–	–	–	–	–	–	+
CIC-rearranged sarcoma[f]	+	–	–	+	–	–	+	Patchy
BCOR-rearranged sarcoma[g]	-	-	-	-	-	-	-	Patchy
Lymphoma or leukemia	–	–	++	–	–	+	–	+
Mesenchymal chondrosarcoma	–	–[d]	–	–	–	–	–	+
Neuroblastoma	–	–[e]	–	–	–	–	–	–
Wilms tumor	–	–	–	–	–	–	++	–
Melanoma	–	++	–	–	–	–	–	–

++, usually or almost always positive (>50%); +, occasionally positive (10% to 50%); −, never or almost never positive (<10%).
[a] CD45, terminal deoxynucleotidyl transferase, CD3, CD20, CD79a (as appropriate).
[b] Stronger and more diffuse in alveolar rhabdomyosarcoma.
[c] Only carboxyl-terminal epitopes in DSRCT.
[d] Except in overtly cartilaginous areas.
[e] Except in schwannian stromal areas.
[f] Consider also ETV4 or DUX4.
[g] Consider CCNB3 or BCOR.

stroma. If such a tumor arises in the abdomen and imaging techniques do not show an organ-specific location, the differential diagnosis of DSRCT is likely to arise. Attention should be paid to subtle morphologic features; fibrosis should not be mistaken for true desmoplasia, and capillary hyperplasia is characteristic of DSRCT. Both entities can share keratin and CD99 expression, although desmin (not myogenin) is usually expressed only in DSRCT. *EWSR1-WT1* fusions present in DSRCT lead to overexpression of the carboxyl-terminal domain of the WT1 protein,[13] which can be detected by immunohistochemistry, although available antibodies show inconsistent results. FISH analysis with commercial *EWSR1* breakapart probes is useless for this differential diagnosis because both entities share gene fusions with *EWSR1* rearrangements. RT-PCR, if frozen tissue is available, or next-generation sequencing are the techniques of choice.

Small cell osteosarcoma (**Fig. 5**) can pose particular diagnostic problems in core biopsy specimens, when osteoid may be scarce or absent. However, even if osteoid deposition is focal, tumor cell nuclei usually have mild variability in their size and shape, an uncommon finding in ES. Expression of STAB2, a nuclear protein shown to be of importance for osteoblastic differentiation, has been reported to be of help to differentiate hyalinized collagen and osteoid.[20] Caution, however, is to be used in the evaluation of STAB2 overexpression in small round cell sarcomas because it is usually positive in *BCOR*-rearranged sarcomas of bone in adolescents. A somewhat similar problem can arise in mesenchymal chondrosarcoma because the cartilaginous component may be missed in small biopsy specimens. Moreover,

CD99 expression is often detected in the cell membrane of the undifferentiated round cell component of mesenchymal chondrosarcoma.[12] Molecular analyses can solve the problem in both situations by confirming the presence of *EWSR1* gene rearrangement and the diagnosis of ES.

ES shares a variable degree of neural differentiation with neuroblastoma. There is a subgroup of schwannian stroma-poor neuroblastomas, designated undifferentiated, which can have small round cell morphologic features overlapping with those of ES. Age is helpful in this situation because this subset of neuroblastomas typically presents in patients younger than 18 months of age, which would be exceptional for ES. Neuroblastoma typically lacks CD99 expression and translocations involving the *EWSR1* gene.

ES can arise in the kidney. At this site, monophasic blastematous Wilms tumors can enter the differential diagnosis. Again, age is of help, because 90% of Wilms tumors arise before 6 years of age, which would be very uncommon for ES. In addition, Wilms tumors lack rearrangements involving the *EWSR1* gene.

PROGNOSIS AND TREATMENT

Prognostic factors in ES include stage, tumor location and volume, age, and response to induction chemotherapy.[21]

Multimodal approaches within clinical trials, using combination chemotherapy and surgery or radiation therapy, have improved 5-year survival rates from less than 10% to close to 80%. All current standard trials use 3 to 6 cycles of initial chemotherapy after biopsy, followed by local

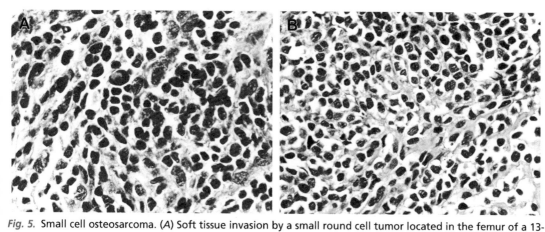

Fig. 5. Small cell osteosarcoma. (*A*) Soft tissue invasion by a small round cell tumor located in the femur of a 13-year-old boy. Mild pleomorphism and nuclear hyperchromasia suggest the diagnosis of small cell osteosarcoma; compare the chromatin quality with **Fig. 3**. (*B*) Osteoid produced by tumor cells was found after thorough sampling of the specimen, confirming the diagnosis of small cell osteosarcoma.

therapy and another 6 to 10 cycles of chemotherapy. Local control is attempted by surgery and radiation therapy if complete surgical resection is impossible, or if histologic response in the surgical specimen was poor (ie, >10% viable tumor cells).[21] Extraskeletal ES patients have a better prognosis than patients with osseous ES, independent of age, ethnic group, or primary site.[5]

PERSPECTIVES REGARDING NEW THERAPIES

It is beyond the scope of this article to detail all innovative therapies in ES. There are several recent comprehensive reviews on the subject.[22,23] Fig. 6 presents these therapies, together with some proposed targets or mechanisms of action. ES is a relatively rare disease (in Europe about 3 new cases per million a year). This generates several problems related to new therapy research:

- The pharmaceutical industry is not particularly interested in research on new therapies in pediatric neoplasms, especially those with a low incidence such as ES.

- From the biological point of view, ES lacks preneoplastic lesions. Moreover, there is no normal tissue counterpart. This happens in most sarcomas and does not help prevention as well as hampers the research on sarcomagenesis and tumor progression.
- Translocations and gene fusions of ES seem, at least in theory, to be the ideal drug target. Nevertheless, subcellular location of these molecules is the nucleus, which might not be easily reachable for many drugs. In addition, most sarcoma translocation-derived gene fusions correspond to chimerical transcription factors. They are actually involved in a complex mesh of protein-protein, protein-DNA, and epigenetic interactions, which represent the actual target. Therefore, the activity of most chimerical proteins cannot be regulated allosterically.
- There is a lack of genetically modified models of ES, in sharp contrast to other translocation-related sarcomas, such as synovial sarcoma or myxoid liposarcoma. Needless to say, such a model would be extremely valuable

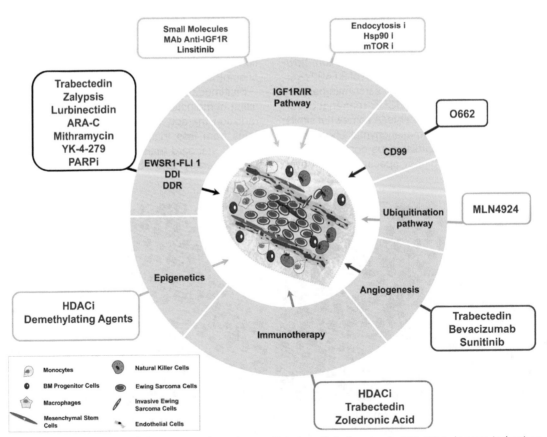

Fig. 6. The main targets and drugs currently under preclinical or clinical research. DDI, DNA damage induction; DDR, DNA damage repair.

to help find pharmacodynamic markers of response to new therapies.

- Clinical samples of ES are very scarce. Samples required include not only primary tumor but also relapsed or metastatic tumor samples, as well as body fluids (ie, plasma for proteomics and circulating biomarkers). A strong need exists for the development of biobanks with well-annotated samples that allow for adequate clinical validation of preclinical studies.
- Another major problem for biomarker validation in ES is that most studies assessing the prognostic value of biomarkers have been performed using small retrospective series of subjects. Several promising biomarkers that have shown prognostic impact in retrospective studies but require careful validation in prospective joint investigation have recently been described by the ES scientific community. A higher degree of clinical evidence would be attainable through the use of prospective studies. Prospectively validated prognostic and/or predictive biomarkers are thus needed to better stratify patients and to provide personalized risk-adapted therapeutic approaches. PROspective VAlidation of Biomarkers in Ewing Sarcoma for personalised

translational medicine (PROVABES), a joint European proposal that aims to cover this need (http://provabes.uni-muenster.de/) has been working on the prospective clinical validation of relevant ES biomarkers using samples and data from the EuroEwing trials.

Many coordinated resources are, therefore, needed to overcome the gap between basic research and clinical validation in ES, especially in understanding of biology and of design of better disease models (**Fig. 7**).

The role of pathologists within a multidisciplinary team in the application of molecular pathology to therapeutic implications cannot be overemphasized. Their involvement is important at least for the following reasons:

- Correct diagnosis or molecular characterization is a mandatory prerequisite to provide tumor samples with a precise histopathological and molecular diagnostic characterization. This is required for further comprehensive characterization of the patient derived biomaterials. Reference pathology panels should review cases to confirm the diagnosis and molecular characteristics of patient samples. The histopathological review provides an accurate diagnosis based on the 2013 WHO

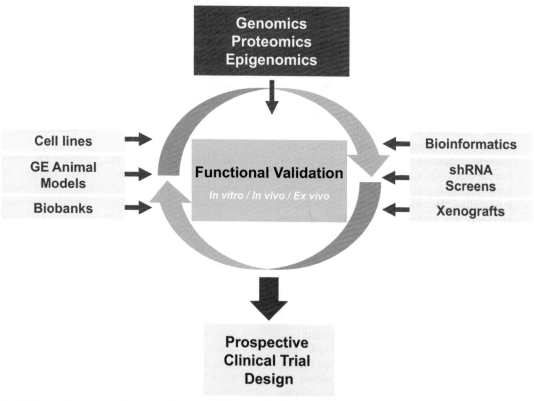

Fig. 7. Perspectives regarding new therapies. GE, genetically engineered.

classification of ES[1] and, together with strict adherence to standard operating procedures (SOPs), ensures the success of the in-depth molecular characterization.

- Pathologists are also required for a careful and comprehensive collection of biomaterials. This is a mandatory backbone for any translational research approach. New sequencing techniques allow a genome-wide assessment of cancer-related genes and pathways. In addition to genetic parameters that may be associated with age, localization, and tumor phenotype, a particular interest focuses on parameters that may be associated with the aggressiveness of the disease. An in-depth characterization of tumor material obtained from clinically well-annotated patients will allow the identification and validation of novel prognostic or predictive biomarkers as well as druggable pathways. The comprehensive characterization of tumor material is necessary to understand the spectrum of distinct alterations in ES to identify patients who are likely to respond to particular therapies, and to facilitate the selection of treatment modalities. It should include identification and characterization of small noncoding RNAs present in tumor tissue by high throughput sequencing, characterization of transcriptome signatures, and genomic and epigenomic variations in ES cells compared with the germline counterpart. SOPs for ES sample collection and banking should, therefore, be available in the Pathology departments of all major reference sarcoma centers. Prognostic biomarker studies traditionally focus on investigations in primary tumor, although disseminated disease and genetic variation in drug metabolism and transport will contribute to a patients' response to treatment and outcome. Furthermore, for real-time monitoring of patient response and disease course, clinically informative biomarkers that can be detected in blood are particularly attractive because blood is a minimally invasive compartment for sampling. In cases in which such changes predict Efent-free survival (EFS) or Overall survival (OS), circulating biomarkers may be useful to inform the selection of optimal therapy for individual patients and are especially attractive in cancer types such as ES in which viable tumor at diagnosis can be limited.
- Prospective tissue microarray (TMA) sets should be performed by the reference Pathology centers. The use of TMAs allows the processing of hundreds of tumor samples with a variety of techniques; that is, immunohistochemistry and fluorescent in situ hybridization at the same time. The TMA collections established within the biobank are among the most crucial resources for discovering and validating potential biomarkers. Because representativeness of the tissue cores may be a disadvantage compared with full sections, a careful production of TMA by experienced reference pathologists is mandatory to achieve representative results. The TMA panels are used to prospectively validate markers that have been previously described and for future studies on markers that may be identified within these tasks.
- Biomarkers include pharmacodynamic markers, which allow the assessment of the actual response to drugs by in situ evaluation of the response of its targets. Some of them are actually detected by immunohistochemistry, a robust approach familiar to almost all pathologists. Image analysis can be applied at pathology departments to provide an objective measure and quantification of response to drugs.
- Pathologists can also play an important role in animal model characterization. This includes processing and characterization of tumor xenografts, including TMA construction and pharmacodynamics, as previously described, and morphologic and molecular characterization of genetically modified animal models. Another interesting resource is the generation of patient-derived xenografts from the primary small round cell tumor samples because they represent a closer model to the clinical setting than regular cell line xenografts[24]

REFERENCES

1. de Alava E, Lessnick SL, Sorensen PH. Ewing sarcoma. In: Fletcher CDM, Bridge JA, Hogendoorn PCW, et al, editors. World Health Organization classification of tumours: pathology and genetics of tumours of soft tissue and bone. Lyon (France): IARC Press; 2013. p. 306–9.
2. Sheffield NC, Pierron G, Klughammer J, et al. DNA methylation heterogeneity defines a disease spectrum in Ewing sarcoma. Nat Med 2017;23:386–95.
3. Tirode F, Laud-Duval K, Prieur A, et al. Mesenchymal stem cell features of Ewing tumors. Cancer Cell 2007;11:421–9.
4. von Levetzow C, Jiang X, Gwye Y, et al. Modeling initiation of Ewing sarcoma in human neural crest cells. PLoS One 2011;6:e19305.
5. Cash T, McIlvaine E, Krailo MD, et al. Comparison of clinical features and outcomes in patients with extraskeletal versus skeletal localized Ewing sarcoma: a

report from the Children's Oncology Group. Pediatr Blood Cancer 2016;63(10):1771–9.

6. Gaspar N, Hawkins DS, Dirksen U, et al. Ewing sarcoma: current management and future approaches through collaboration. J Clin Oncol 2015;33:3036–46.

7. de Alava E, Pardo J. Ewing tumor: tumor biology and clinical applications. Int J Surg Pathol 2001;9:7–17.

8. Nascimento AG, Unni KK, Pritchard DJ, et al. A clinicopathologic study of 20 cases of large-cell (atypical) Ewing's sarcoma of bone. Am J Surg Pathol 1980;4:29–36.

9. Antonescu CR, Owosho AA, Zhang L, et al. Sarcomas with CIC-rearrangements are a distinct pathologic entity with aggressive outcome: a clinico-pathologic and molecular study of 115 cases. Am J Surg Pathol 2017, [Epub ahead of print].

10. Kang LC, Dunphy CH. Immunoreactivity of MIC2 (CD99) and terminal deoxynucleotidyl transferase in bone marrow clot and core specimens of acute myeloid leukemias and myelodysplastic syndromes. Arch Pathol Lab Med 2006;130:153–7.

11. Righi A, Gambarotti M, Longo S, et al. Small cell osteosarcoma: clinicopathologic, immunohistochemical, and molecular analysis of 36 cases. Am J Surg Pathol 2015;39:691–9.

12. Granter SR, Renshaw AA, Fletcher CD, et al. CD99 reactivity in mesenchymal chondrosarcoma. Hum Pathol 1996;27:1273–6.

13. Gerald WL, Ladanyi M, de Alava E, et al. Clinical, pathologic, and molecular spectrum of tumours associated with t(11;22)(p13;q12): desmoplastic small round-cell tumor and its variants. J Clin Oncol 1998;16:3028–36.

14. Hasegawa T, Hirose T, Ayala AG, et al. Adult neuroblastoma of the retroperitoneum and abdomen: clinicopathologic distinction from primitive neuroectodermal tumour. Am J Surg Pathol 2001;25:918–24.

15. Hornick JL. Novel uses of immunohistochemistry in the diagnosis and classification of soft tissue tumors. Mod Pathol 2014;27:S47–63.

16. Antonescu C. Round cell sarcomas Ewing: emerging entities. Histopathology 2014;64:26–37.

17. Chen S, Deniz K, Sung YS, et al. Ewing sarcoma with ERG gene rearrangements: a molecular study focusing on the prevalence of FUS-ERG and common pitfalls in detecting EWSR1-ERG fusions by FISH. Genes Chromosomes Cancer 2016;55(4):340–9.

18. Machado I, Noguera R, Pellin A, et al. Molecular diagnosis of Ewing sarcoma family of tumors: a comparative analysis of 560 cases with FISH and RT-PCR. Diagn Mol Pathol 2009;18:189–99.

19. Marino-Enriquez A. Advances in the molecular analysis of soft tissue tumors and clinical implications. Surg Pathol Clin 2015;8:525–37.

20. Conner JR, Hornick JL. SATB2 is a novel marker of osteoblastic differentiation in bone and soft tissue tumours. Histopathology 2013;63:36–49.

21. Casali PG, Blay JY, Bertuzzi A, et al, ESMO Guidelines Working Group. Bone sarcomas: ESMO Clinical Practice Guidelines for diagnosis, treatment and follow-up. Ann Oncol 2014;25(Suppl 3):iii113–23.

22. Kovar H, Amatruda J, Brunet E, et al. The second European interdisciplinary Ewing sarcoma research summit–a joint effort to deconstructing the multiple layers of a complex disease. Oncotarget 2016;7:8613–24.

23. Amaral AT, Ordóñez JL, Otero-Motta AP, et al. Innovative therapies in Ewing Sarcoma. Adv Anat Pathol 2014;21:44–62.

24. Ordóñez JL, Amaral AT, Carcaboso AM, et al. The PARP inhibitor olaparib enhances the sensitivity of Ewing sarcoma to trabectedin. Oncotarget 2015;6(22):18875–90.

Update on Families of Round Cell Sarcomas Other than Classical Ewing Sarcomas

 CrossMark

Francois Le Loarer, MD, PhD[a,b,*], Daniel Pissaloux, PhD[c],
Jean Michel Coindre, MD[a,b], Franck Tirode, PhD[d,e],
Dominique Ranchere Vince, MD[c]

KEYWORDS

- Ewing sarcoma • Ewing-like sarcoma • Atypical Ewing sarcoma • Round cell sarcoma • BCOR
- Fusion genes • Sarcoma • *CIC*

Key points

- The family of Ewing sarcomas refers to sarcomas with round cell phenotype underlined by EWSR1/FUS rearrangements with members of the ETS family of transcription factors.

- Round cell sarcomas negative for EWSR1 and FUS rearrangements with members of the ETS family of transcription factors were referred to as "Ewing-like tumors," which can be subdivided into 3 distinct families, namely EWSR1–non-ETS round cell sarcomas, CIC-rearranged and BCOR-rearranged sarcomas.

- These sarcomas often display atypical features, hence their name of "atypical Ewing sarcomas."

- Morphologic clues pointing toward their diagnosis include cell spindling, nuclear atypia, and stromal changes.

ABSTRACT

This article focuses on families of round cell sarcomas other than classical Ewing sarcomas. Until recently, these tumors were referred to as so-called Ewing-like tumors, as they morphologically resemble Ewing sarcomas but are negative for canonical fusion transcripts of Ewing sarcomas involving gene members of the ETS family of transcription factors. Clinicopathologic and molecular evidence has dramatically influenced the diagnostic approach of these tumors in recent years. Molecular data that support these sarcoma subtypes are biologically distinct from those of Ewing sarcomas, thereby advocating discarding the all-embracing and confusing terminology of "Ewing-like tumors."

OVERVIEW

Round cell sarcomas negative for *EWSR1* and *FUS* fusions to members of the E26 transformation-specific (ETS) family of transcription factors have been long called "Ewing-like

Disclosure Statement: The authors have no commercial or financial conflict of interest to declare.
Financial Support: F. Le Loarer has received financial support from La Ligue contre le cancer de Savoie.
[a] Department of Pathology, Institut Bergonie, 229 cours de l'argonne, Bordeaux 33000, France; [b] Université de Bordeaux, Campus Carreire, Bordeaux 33000, France; [c] Departement de Biopathologie, Centre Leon Berard, Cheney B, 24 rue Laennec, Lyon 69000, France; [d] Cancer Research Center of Lyon, 24 rue Laennec, Lyon 69000, France; [e] Laboratoire de recherche translationnelle, Centre Leon Berard, Cheney B, 3e etage, 24 rue Laennec, Lyon 69000, France
* Corresponding author.
E-mail address: f.le-loarer@bordeaux.unicancer.fr

Surgical Pathology 10 (2017) 587–620
http://dx.doi.org/10.1016/j.path.2017.04.002
1875-9181/17/

tumors." As a whole, they represent the second most frequent category of round cell sarcomas (11%), just after Ewing sarcoma (ES) (which account for 80%).[1] Most of Ewing-like tumors were previously classified as "Ewing sarcoma" or "unclassified round cell sarcoma" before the implementation of molecular testing in routine practice.

ES is underlined by *EWSR1* or *FUS* fusions to members of the ETS family of transcription factors.[2] Typical ES is composed of monomorphic round cells with scant clear cytoplasm and ill-defined borders; displaying monotonous nuclei with smooth nuclear contours. However, a subset of ES presents with atypical features consisting of a higher degree of cytologic variability, which subset is referred to as "atypical ES." In this setting,

tumor cells display variations in size and shape of their nuclei, coarse chromatin, distinct nucleoli, slightly more abundant cytoplasm, cell spindling, and presence of stromal changes (**Fig. 1**). Although these atypical features may be rarely seen in bona fide ES, they are much more common in so-called "Ewing-like tumors." Therefore, there is a significant overlap between "atypical ES" and "Ewing-like tumors."

"Ewing-like tumors" can be subdivided into 4 categories of tumors, which include sarcomas with *EWSR1* fusions to non-ETS family members, capicua transcriptional repressor (*CIC*)-rearranged sarcomas, Bcl6 corepressor (*BCOR*)-rearranged sarcomas, and unclassified round cell sarcomas.[1] Most of these categories display subtle recurrent

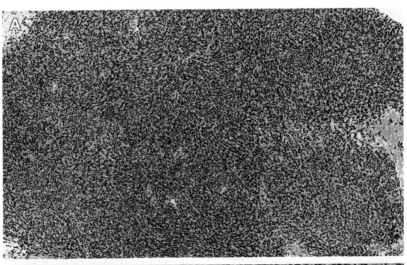

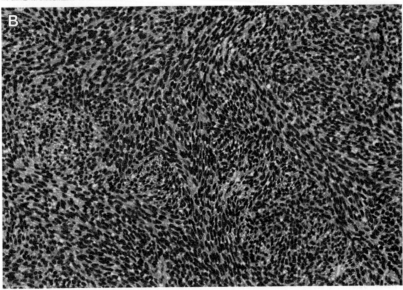

Fig. 1. "Atypical" ES with spindle cell phenotype. (*A*) Spindle cell proliferation arranged in intersecting fascicles. (*B*) Tumor cells display ovoid monomorphic nuclei with smooth chromatin. This tumor was associated with a *EWSR1-FLI1* fusion transcript (H&E, original magnification, [*A*] ×2.5; [*B*] ×10).

morphologic features that, although not pathognomonic, help stratify the diagnostic approach of these lesions when combined with surrogate immunostainings. Nonetheless, considering the substantial morphologic overlap and the relatively recent description of these entities, molecular typing is still mandatory to classify these neoplasms with certainty.[3] Molecular data support they are biologically distinct from ES. Nonetheless, they have not yet been endorsed as independent sarcoma subtypes in the last 2013 World Health Organization (WHO) classification[4] (Table 1).

ROUND CELL SARCOMAS WITH EWSR1-REARRANGEMENTS INVOLVING NON–E26 TRANSFORMATION-SPECIFIC FUSION PARTNERS (EWSR1-non ETS TRANSFORMATION-SPECIFIC REARRANGED ROUND CELL SARCOMAS)

A subset of EWSR1-rearranged round cell sarcomas involves fusion partners that are not members of the ETS family of transcription factors, in contrast to those involved in bona fide ES (namely FLI1, ERG, ETV1/4, and FEV, all of them belonging to the ETS family). Definitive evidence is still lacking as to whether they represent variants of ES

or biologically distinct subtypes of round cell sarcomas.

CLINICAL FEATURES

Affected patients seem to be significantly older than patients with ES. EWSR1-PATZ1 round cell sarcomas have been reported in the chest wall,[5] whereas EWSR1-NFATc2 round cell sarcomas occur preferentially in bone.[6]

MICROSCOPIC AND IMMUNOHISTOCHEMICAL FEATURES

This category has not been systematically studied in clinicopathological series, available data being mostly limited to isolated reports. Nonetheless, atypical features are a common finding. For instance, sarcomas with EWSR1-NFATc2 rearrangements harbor distinct nucleoli, increased pleomorphism, and tumor cells may arrange in nests[6] (Fig. 2A–C). CD99 is positive in most of these tumors, as seen in ES.

EWSR1 REARRANGEMENTS

EWSR1 is rearranged but fused to genes that are not members of the ETS family. Nuclear factor of activated T-cells, calcineurin-dependent 2

Table 1
Immunostainings used as surrogate markers in sarcomas with round cell phenotype

Staining	Ewing Sarcoma	Sarcomas with EWSR1–Non-ETS Partners Fusions	CIC-Sarcomas	BCOR-Sarcomas	Potential Mimicker
CD99	Diffuse membranous pattern	Variable positivity	Focal	Focal	Lymphoma
ETV4	Focal, 10%	Negative (LE)	Nuclear pattern (93%)	Negative	DSRCT, melanoma
WT1cTer	Negative	LE	Nuclear (75%)	Negative	DSRCT
CCNB3	Negative	LE	Negative	Positive in BCOR-CCNB3 sarcomas	Cytoplasmic background in SS, ES
BCOR	Rare	LE	Rare	Positive in sarcoma with any BCOR alteration	SS (50%)
DUX4	Negative	LE	Positive in CIC-DUX4 sarcomas	Negative (1 case)	NT
TLE1	Negative	LE	Negative	Negative	SS

Abbreviations: BCOR, Bcl6 corepressor; CIC, capicua transcriptional repressor; DSRCT, desmoplastic small round cell tumor; ES, Ewing sarcomas; LE, limited evidence available; NT, not tested; SS, synovial sarcoma.

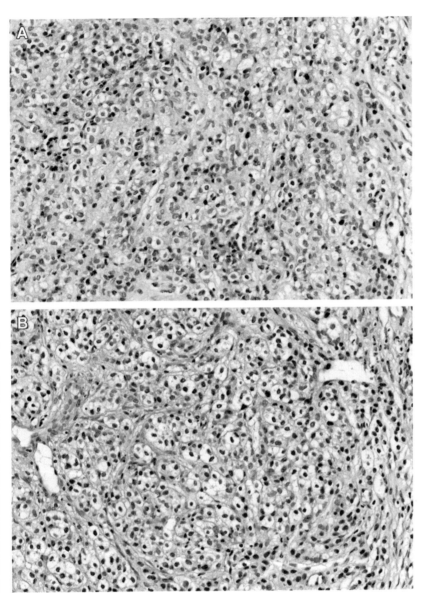

Fig. 2. Sarcoma with *EWSR1-NFATc2* fusion in a 29-year-old man, located in tibia with extension into adjacent soft tissue. (*A*) Small round cells with variable clear cytoplasm, embedded in a hyaline stroma. (*B*) Focal area with hyaline stroma with nested pattern (H&E, original magnification, [*A*] ×10; [*B*] ×15).

(NFATc2), located in 20q13, was the first non-ETS fusion partner identified and described on a small series.[6] As in classic ES, this fusion preserves the transactivation domain of *EWSR1* but is unbalanced associated with gain/amplification of 20q and/or 22q regions nearing the breakpoints (see **Fig. 2D**).

Other non-ETS fusion partners have been described in isolated reports, including *SP3*,[7] *PATZ1*,[5] and *SMARCA5*.[8] Although these tumors share *EWSR1* rearrangements, it remains to be seen whether they account for a biologically homogeneous group, as these fusion partners are not functionally related to one another. *EWSR1-PATZ1* fusions involve a 22-intrachromosomal inversion, both genes being located in 22q12, separated by approximately 2 Mb. As a consequence, this fusion may be inconspicuous or difficult to diagnose with an *EWSR1* breakapart fluorescence in situ hybridization (FISH) (**Fig. 3**).

Altogether, these tumors involve rare fusion transcripts that are not targeted by most multiplexed reverse-transcriptase polymerase chain

Fig. 2. (continued). (C) Significant nuclear atypia with variations in size and shape, and hyperchromatic chromatin (H&E, original magnification, [C] ×20). (D) FISH with a *EWSR1* break-apart probe (green and red probes are respectively located in 3′/telomeric and 5′ parts of *EWSR1*). Most tumor cells display one normal fused signal and an increased number of the second red signal clustering together, whereas no second green spot is seen. This finding suggests a *EWSR1* break associated with an amplification of the 5′ part and a probable deletion of the 3′ part. This pattern is common in *EWSR1-NFATc2* sarcomas ([D] DAPI counterstain).

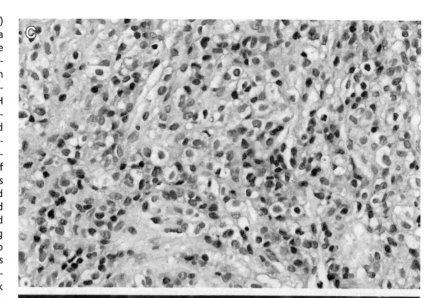

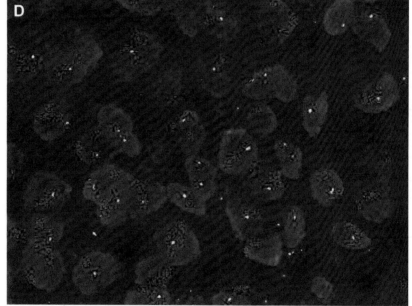

reaction (RT-PCR) used in routine practice. Their diagnosis mostly relies in identification of *EWSR1* rearrangements by FISH. This finding is poorly specific, explaining why these subtypes have been mainly characterized with single case reports. RNA-sequencing screening will certainly facilitate their diagnosis in routine practice in the future and may certainly help better delineate their clinicopathological features.

DIFFERENTIAL DIAGNOSIS

- These tumors may be confused with ES. There is both morphologic and genetic overlap, as *EWSR1* rearrangements are involved in both categories.
- Cell spindling may raise suspicion for poorly differentiated synovial sarcoma (SS). TLE1 immunostaining is a useful surrogate marker with diffuse nuclear expression in SS. *SS18*

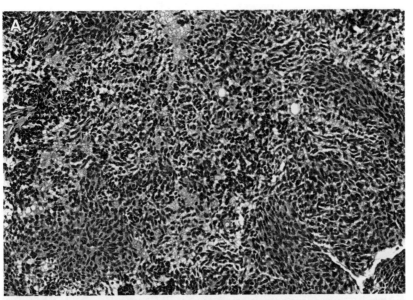

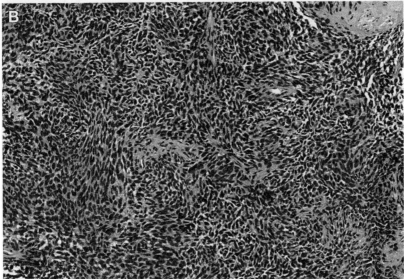

Fig. 3. Round cell sarcoma with *EWSR1-PATZ1* fusion in a 55-year-old man located in anterior mediastinum with lysis of sternum. (*A*) Monomorphic proliferation with a mixed round to spindled growth pattern with minimal stroma. (*B*) Densely cellular and basophilic proliferation reminiscent of a poorly differentiated SS (H&E, original magnification, [*A, B*] ×10).

rearrangements can be evidenced by FISH or RT-PCR to confirm the diagnosis of SS.

CAPICUA TRANSCRIPTIONAL REPRESSOR-REARRANGED ROUND CELL SARCOMAS (CAPICUA TRANSCRIPTIONAL REPRESSOR-SARCOMAS)

CIC-rearranged sarcomas represent the most frequent subtype of "Ewing-like tumors." They are associated with recurrent rearrangements of *capicua transcriptional repressor* (*CIC*) located on chromosome 19p13.2. Translocations involving its locus had been reported in early cytogenetic studies[9] but were not genetically characterized until 2006.[10] *CIC* rearrangements represent the second most frequent genetic event in round cell sarcomas after *EWSR1* translocations.[1,11] Since their identification, the clinicopathological features of this tumor subtype have been better delineated in two series, and their molecular spectrum has

Fig. 3. (continued). (*C*) Nuclear atypia with variations in size and shape and smudged chromatin (H&E, original magnification, [*C*] ×15). (*D*) FISH with *EWSR1* break-apart probe (green and red probes are respectively located in 3'/telomeric and 5' parts of *EWSR1*). Most tumor cells display a normal fused signal along with a split signal with minimal gap separating the probes. An *EWSR1-PATZ1* transcript fusion was identified by RT-PCR. This fusion involves an intrachromosomic inversion ([*D*] DAPI counterstain).

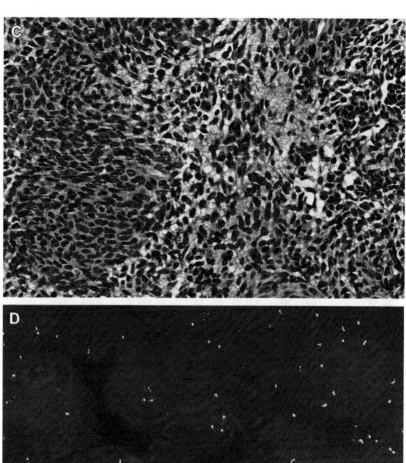

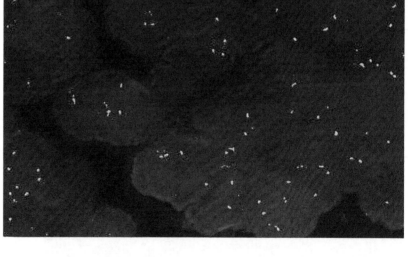

been expanded. These sarcomas are not yet acknowledged as a distinct subgroup in the 2013 WHO classification, but recent evidence suggests they constitute a distinct sarcoma subtype.

CLINICAL FEATURES

These tumors have a predilection for children and young adults, with a median age of 29 years, with a wide age distribution ranging from 6 to 73 years.[11] These sarcomas are primarily located in deep soft tissue, with limbs representing half of cases. They may also locate in superficial soft tissue and viscera.[12,13] Primary bone locations are rare, but bones are a frequent dissemination site at advanced stages.[14]

RADIOLOGICAL AND GROSS FEATURES

No specific radiologic nor macroscopic features have been reported. Necrosis and hemorrhage are common.[11]

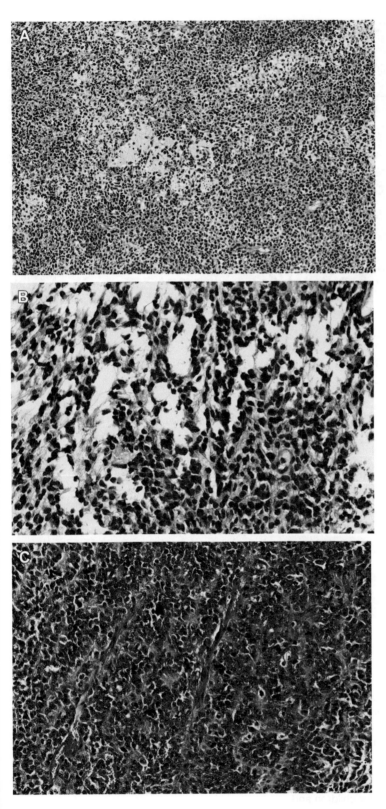

Fig. 4. *CIC-DUX4* sarcoma. (*A*) Dense proliferation arranged in solid sheets with focally myxoid stroma. (*B*) Strand or reticular pattern. (*C*) Fibrous intervening stroma (H&E, original magnification, [*A*] ×5; [*B*] ×15; [*C*] ×15).

Fig. 4. (continued). (D) Areas of necrosis and hemorrhage. (E) Marked nuclear atypia with variation of size and shape. (F) Nuclear atypia with distinct nucleoli (H&E, original magnification, [D] ×5; [E] ×15; [F] ×15).

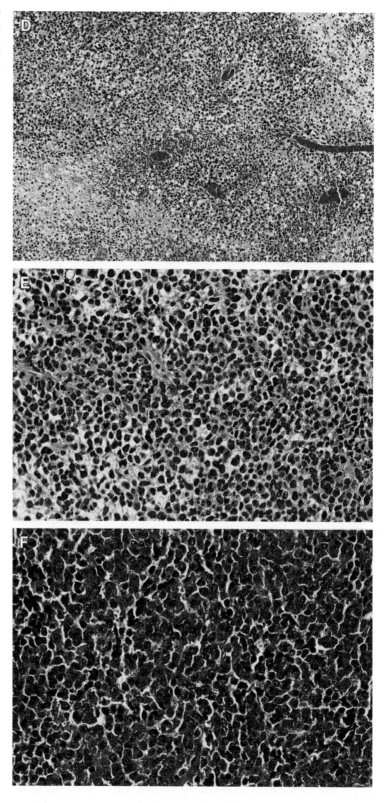

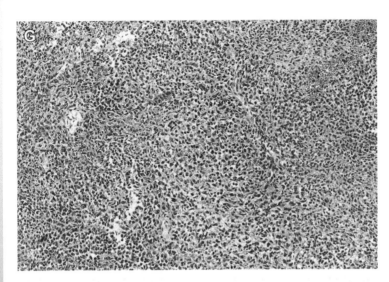

Fig. 4. (continued). (G) Focal spindling is a common finding in CIC-rearranged sarcomas (H&E, original magnification, [G] ×5).

MICROSCOPIC FEATURES

CIC-rearranged sarcomas are round cell sarcomas with a less monotonous appearance than that of ES, although they may be focally indistinguishable from bona fide ES.[14] Tumor cells are small to medium-sized with ill-defined borders with variable eosinophilic to amphophilic cytoplasm (Fig. 4A–C). Their nuclei are relatively heterogeneous with variations in size and shape, commonly displaying coarse chromatin dotted with distinct nucleoli (see Fig. 4D–F). Tumor cells are mostly arranged in solid sheets, although other growth patterns may be focally seen, including spindled or reticular architecture (see Fig. 4G). Rosette formation is uncommon.[14] There is minimal intervening stroma, but myxoid stromal changes are frequent, as well as necrosis and hemorrhage.[13] They display high mitotic rate, commonly more than 10 mitoses per 10 high-powered fields.

IMMUNOHISTOCHEMICAL FEATURES

CD99 membranous staining is present in up to 85% of cases, but is heterogeneous and mostly focal, contrasting with the diffuse staining seen in most ES.[13] ETV4 is diffusely expressed with a nuclear pattern in 93% of cases; rare cases displaying patchy or negative staining (3.5%, each).[15,16] ETV4 is not entirely specific, staining focally 10% of ES and occasionally desmoplastic small round cell tumors, rhabdomyosarcomas, and melanomas.[15,16] ETV4 RNA in situ hybridization has also been proposed, although its sensitivity and specificity have not been compared with ETV4 immunostaining.[17] ERG and FLI1 are frequently expressed and not helpful to discriminate CIC-rearranged sarcomas from ES.[18] Nuclear WT1 expression has been reported in 75% of cases, both with antibodies targeting the N and C terminus[13,15,16] (Fig. 5). Focal expression of desmin, S100 protein, MUC4, epithelial membrane antigen (EMA), cytokeratins, and calretinin have been occasionally reported.[11,15,19] C-MYC nuclear expression has been described in a small series.[18] DUX4 immunostaining has been pointed out as a sensitive marker for tumors associated with CIC-DUX4 fusions.[20]

CAPICUA TRANSCRIPTIONAL REPRESSOR REARRANGEMENTS

CIC encodes a transcriptional repressor with a high mobility group box located on 19p13.2.

DUX4 represents its most common fusion partner.[11] DUX4 is a double homeodomain gene, containing a 3.3-kb tandem repeat sequence located in the subtelomeric regions of the long arms of chromosomes 4 and 10.[21] CIC may be fused either to DUX4 in 4q35 or its paralog in 10q26, accounting for translocations t(4;19) (q35;q13) and t(10;19) (q26;q13). The CIC-DUX4 chimeric protein retains most of CIC fused in frame to the C-terminus of DUX4. It acts as an oncogenic transcription factor inducing upregulation of polyoma enhancer activator 3 (PEA3) family of genes.[10] PEA3 is part of the family of ETS-related transcription factors that include ETV4 (also known as E1AF or PEA3),

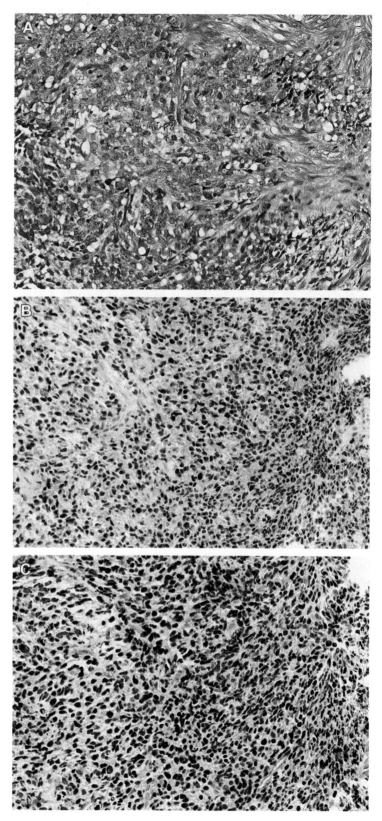

Fig. 5. Immunohistochemical features of *CIC-DUX4* sarcoma in a 15-year-old girl. (*A*) Ovoid monomorphic nuclei with distinct nucleoli. (*B*) Diffuse nuclear staining with ETV4 and (*C*) antibody targeting the C-terminal portion of WT1 (H&E, original magnification, [*A–D*] ×10; [*E*] ×5).

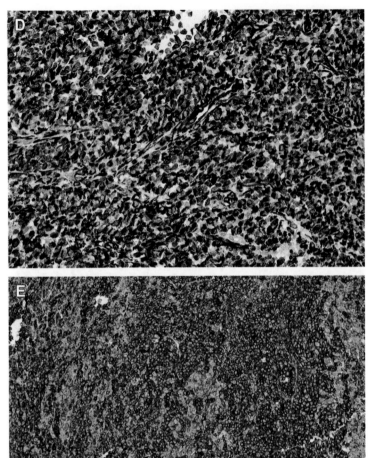

Fig. 5. (*continued*). (*D*) Nonspecific cytoplasmic staining with antibody targeting N-terminal part of WT1. (*E*) Heterogeneous membranous staining for CD99 distinct from the typical diffuse and complete staining seen in ES (H&E, original magnification, [*A–D*] ×10; [*E*] ×5).

ETV1, and ETV5. Interestingly, ETV1 and ETV4 are rare fusion partners of *EWSR1* in ES.[22,23]

Fusion partners alternative to *DUX4* have been more recently identified, including *FOXO4*[24] and *NUT midline carcinoma family member 1* (*NUTM1*).[25] Although only 2 case reports of *CIC-FOXO4* sarcomas are available, they seem to display morphologic and immunophenotypic features similar to those seen in *CIC-DUX4* sarcomas.[24,26] *CIC-NUTM1* sarcomas have been originally described in a central nervous system (CNS) location[25] (**Fig. 6**). A study focused on CNS tumors has shown the transcriptional and methylation profiles of these 2 variants are distinct from those of ES.[25] In keeping with this evidence, soft tissue *CIC-DUX4* sarcomas display expression profiles consistently different from those of ES.[13]

MOLECULAR TESTING

Molecular confirmation is still required to render a definitive diagnosis.

FISH with *CIC* break-apart probe screens for all *CIC* rearrangements, whatever gene partner is involved but may miss cryptic rearrangements (**Fig. 7**A, B).

Alternatively, RT-PCR can identify *CIC-DUX4* fusion transcript, as there are few variations in positions of genomic breakpoints.[11] However, this technique may render false-negative results in case of the position of genomic breakpoints varies or if alternative fusion partners are involved.

Of note, the use of FISH and RT-PCR techniques imply a sequential screening approach, whereas "one-shot" methods based on next-generation sequencing (NGS) technologies can

Fig. 6. Sarcoma with *CIC-NUTM1* fusion of temporal bone with features similar to those of *CIC-DUX4* sarcoma. (A)Tumor cells arranged in solid sheets with vague spindling. (*B*) Monotonous round to ovoid nuclei with atypical features (H&E, original magnification, [*A*] ×5; [*B*] ×10).

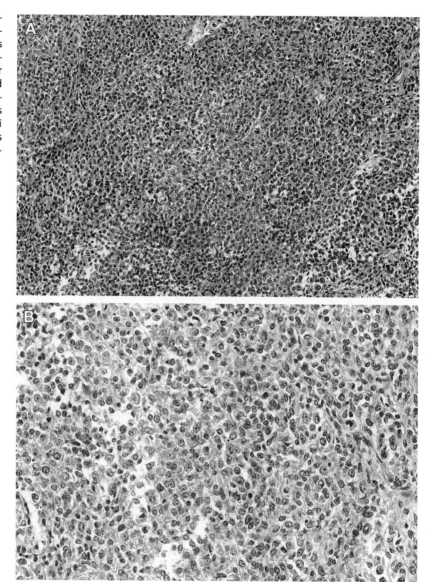

now be used with formalin-fixed, paraffin-embedded specimens, enabling to screen simultaneously for hundreds of fusion genes. These methods rely on a targeted approach using anchored multiplex PCR or probe hybridization before sequencing. Their use is particularly relevant in the setting of round cell sarcomas due to the significant morphologic overlap displayed by these tumors. Conversely, FISH remains extremely useful when dealing with scant specimens, as it can be performed with 1 slide and enables a morphologic correlation. Conventional cytogenetics and array-comparative genomic hybridization (aCGH) (the former having been replaced by aCGH in most laboratories) may tip toward the diagnosis in some cases. Typically, *CIC*-rearranged sarcomas display simple genetic profiles in keeping with underlying balanced translocation as seen in ES.[9,27] Occasionally, they may display more complex genetics with unbalanced translocations associated with copy number alterations (CNA) at sites of breakpoints[10,11] (see **Fig. 7**C, D). Gains and trisomy of chromosome 8 seem to be common,[25] occasionally translating into genomic amplification and overexpression of C-MYC according to a single study.[18] In line with their simple genetic background, *CIC*-rearranged sarcomas display low mutational burden.[28]

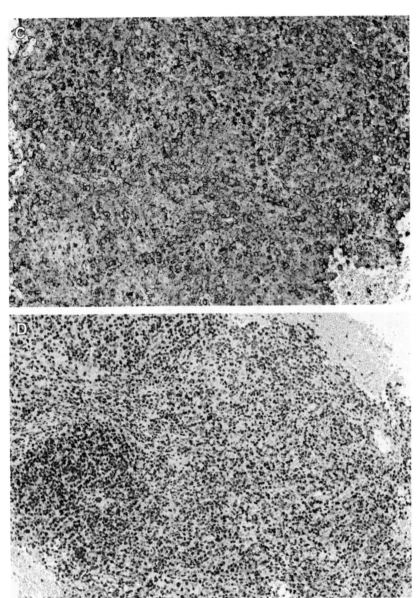

Fig. 6. (continued). (*C*) CD99 heterogeneous membranous staining. (*D*) Diffuse nuclear staining with ETV4 (H&E, original magnification, [*C, D*] ×5).

DIFFERENTIAL DIAGNOSIS

- ES represents the main differential diagnosis. Although the presence of atypical cytologic features favor a *CIC*-rearranged sarcoma, atypia may be present in bona fide ES.[29] Presence of myxoid stromal changes is reminiscent of *CIC* sarcoma. ETV4 diffuses expression along with CD99 heterogeneous or negative staining also favors a *CIC*-rearranged sarcoma. Molecular screening is required to assert definitively this differential. Notably, ES with atypical features is more commonly associated with translocation variants involving non-ETS transcription factors, thereby rendering their molecular diagnosis more difficult. FISH screening with *EWSR1* break-apart probe represents a sensitive screening strategy, albeit poorly specific.

- Reticular architecture and myxoid changes may raise suspicion for extraskeletal myxoid chondrosarcoma (EMC) or myoepithelial tumors; however, these patterns are mostly focal in *CIC*-sarcomas (Fig. 8). High-grade nuclear features seen in *CIC*-sarcomas are rare in EMC.

Fig. 7. Molecular findings in *CIC*-rearranged sarcomas. (*A*) FISH with a *CIC* break-apart probe showing in each cell 1 normal fused signal and 1 split signal indicative of *CIC* rearrangement. (*B*) FISH with a *CIC* break-apart probe showing 2 fused signals rendered as negative. However, one of the signals presents with minimal gap with one of the green 3′ signals decreased in size, which may raise suspicion for an unbalanced rearrangement ([*A, B*] DAPI counterstain).

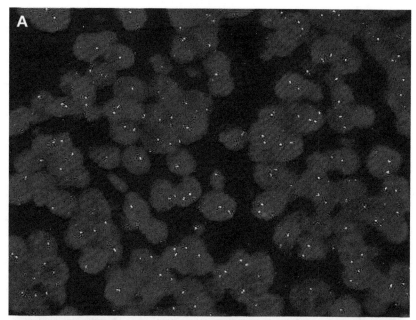

Aggressive EMCs display a solid growth pattern with an epithelioid to rhabdoid cell appearance.[30] The expression of ETV4 has not been assessed in EMC. Screening for *NR4A3* rearrangement can be performed to support the differential diagnosis in difficult cases.

- Malignant myoepithelial tumor may be suspected considering the high-grade nuclear features of *CIC*-sarcomas. *CIC*-sarcomas may express focally cytokeratins and S100 protein. SOX10 expression has not been

assessed yet in *CIC*-sarcomas but is consistently expressed by myoepithelial tumors. SMARCB1/INI1 nuclear expression is lost in 20% of malignant myoepithelial tumors, related to homozygous deletions in 22q12. Screening for *EWSR1* might be helpful in difficult cases, although rearrangements are present in only 50% of cases and is poorly specific in this morphologic setting.

- Sclerosing epithelioid fibrosarcoma (SEF) may occur in bones. SEF presents with

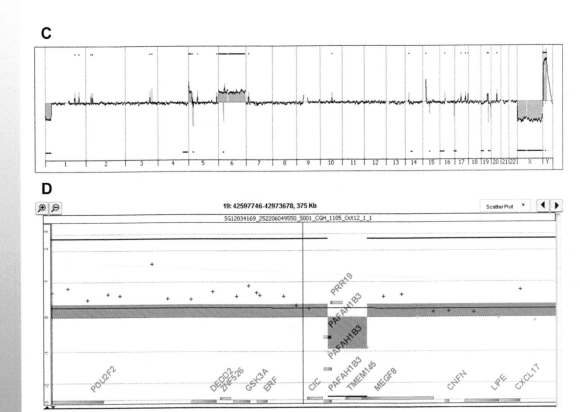

C

D

19: 42597746-42973678, 375 Kb

SG12034169_252206049550_S001_CGH_1105_Oct12_1_1

Fig. 7. (*continued*). (*C*) aCGH profiling evidenced a few CNAs, including chromosome 6 and 5qter gains, 1pter loss. Chromosomes 1 to 22 are plotted on the x-axis. Log2 ratio values are indicated on the y-axis. (*D*) Chromosomal view of aCGH profile on 19p13 locus. Presence of a breakpoint in 19q13 involving *CIC* locus with a genomic loss of the 3' part of the gene. This genomic loss accounts for the false-negative result obtained with FISH. RT-PCR evidenced a *CIC-DUX4* fusion transcript.

monomorphic rounded tumor cells embedded in a sclerosing/hyaline stroma that may raise suspicion for round cell sarcoma (**Fig. 9**). SEF may be pure or admixed with areas of low-grade fibromyxoid sarcoma (LGFMS), which are less cellular and display a fibromyxoid stroma. SEFs display MUC4 nuclear expression in 70% of cases.[31] They are associated with *EWSR1-CREB3L1* rearrangements.[32]

- Epithelioid angiosarcoma may enter in the differential diagnosis. These tumors may lack vasoformation and present with a solid growth pattern (**Fig. 10**). They consistently express vascular markers ERG and CD31, but CD31 can be difficult to assess due to histiocytic infiltration. ERG can be expressed by *CIC*-rearranged sarcoma, mostly focally. Molecular testing may add confusion to the matter, as *CIC* rearrangements have been identified in a subset of angiosarcomas involving a different partner, *LEUTX*.[33] Intriguingly, *LEUTX* belongs to the same class of homeobox genes as *DUX4* and angiosarcomas with

CIC-LEUTX fusions display significant transcriptional overlap with upregulation of the PEA3 family of ETS genes, including ETV4 similar to that seen in *CIC*-rearranged round cell sarcomas.[33]

- In the clinical setting of an abdominal mass, desmoplastic small round cell tumor (DSRCT) may be considered. The stromal desmoplasia harbored by DSRCT may be reduced or absent in rare cases. These tumors have a notable immunophenotypic overlap with *CIC*-sarcomas sharing expression of cytokeratins, desmin, and WT1cter at variable levels. Conversely, a subset of DSRCTs have limited expression of desmin and may express ETV4.[15,16] Expression of WT1cter in DSRCT is related to underlying *EWSR1-WT1* fusions.
- SMARCA4-deficient thoracic sarcomas (SMARCA4-DTS) can mimic *CIC*-sarcomas.[34] Although they present with thoracic mass in pleura or mediastinum, they may disseminate to bones. These tumors are composed of high-grade round to epithelioid cells arranged

Fig. 8. *CIC*-rearranged sarcoma with myxoid features. (*A*) Tumor cells are arranged in sheets or strands embedded in a myxoid stroma, reminiscent of EMC. (*B*) Formation of cordons, there is significant nuclear atypia. (*C*) Reticular growth pattern reminiscent of EMC and myoepithelial tumors (H&E, original magnification, [*A*] ×5; [*B*] ×15; [*C*] ×2.5).

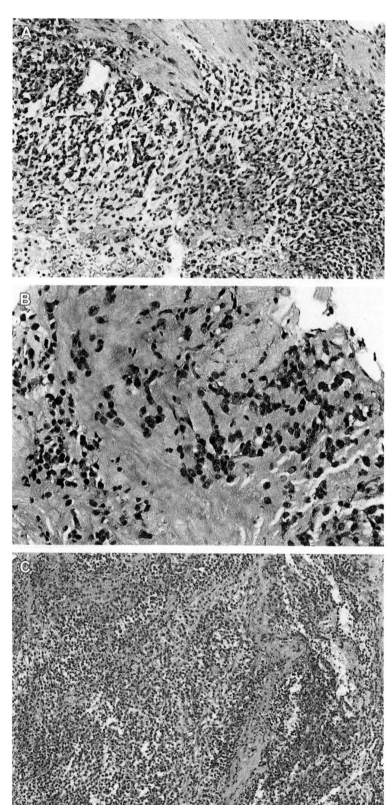

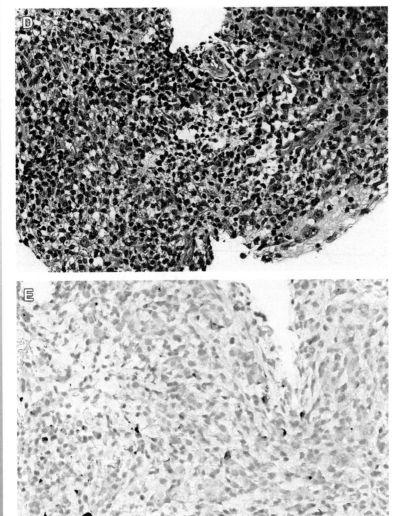

Fig. 8. (continued). (D) Area with dense cellularity and significant nuclear atypia. No NR4A3 and EWSR1 rearrangements were seen but a CIC-DUX4 fusion transcript was found. (E) Focal staining for AE1/E3 along with S100 protein (not shown), which raised suspicion for a malignant myoepithelial tumor in this case. ETV4 was diffusely expressed and a rearrangement of CIC was seen by FISH (H&E, original magnification, [D] ×10; [E] ×12.5).

in solid sheets. They stain for AE1/E3 or EMA at least focally in virtually all cases, CD34 in 80% of cases, and always lose SMARCA4 nuclear expression (Fig. 11).

- Rhabdomyosarcomas, lymphomas, and SSs should always enter in the differential diagnosis of round cell sarcomas, especially in young patients. Immunohistochemical panel should therefore include desmin, myogenin/MYOD1, CD3, CD20, and TLE1 in the first place. SMARCB1 antibody should be included in the panel to explore round cell tumors in infants.

MANAGEMENT AND PROGNOSIS

Clinical data are still limited, mainly based on small retrospective series. Nonetheless, these tumors display an aggressive course with metastatic rates close to 50%.[11] Investigators have reported a lower sensitivity to ES-type chemotherapy regimens (using doxorubicin-ifosfamide or multicombination vincristine-doxorubicin-cyclophosphamide-ifosfamide-etoposide).[11,35] Although there is no consensus regarding the management of Ewing-like tumors and undifferentiated round cell sarcomas, most institutions follow ES treatment

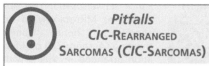

Pitfalls
CIC-REARRANGED SARCOMAS (CIC-SARCOMAS)

! Atypical morphologic features are common in CIC-rearranged sarcomas.

! CIC-sarcomas in bones correspond to secondary sites, whereas bone primary location seems exceptional if ever present.

! CIC-sarcomas display nuclear expression of WT1 C-terminal, which may raise suspicion for DSRCT in the setting of an intra-abdominal mass.

! A subset of ESs associated with bona fide EWSR1-FLI1 fusions or rare variants, such as EWSR1-PATZ1, display consistent atypia and high-grade features similar to those observed in CIC-rearranged sarcomas.

! Calretinin and cytokeratin expression may be occasionally seen, which may raise suspicion for the bone metastases of a carcinoma.

! ERG and FLI1 stainings do not discriminate CIC-sarcomas from ES.

guidelines to manage pediatric patients, whereas adult patients would receive only adjuvant chemotherapy in case of disseminated disease.[11]

BCL6 COREPRESSOR-REARRANGED ROUND CELL SARCOMAS (BCL6 COREPRESSOR-ROUND CELL SARCOMAS)

BCOR-round cell sarcomas were first identified in 2012 through an RNA-sequencing screen conducted in fusion-negative tumors suspicious for ES. They account for approximately 4% of round cell sarcomas, being less common than CIC-rearranged sarcomas.[36] The initial study pointed out intrachromosomal fusions of Bcl6 corepressor (BCOR) to testis-specific cyclin B3 (CCNB3). Alternative BCOR rearrangements have been evidenced since then.[25,37,38] These tumors affect mainly adolescents and young adults and have a predilection for bones. Microscopically, they display features intermediate between SS and ES. BCOR-sarcomas differ substantially from ES from morphologic, genomic, and transcriptional standpoints. Although BCOR rearrangements delineate a distinct group of round cell sarcomas, they are not restricted to this tumor subtype, as previously exemplified with EWSR1 fusions.

CLINICAL FEATURES

BCOR-round cell sarcomas affect predominantly adolescents and young adults with a median age of 15 years, although age distribution is wide, ranging from 2 to 70 years.[39] There is a striking male predominance, higher than that is seen in ES. BCOR-CCNB3 sarcomas develop in bones in 85% of cases, affecting both long and flat bones.[36,40] Sarcomas with alternative BCOR alterations tend to locate more commonly in deep soft tissue or viscera, affecting slightly older individuals.[37] Most patients present with local disease.[39]

RADIOLOGICAL AND GROSS FEATURES

BCOR-round cell sarcomas may develop in any type of bones with a slight predilection for meta-diaphysis of long bones or spine.[39] Radiological features are not specific, reflecting the aggressiveness of these tumors with periosteal reaction in long bones and cortical destruction. Surrounding soft tissues are virtually always invaded.[39] No specific macroscopic features have been reported.[40]

MICROSCOPIC FEATURES

BCOR-round cell sarcomas are composed of uniform medium-sized cells with a mixed rounded to spindled appearance in 45% of cases. Alternatively, they display exclusive round or spindled patterns in 40% and 15% of cases, respectively.[39] Tumor cells are arranged in sheets or fascicles (**Fig. 12**). Short fascicles with whorling pattern, reminiscent of SS, are present in 40% of cases. They also may arrange in long fascicles with a herringbone pattern. Cell nuclei are dotted with stippled chromatin. Tumor cells may sometimes associate with fibrous or myxoid stroma. Necrosis or hemorrhage are present in two-thirds of cases. Mitotic index is high in most cases (median of 30 mitoses).[39] Metastatic or recurring tumors display a higher degree of pleomorphism and increased cellularity.[40]

IMMUNOHISTOCHEMICAL FEATURES

CD99 expression is heterogeneous, focally expressed in 27% of cases.[39–41] BCOR-CCNB3 fusion leads to reexpression of CCNB3 in tumor cell nuclei.[36] CCNB3 stains virtually all BCOR-CCNB3 sarcomas, although its expression is focal and patchy in a small subset of cases.[40] CCNB3 staining is highly specific but cytoplasmic staining may be seen in a subset of tumors including ES, SSs, and alveolar rhabdomyosarcomas.[36,40] It is notable as CCNB3 expression may be difficult to interpret due to variable cytoplasmic background

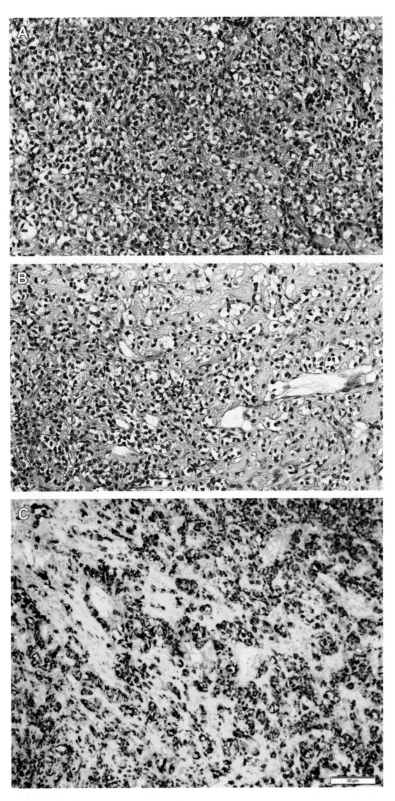

Fig. 9. SEF versus round cell sarcoma. (*A*) Microbiopsy of an aggressive bone tumor showing (*A*) round cell proliferation arranged in sheets with variable amount of stroma. (*B*) Focally, tumor cells are embedded in a sclero-hyaline matrix, with a nested pattern. (*C*) Diffuse nuclear staining for MUC4. Molecular testing evidenced a *EWSR1-CREB3L1* fusion transcript (H&E, original magnification, [*A–D*] ×5). (*Courtesy of* Dr N. Weingertner, CHU Strasbourg, France.)

Fig. 9. (continued). (D, E) CIC-rearranged sarcoma invading bone mimicking SEF. Tumor cells display round to ovoid nuclei with variable atypia and prominent necrosis (H&E, original magnification, [A–D] ×5; [E] ×10).

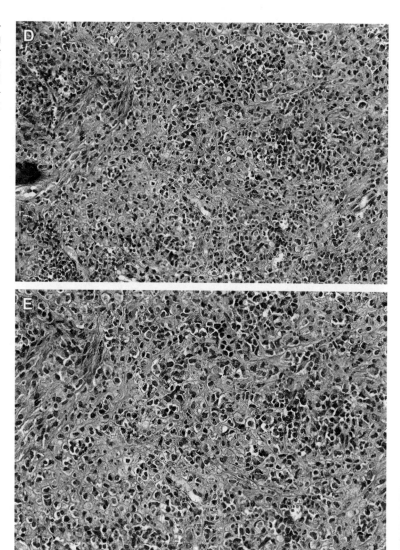

(Fig. 13). CCNB3 expression also can be patchy or negative in posttreatment samples, although the fusion transcript is still present.[40,41]

BCOR staining has been recently shown as a sensitive marker of *BCOR*-round cell sarcomas.[42] However, ES, *CIC*-sarcomas, and SS occasionally stain for BCOR (amounting to half of cases in the latter).[42] CD117 can be expressed.[40] No desmin or cytokeratin expression has been reported.[40] Notably, SATB2 is expressed by 75% of BCOR-sarcomas, which might raise suspicion for small cell osteosarcoma when dealing with small biopsy specimens.[42]

BCL6 COREPRESSOR REARRANGEMENTS

BCOR-CCNB3 fusions account for approximately 60% of *BCOR* alterations. Both genes are located on chromosome X, their fusion involving a paracentric inversion that induces ectopic deregulated expression of CCNB3.[36] BCOR is a transcriptional corepressor, part of a Polycomb complex that binds to BCL6 oncoprotein.[43] Moreover, *BCOR* is an epigenetic regulator of adult stem cell function.[44]

Alternative *BCOR* rearrangements have been identified more recently, including *BCOR-MAML3* and *ZC3H7B-BCOR*. These genetic variants seem to share similar morphologic features to that of *BCOR-CCNB3* sarcomas.[37] These fusions account for approximately 1% to 2% of round cell sarcomas, each.[37] *MAML3* is a member of the mastermindlike family of transcriptional coactivators. Regarding *ZC3H7B-BCOR* fusion, *BCOR* is involved as the 3′ partner to *Zinc finger CCCH domain-containing protein 7B (ZC3H7B)*.[37] This

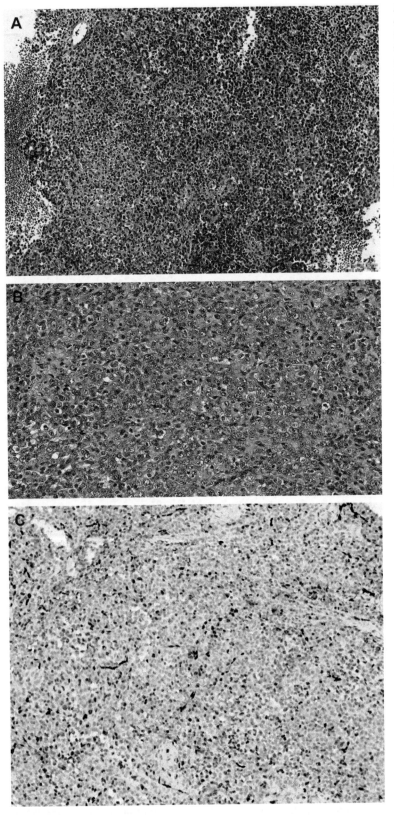

Fig. 10. *CIC*-rearranged sarcoma with epithelioid features. (*A*) Tumor cells are arranged in solid sheets with notable hemorrhagic foci. (*B*) Cells display more abundant cytoplasm giving an epithelioid appearance. (*C*) Focal staining for ERG is not sufficient to render a diagnosis of epithelioid angiosarcoma. CD31 was negative in this case (not shown) (H&E, original magnification, [*A*] ×5; [*B*] ×8; [*C*] ×5).

Fig. 11. *SMARCA4*-deficient thoracic sarcoma. (*A*) High-grade round cell proliferation with abrupt hemorrhage and necrosis. (*B*) Diffuse CD34 staining. (*C*) Loss of nuclear expression of SMARCA4 (H&E, original magnification, [*A–C*] ×8).

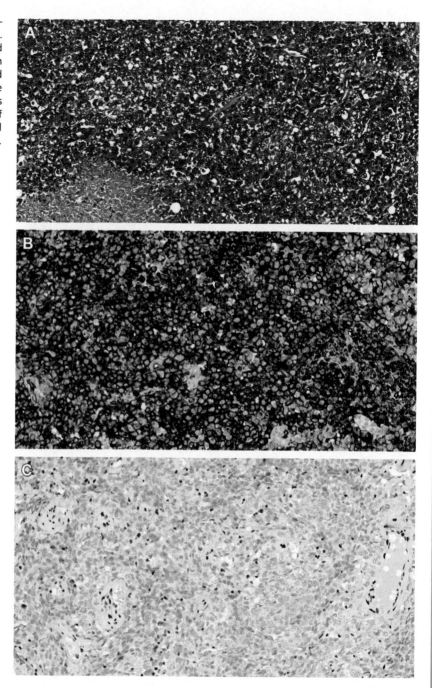

same fusion has been reported in seemingly unrelated mesenchymal lesions, including ossifying fibromyxoid tumor[45] and endometrial stromal sarcoma.[46]

Additionally, *BCOR* internal tandem duplication (ITD) has been described in undifferentiated round cell sarcomas of infancy,[38] which subtypes partially overlap with the former category of primitive myxoid mesenchymal tumor of infancy.[47]

This subset of tumors seems restricted to soft tissue so far, with a predilection for infants. *BCOR*-ITD sarcomas seem transcriptionally close to *BCOR-MAML3* and *BCOR-ZC3H7B* tumors.[38] The translocation partner of *BCOR* remains unknown in 20% of cases.[37]

Array profiling studies have shown that *BCOR-CNNB3* sarcomas are enriched in homeobox genes but not in *EWSR1-FLI1* target genes, as

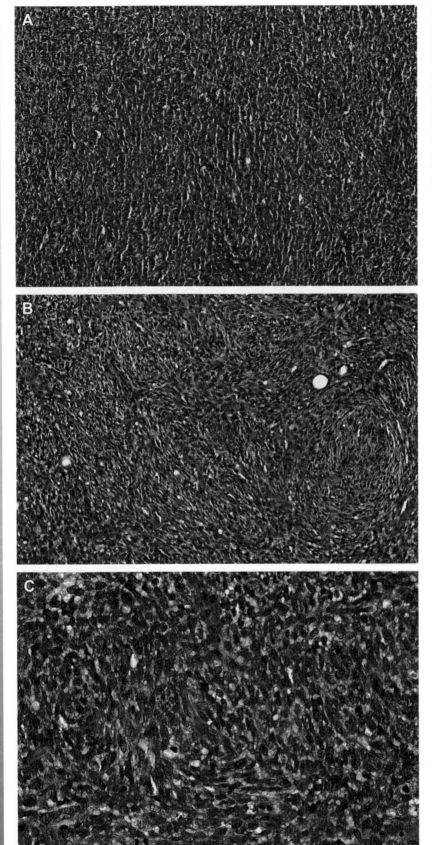

Fig. 12. Sarcoma with BCOR-CCNB3 fusion. (A) Highly cellular proliferation with basophilic appearance. (B) Tumor cells are arranged in short intersecting fascicles with focal whorling. (C) Cells display monomorphic ovoid nuclei with brisk mitotic activity (H&E, original magnification, [A] ×5; [B] ×7; [C] ×10).

Fig. 12. (continued). (D)
Case with diffuse round
cell appearance. (*E*) Tumor cells harbor monoto-
nous round nuclei
reminiscent of ES. (*F*) Variable amount of stroma
with focal hyalinization
(H&E, original magnifica-
tion, [*D*] ×5; [*E*] ×10;
[*F*] ×8).

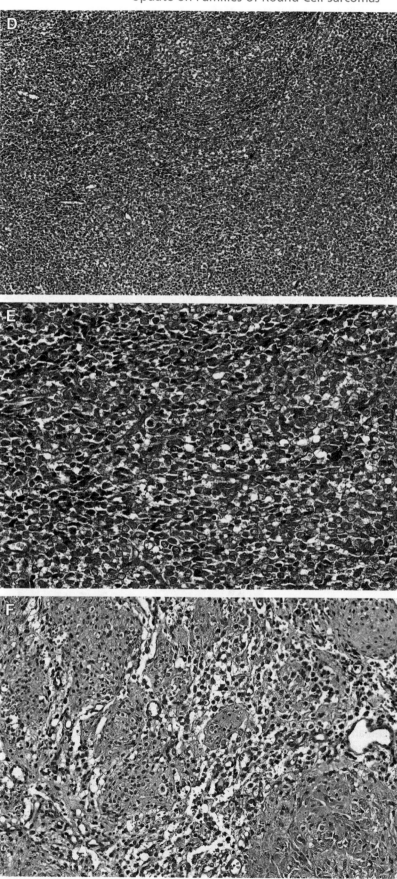

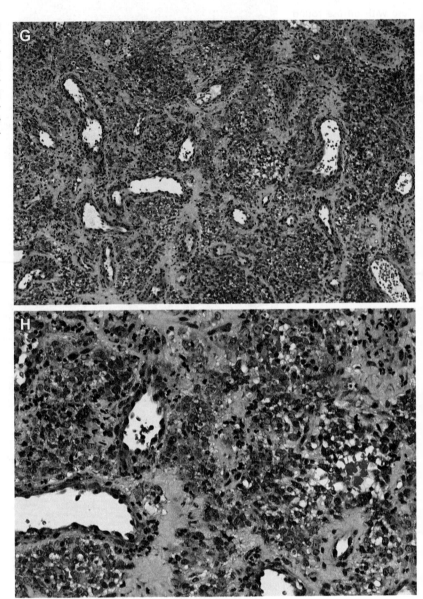

Fig. 12. (continued). (*G*) Prominent hemangiopericytomatous vascular network. (*H*) Round cell tumors with atypical nuclear features including distinct nucleoli and variations in size and shape (H&E, original magnification, [*G*] ×5; [*H*] ×10).

seen in ES.[36] Furthermore, *BCOR*-rearranged sarcomas have transcriptional profiles distinct from *CIC*-rearranged sarcomas and ES,[13,25] supporting *BCOR*-rearranged sarcomas representing a distinct sarcoma subtype.

MOLECULAR TESTING

The screening strategy to adopt depends on the type of underlying *BCOR* alteration and of the fusion partner involved as molecular techniques,

save for NGS or RNA-sequencing testing, do not cover simultaneously the array of possible *BCOR* alterations.

Fluorescence In Situ Hybridization

BCOR-CCNB3 fusions can be evidenced only by dual-fusion *FISH* (**Fig. 14**). *BCOR* and *CCNB3* are both located on chromosome X at Xp11.4 and Xp11.22 loci, respectively. Conversely, interchromosomic translocations involving *MAML3* (located on 4q31.1) and *ZC3H7B* can be

Fig. 13. Immunohistochemical features of *BCOR-CCNB3* sarcoma. (*A*) CD99 staining with a heterogeneous incomplete membranous staining that should be considered as negative. (*B*) Diffuse nuclear staining for CCNB3 and (*C*) BCOR. (*D*) CCNB3 staining in ES. There is a high cytoplasmic background and focal nuclear staining; this staining pattern should be considered negative (H&E, original magnification, [*A*] ×10; [*B*] ×5; [*C, D*] ×8).

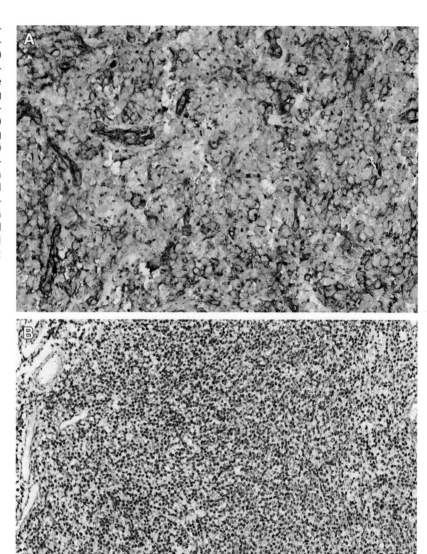

evidenced with *BCOR* break-apart FISH. Presence of *BCOR* rearrangement is not diagnostic per se of *BCOR*-rearranged round cell sarcoma, as it also occurs in other mesenchymal tumors, including ossifying fibromyxoid tumors and endometrial stromal sarcoma.[45,46]

Reverse-Transcriptase Polymerase Chain Reaction

RT-PCR only screens for known fusion transcript. *BCOR-CCNB3* fusion links *BCOR* exon 15 to *CCNB3* exon 5 with variable genomic breakpoints.

BCOR-MAML3 fusion transcript contains exons 2 to 5 of *MAML3*. The use of targeted RNA-sequencing methods is especially relevant with *BCOR*-sarcomas due to the heterogeneity of *BCOR* alterations displayed by these tumors.

Array-Comparative Genomic Hybridization

BCOR-round cell sarcomas harbor mostly balanced genomic profiles.[25,36] One-third of cases display a few recurrent CNAs, including 17p and 10q deletions. These CNAs are different from those present in ES, which display gains of chromosome 8, 1q, 12, and 16q loss.[48]

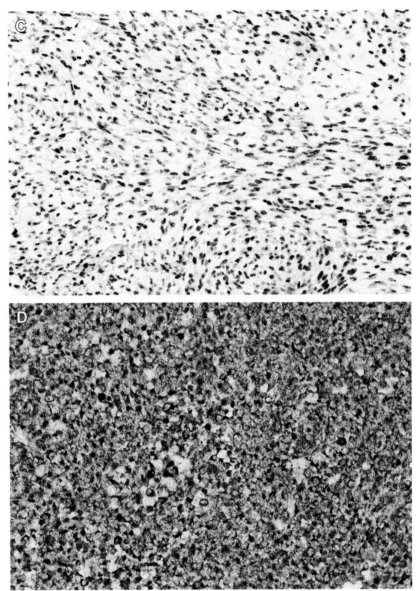

Fig. 13. (*continued*).

DIFFERENTIAL DIAGNOSIS

- ES is a key differential diagnosis. Spindling is an unusual feature in ES, mostly focal and correlates with fusions involving non-ETS transcription factors, such as *EWSR1-PATZ1*. Diffuse expression of CD99 is unusual in BCOC sarcoma and CCNB3 and BCOR positivity tip toward a BCOR-sarcoma.
- SS was one the most frequent diagnoses rendered before the identification of *BCOR-*round cell sarcomas considering the monotonous and spindled presentation of these tumors (**Fig. 15**). TLE1 expression tips toward a diagnosis of SS, although its expression has not been comprehensively assessed in *BCOR*-round cell sarcomas. Identification of *SYT/SS18* rearrangement is confirmatory of SS.
- LGFMS/SEF, see differential diagnosis section of CIC-sarcomas (see **Fig. 9**).

Fig. 14. Molecular findings in *BCOR-CCNB3* sarcoma. (*A*) Design of dual-fusion probes to assay *BCOR-CCNB3* fusions. Tel indicates telomere; Cen, centromere. (*B*) Dual-fusion FISH in a female patient. Genes involved in this fusion are located on chromosome X. In female individuals, tumor cells present with a split signal (normal chromosome X) and a fused signal (allele with BCOR-CCNB3 fusion). (*C*) Dual-fusion FISH in a male patient. Tumor cells display one fused signal indicating a *BCOR-CCNB3* rearrangement ([*B, C*] DAPI counterstain).

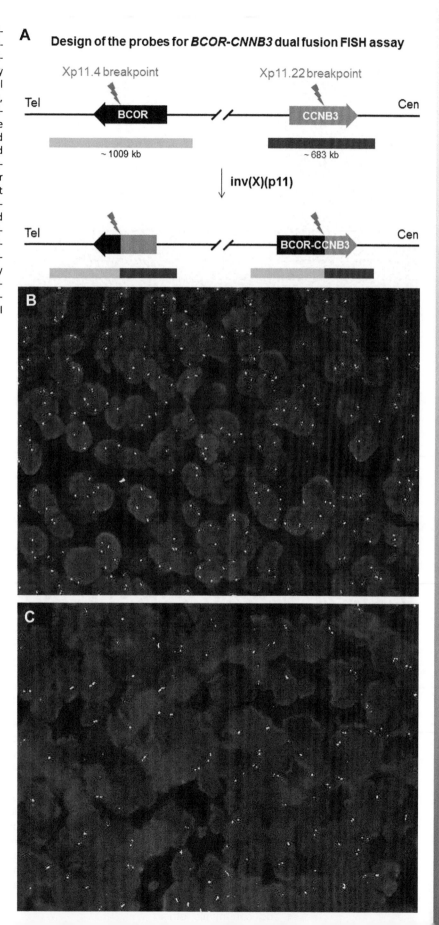

Design of the probes for *BCOR-CNNB3* dual fusion FISH assay

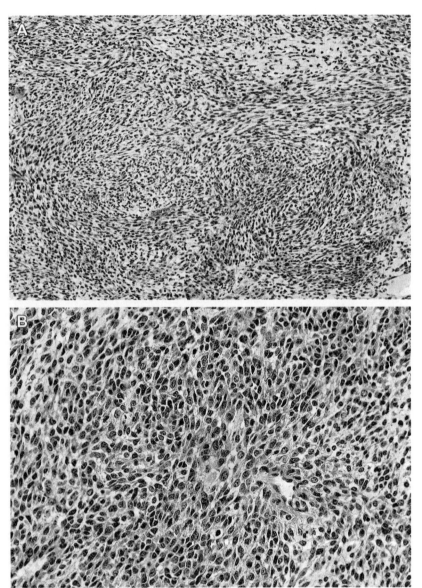

Fig. 15. SS. (A) Spindled monomorphic proliferation. (B) Focal rounded to epithelioid area (H&E, original magnification, [A] ×5; [B] ×10).

- Malignant peripheral nerve sheath tumors may rarely develop in bones. These tumors may present with monomorphic herringbone fascicles resembling SS and BCOR-sarcomas. The clinical setting of neurofibromatosis type 1 helps secure the diagnosis. S100 protein and SOX10 stainings are mostly focal. SOX10 staining has not been assessed in BCOR-sarcomas.
- Spindle cell rhabdomyosarcoma also may develop in bones. Desmin and myogenin/MYOD1 stainings should be performed when facing a spindle cell proliferation, especially in young patients.

MANAGEMENT AND PROGNOSIS

Based on retrospective data, BCOR-rearranged sarcomas seem to display high chemosensitivity in patients who received preoperative chemotherapy.[39] Most patients present with local disease.[39]

Pediatric patients are mostly treated in accordance with ES therapeutic guidelines. Sustained remission has been observed among patients treated with an ifosfamide-anthracycline regimen combined with local treatment, as recommended in ES.[39] Other studies have discussed the pejorative prognosis portended by axial locations.[40]

Fig. 15. (*continued*). (*C*) Diffuse nuclear expression of TLE1 and (*D*) BCOR (H&E, original magnification, [*C, D*] ×5).

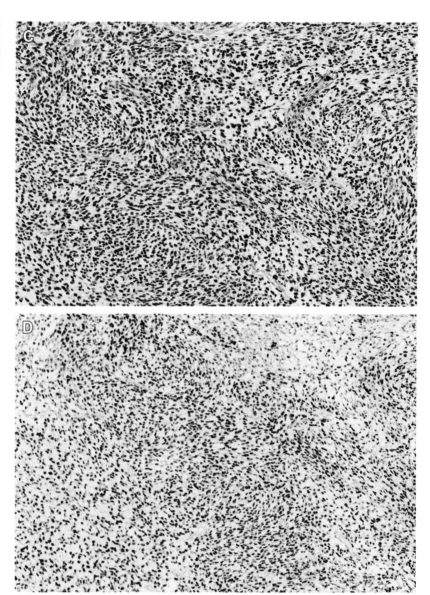

Pitfalls
BCOR-REARRANGED SARCOMAS

! The spindle cell component may predominate, raising suspicion for SSs leading to overlook round cell sarcoma differentials, such as BCOR-sarcomas and rare spindled variant of ESs.

! BCOR immunostaining is positive in 50% of SSs.

! CCNB3 staining may be difficult to interpret due to variable cytoplasmic background. It screens only BCOR-CCNB3 sarcomas. CCNB3 expression may lack in posttreatment samples.

! Molecular testing for BCOR abnormalities should be tailored to an underlying suspected mechanism, unless an NGS-based approach is used. BCOR-CCNB3 fusions can be evidenced by specific dual-fusion FISH or RT-PCR whereas BCOR interchromosomic translocations can be evidenced by BCOR break-apart FISH or RT-PCR. BCOR ITD requires PCR or RNA-sequencing.

UNDIFFERENTIATED/UNCLASSIFIED SMALL ROUND CELL SARCOMAS

Currently, approximately 11% of round cell sarcomas remain unclassified after completion of the panel of gene fusions involved in sarcomas.[1] This diagnostic category of "unclassified round cell sarcomas" keeps reducing with the use of more sensitive molecular techniques, such as RNA-sequencing in the diagnostic workup of these lesions. RNA-sequencing enables identification of cryptic rearrangements or fusion variants, not detected by FISH or RT-PCR (for example, due to a change of the exon involved in the translocation or involving a formerly unknown partner).

It enables also identification of formerly unknown recurrent translocations.[36] Conversely, its widespread use has also led to the identification of nonrecurrent so-called "private fusion genes," which biologic and clinical significance is unknown. The diagnostic implications of private fusions will certainly represent a major challenge to address. Furthermore, the application of NGS technologies to many cancer samples has revealed that the genomes of most carcinomas contain 10 fusion genes on average, all of which (and maybe none) consisting of translocation driving the tumorigenic process.[49] The integration of morphologic and molecular data therefore remains necessary to reach accurate and clinically meaningful diagnosis.

Key Features
OF FAMILIES OF ROUND CELL SARCOMAS

	Sarcomas with EWSR1–non-ETS Fusions	CIC-Sarcomas	BCOR-Sarcomas	Unclassified Round Cell Sarcomas
Fusion partners	NFATc2, PATZ1, SP3, SMARCA5	DUX4, FOXO4, NUTM1	CCNB3, BCOR-ITD, MAML3, ZC3H7B	Unknown
Patient demographics	Older than ES patients	Peak in AYA Wide age distribution	Male predominance Mainly AYA	
Location	Chest wall if PATZ1 Bone if NFATc2	Limbs in 50% Uncommon in bone	Bone with involvement of adjacent soft tissue	
Microscopy	Atypical features Nested pattern if NFATc2	Round cell sarcoma with atypical features, myxoid stromal changes, geographic necrosis	Monomorphic, spindling present in 60% of cases	Round cell phenotype
CD99	Diffuse positivity (LD)	Variable	Positive (2/3)	Variable
Surrogate markers		ETV4, WT1 cTer, DUX4 (if CIC-DUX4)	BCOR (any BCOR rearrangement) CCNB3 (if BCOR-CCNB3)	
Molecular pitfalls	False negative by EWSR1 break-apart FISH if PATZ1 is involved		BCOR-CCNB3: dual-fusion probe FISH BCOR-ITD: RT-PCR Other BCOR fusions: BCOR Break-apart FISH	RNA-seq discovery
Genomic features	Genomic amplification near breakpoints if NFATc2 is involved	Gain/trisomy of chrom 8 (C-MYC)	17p and 10q deletions in 33%	
Survival	LD	At least as aggressive as ES	75% and 55% survival at 5 and 10 y	

Abbreviations: AYA, adolescents and young adults; BCOR, Bcl6 corepressor; chrom, chromosome; CIC, capicua transcriptional repressor; ES, Ewing sarcoma; ITD, internal tandem duplication; LD, limited data.

SUMMARY

Ewing-like tumors refer to a heterogeneous group of round cell sarcomas negative for known fusion genes involved in ESs. Their dismantling has been enabled by the development of RNA-sequencing technologies and the collaborative effort to correlate genetic and morphologic data, yielding to the identification of new sarcoma entities in recent years, such as *CIC*-rearranged and *BCOR*-rearranged sarcomas. Molecular studies strongly support that they represent biologically homogeneous sarcoma subtypes, distinct from ESs.

REFERENCES

1. Machado I, Navarro L, Pellin A, et al. Defining Ewing and Ewing-like small round cell tumors (SRCT): the need for molecular techniques in their categorization and differential diagnosis. A study of 200 cases. Ann Diagn Pathol 2016;22:25–32.

2. Delattre O, Zucman J, Plougastel B, et al. Gene fusion with an ETS DNA-binding domain caused by chromosome translocation in human tumours. Nature 1992;359(6391):162–5.

3. Machado I, Noguera R, Mateos EA, et al. The many faces of atypical Ewing's sarcoma. A true entity mimicking sarcomas, carcinomas and lymphomas. Virchows Arch 2011;458(3):281–90.

4. Fletcher CDM, Bridge JA, Hogendoorn PCW, et al. WHO classification of tumours of soft tissue and bone. 4th edition. Lyon (France): IARC press; 2013.

5. Mastrangelo T, Modena P, Tornielli S, et al. A novel zinc finger gene is fused to EWS in small round cell tumor. Oncogene 2000;19(33):3799–804.

6. Szuhai K, Ijszenga M, de Jong D, et al. The NFATc2 gene is involved in a novel cloned translocation in a Ewing sarcoma variant that couples its function in immunology to oncology. Clin Cancer Res 2009; 15(7):2259–68.

7. Wang L, Bhargava R, Zheng T, et al. Undifferentiated small round cell sarcomas with rare EWS gene fusions: identification of a novel EWS-SP3 fusion and of additional cases with the EWS-ETV1 and EWS-FEV fusions. J Mol Diagn 2007;9(4):498–509.

8. Sumegi J, Nishio J, Nelson M, et al. A novel t(4;22)(q31;q12) produces an EWSR1-SMARCA5 fusion in extraskeletal Ewing sarcoma/primitive neuroectodermal tumor. Mod Pathol 2011;24(3):333–42.

9. Richkind KE, Romansky SG, Finklestein JZ. t(4;19)(q35;q13.1): a recurrent change in primitive mesenchymal tumors? Cancer Genet Cytogenet 1996;87(1):71–4.

10. Kawamura-Saito M, Yamazaki Y, Kaneko K, et al. Fusion between CIC and DUX4 up-regulates PEA3 family genes in Ewing-like sarcomas with

11. Italiano A, Sung YS, Zhang L, et al. High prevalence of CIC fusion with double-homeobox (DUX4) transcription factors in EWSR1-negative undifferentiated small blue round cell sarcomas. Genes Chromosomes Cancer 2012;51(3):207–18.

12. Machado I, Cruz J, Lavernia J, et al. Superficial EWSR1-negative undifferentiated small round cell sarcoma with CIC/DUX4 gene fusion: a new variant of Ewing-like tumors with locoregional lymph node metastasis. Virchows Arch 2013;463(6):837–42.

13. Specht K, Sung YS, Zhang L, et al. Distinct transcriptional signature and immunoprofile of CIC-DUX4 fusion-positive round cell tumors compared to EWSR1-rearranged Ewing sarcomas: further evidence toward distinct pathologic entities. Genes Chromosomes Cancer 2014;53(7):622–33.

14. Yoshida A, Goto K, Kodaira M, et al. CIC-rearranged sarcomas: a study of 20 cases and comparisons with Ewing sarcomas. Am J Surg Pathol 2016; 40(3):313–23.

15. Le Guellec S, Velasco V, Pérot G, et al. ETV4 is a useful marker for the diagnosis of CIC-rearranged undifferentiated round-cell sarcomas: a study of 127 cases including mimicking lesions. Mod Pathol 2016;29:1523–31.

16. Hung YP, Fletcher CD, Hornick JL. Evaluation of ETV4 and WT1 expression in CIC-rearranged sarcomas and histologic mimics. Mod Pathol 2016;29: 1324–34.

17. Smith SC, Palanisamy N, Martin E, et al. The utility of ETV1, ETV4 and ETV5 RNA in-situ hybridization in the diagnosis of CIC-DUX sarcomas. Histopathology 2016;70:657–63.

18. Smith SC, Buehler D, Choi EY, et al. CIC-DUX sarcomas demonstrate frequent MYC amplification and ETS-family transcription factor expression. Mod Pathol 2015;28(1):57–68.

19. Graham C, Chilton-MacNeill S, Zielenska M, et al. The CIC-DUX4 fusion transcript is present in a subgroup of pediatric primitive round cell sarcomas. Hum Pathol 2012;43(2):180–9.

20. Siegele B, Roberts J, Black JO, et al. DUX4 immunohistochemistry is a highly sensitive and specific marker for CIC-DUX4 fusion-positive round cell tumor. Am J Surg Pathol 2016;41:423–9.

21. van Geel M, Dickson MC, Beck AF, et al. Genomic analysis of human chromosome 10q and 4q telomeres suggests a common origin. Genomics 2002; 79(2):210–7.

22. Jeon IS, Davis JN, Braun BS, et al. A variant Ewing's sarcoma translocation (7;22) fuses the EWS gene to the ETS gene ETV1. Oncogene 1995;10(6):1229–34.

23. Kaneko Y, Yoshida K, Handa M, et al. Fusion of an ETS-family gene, EIAF, to EWS by t(17;22)(q12;q12) chromosome translocation in an undifferentiated

sarcoma of infancy. Genes Chromosomes Cancer 1996;15(2):115–21.

24. Sugita S, Arai Y, Tonooka A, et al. A novel CIC-FOXO4 gene fusion in undifferentiated small round-cell sarcoma: a genetically distinct variant of Ewing-like sarcoma. Am J Surg Pathol 2014;38(11):1571–6.

25. Sturm D, Orr BA, Toprak UH, et al. New brain tumor entities emerge from molecular classification of CNS-PNETs. Cell 2016;164(5):1060–72.

26. Solomon DA, Brohl AS, Khan J, et al. Clinicopathologic features of a second patient with Ewing-like sarcoma harboring CIC-FOXO4 gene fusion. Am J Surg Pathol 2014;38(12):1724–5.

27. Rakheja D, Goldman S, Wilson KS, et al. Translocation (4;19)(q35;q13.1)-associated primitive round cell sarcoma: report of a case and review of the literature. Pediatr Dev Pathol 2008;11(3):239–44.

28. Lazo de la Vega L, Hovelson DH, Cani AK, et al. Targeted next-generation sequencing of CIC-DUX4 soft tissue sarcomas demonstrates low mutational burden and recurrent chromosome 1p loss. Hum Pathol 2016;58:161–70.

29. Nascimento AG, Unii KK, Pritchard DJ, et al. A clinicopathologic study of 20 cases of large-cell (atypical) Ewing's sarcoma of bone. Am J Surg Pathol 1980;4(1):29–36.

30. Agaram NP, Zhang L, Sung YS, et al. Extraskeletal myxoid chondrosarcoma with non-EWSR1-NR4A3 variant fusions correlate with rhabdoid phenotype and high-grade morphology. Hum Pathol 2014;45(5):1084–91.

31. Doyle LA, Wang WL, Dal Cin P, et al. MUC4 is a sensitive and extremely useful marker for sclerosing epithelioid fibrosarcoma: association with FUS gene rearrangement. Am J Surg Pathol 2012;36(10):1444–51.

32. Arbajian E, Puls F, Magnusson L, et al. Recurrent EWSR1-CREB3L1 gene fusions in sclerosing epithelioid fibrosarcoma. Am J Surg Pathol 2014;38(6):801–8.

33. Huang SC, Zhang L, Sung YS, et al. Recurrent CIC gene abnormalities in angiosarcomas: a molecular study of 120 cases with concurrent investigation of PLCG1, KDR, MYC, and FLT4 gene alterations. Am J Surg Pathol 2016;40(5):645–55.

34. Le Loarer F, Watson S, Pierron G, et al. SMARCA4 inactivation defines a group of undifferentiated thoracic malignancies transcriptionally related to BAF-deficient sarcomas. Nat Genet 2015;47(10):1200–5.

35. Choi EY, Thomas DG, McHugh JB, et al. Undifferentiated small round cell sarcoma with t(4;19)(q35;q13.1) CIC-DUX4 fusion: a novel highly aggressive soft tissue tumor with distinctive histopathology. Am J Surg Pathol 2013;37(9):1379–86.

36. Pierron G, Tirode F, Lucchesi C, et al. A new subtype of bone sarcoma defined by BCOR-CCNB3 gene fusion. Nat Genet 2012;44(4):461–6.

37. Specht K, Zhang L, Sung YS, et al. Novel BCOR-MAML3 and ZC3H7B-BCOR gene fusions in undifferentiated small blue round cell sarcomas. Am J Surg Pathol 2016;40(4):433–42.

38. Kao YC, Sung YS, Zhang L, et al. Recurrent BCOR internal tandem duplication and YWHAE-NUTM2B fusions in soft tissue undifferentiated round cell sarcoma of infancy: overlapping genetic features with clear cell sarcoma of kidney. Am J Surg Pathol 2016;40(8):1009–20.

39. Cohen-Gogo S, Cellier C, Coindre JM, et al. Ewing-like sarcomas with BCOR-CCNB3 fusion transcript: a clinical, radiological and pathological retrospective study from the Société Française des Cancers de L'Enfant. Pediatr Blood Cancer 2014;61(12):2191–8.

40. Puls F, Niblett A, Marland G, et al. BCOR-CCNB3 (Ewing-like) sarcoma: a clinicopathologic analysis of 10 cases, in comparison with conventional Ewing sarcoma. Am J Surg Pathol 2014;38(10):1307–18.

41. Peters TL, Kumar V, Polikepahad S, et al. BCOR-CCNB3 fusions are frequent in undifferentiated sarcomas of male children. Mod Pathol 2015;28(4):575–86.

42. Kao YC, Sung YS, Zhang L, et al. BCOR overexpression is a highly sensitive marker in round cell sarcomas with BCOR genetic abnormalities. Am J Surg Pathol 2016;40:1670–8.

43. Gearhart MD, Corcoran CM, Wamstad JA, et al. Polycomb group and SCF ubiquitin ligases are found in a novel BCOR complex that is recruited to BCL6 targets. Mol Cell Biol 2006;26(18):6880–9.

44. Fan Z, Yamaza T, Lee JS, et al. BCOR regulates mesenchymal stem cell function by epigenetic mechanisms. Nat Cell Biol 2009;11(8):1002–9.

45. Antonescu CR, Sung YS, Chen CL, et al. Novel ZC3H7B-BCOR, MEAF6-PHF1, and EPC1-PHF1 fusions in ossifying fibromyxoid tumors–molecular characterization shows genetic overlap with endometrial stromal sarcoma. Genes Chromosomes Cancer 2014;53(2):183–93.

46. Panagopoulos I, Thorsen J, Gorunova L, et al. Fusion of the ZC3H7B and BCOR genes in endometrial stromal sarcomas carrying an X;22-translocation. Genes Chromosomes Cancer 2013;52(7):610–8.

47. Alaggio R, Ninfo V, Rosolen A, et al. Primitive myxoid mesenchymal tumor of infancy: a clinicopathologic report of 6 cases. Am J Surg Pathol 2006;30(3):388–94.

48. Armengol G, Tarkkanen M, Virolainen M, et al. Recurrent gains of 1q, 8 and 12 in the Ewing family of tumours by comparative genomic hybridization. Br J Cancer 1997;75(10):1403–9.

49. Vogelstein B, Papadopoulos N, Velculescu VE, et al. Cancer genome landscapes. Science 2013;339(6127):1546–58.

Vascular Tumors of Bone
The Evolvement of a Classification Based on Molecular Developments

David G.P. van IJzendoorn, BSc, Judith V.M.G. Bovée, MD, PhD*

KEYWORDS

- Epithelioid hemangioma • Epithelioid hemangioendothelioma • Vascular tumor • Angiosarcoma
- Pseudomyogenic hemangioendothelioma

Key points

- Vascular tumors with primary bone localization include hemangioma, epithelioid hemangioma, pseudomyogenic (epithelioid sarcoma-like) hemangioendothelioma, epithelioid hemangioendothelioma, and angiosarcoma.

- A panel of vascular markers should be used to confirm endothelial differentiation (including ERG, CD31, and CD34).

- Epithelioid hemangioendothelioma is characterized by WWTR1-CAMTA1 fusions, whereas epithelioid hemangioma and pseudomyogenic hemangioendothelioma carry alterations within the FOS family (FOS and FOSB). Molecular analysis or immunohistochemistry for CAMTA1 or FOSB can help in the differential diagnosis.

- Angiosarcoma of bone is highly aggressive, often epithelioid, and without recurrent genetic alterations.

ABSTRACT

The classification of vascular tumors of bone has been under debate over time. Vascular tumors in bone are rare, display highly overlapping morphology, and, therefore, are considered difficult by pathologists. Compared with their soft tissue counterparts, they are more often multifocal and sometimes behave more aggressively. Over the past decade, with the advent of next-generation sequencing, recurrent molecular alterations have been found in some of the entities. The integration of morphology and molecular changes has led to a better characterization of these separate entities.

OVERVIEW

The common denominator of vascular tumors consists of their endothelial differentiation, with a variable capability of forming mature or immature vessels. Literature on the cell of origin for vascular tumors (other than infantile hemangioma) is scarce and points to an endothelial precursor cell or a hematopoietic precursor cell along its path of endothelial differentiation, for canine and murine hemangioma/angiosarcoma.[1,2] The definition of these cells in mice and humans, however, is controversial.[3,4]

The classification of vascular tumors of bone has been a matter of discussion over time.[5-7] With the rapid elucidation of molecular changes in tumors using next-generation sequencing, however, which also included vascular tumors of bone, the classification has evolved and morphology and molecular changes were integrated to better define the separate entities[8] that are sometimes extremely difficult to distinguish based on morphology alone. Like in soft tissue, the entity of hemangiopericytoma of bone is no longer recognized, because these lesions are rare presentations of synovial sarcoma, solitary fibrous tumor, and myofibroma primary of bone.[9] Moreover, although in the past there has

---

Disclosures Statement: The authors report no conflicts of interest.
Department of Pathology, Leiden University Medical Center, Postzone L1-Q, Postbus 9600, Leiden 2300 RC, The Netherlands
* Corresponding author.
E-mail address: J.V.M.G.bovee@lumc.nl

Surgical Pathology 10 (2017) 621–635
http://dx.doi.org/10.1016/j.path.2017.04.003
1875-9181/17/© 2017 Elsevier Inc. All rights reserved.

Table 1
Summary of prognosis and treatment of vascular bone tumors

Classification	Entity	Prognosis	Treatment
Benign	Hemangioma	100% survival, 0% metastasis	Treat symptoms
Intermediate	Epithelioid hemangioma	100% survival, 2% metastases, 9% local recurrence	Curettage or marginal excision
	Pseudomyogenic hemangioendothelioma	Limited follow-up, stable or progressive osseous disease	
Malignant	Epithelioid hemangioendothelioma	85% survival, 25% metastases	Wide resection
	Angiosarcoma	30% survival	Wide resection, consider systemic therapy

been ample discussion about hemangioendothelioma of bone as a separate entity,[10] it is now generally accepted that the previously reported cases represent epithelioid hemangioma of bone,[8,9,11] and with the elucidation of specific genetic alterations in epithelioid hemangioma of bone[12,13] this discussion may be definitively resolved in the future.

Now that the different vascular tumors have been better characterized, their distinct behavior in bone compared with when they are located in the soft tissues is becoming obvious. Vascular tumors of bone are more frequently multifocal, affecting multiple bones.[6] Also, although histologically and genetically similar, epithelioid hemangioma in soft tissue is considered benign, whereas in bone it behaves as a locally aggressive, rarely metastasizing lesion and is, therefore, considered of the intermediate category.[8] In addition, atypical epithelioid hemangioma has a preference for bone and penile location.[14] Moreover, after the morphologic and molecular characterization of pseudomyogenic (epithelioid sarcoma-like) hemangioendothelioma,[15,16] cases are reported that are exclusively located in bone, with unique histologic findings.[17]

This article discusses the most common vascular tumors of bone. These tumor entities range from the benign hemangioma of bone, with a good prognosis and no metastasis in all patients, to the intermediate epithelioid hemangioma (including the atypical variant) and the pseudomyogenic hemangioendothelioma whose survival is excellent but with some metastasis and recurrences. Epithelioid hemangioendothelioma is considered low-grade malignant, with 85% survival and 25% metastases. Angiosarcoma is high-grade malignant with a very poor survival of only 30% over 5 years (**Table 1**). This review covers the classic presentations of these tumor entities, including the diagnostic pitfalls and immunohistochemistry and discusses the recent developments regarding the genetics and tumorigenesis of these vascular tumors of bone (**Table 2**).

IMMUNOHISTOCHEMISTRY

In all vascular tumors, endothelial differentiation can be highlighted using a panel of immunohistochemical markers, including CD31, CD34, and ERG. ERG positivity can be highly specific for endothelial differentiation, although this is dependent on the clone used: antibodies against the N-terminal part of the protein are more specific compared with antibodies directed against the C-terminal part, which can also be positive in a variety of other mesenchymal tumors.[18] Moreover, approximately 50% of the prostate carcinomas harbor translocations involving ERG and thereby can be positive.[19] FLI1 and von Willebrand factor (VWF), or factor VIII, can also be used. Smooth muscle actin can highlight the pericytes, whereas D2-40 (podoplanin) and Prox1 can demonstrate lymphatic differentiation. A notorious pitfall that pathologists should be aware of, especially in bone where vascular tumors are often epithelioid (93%–100%[20,21]), is the expression of keratin in a significant percentage of vascular tumors.[20,22,23]

HEMANGIOMA

DEFINITION, EPIDEMIOLOGY, AND CLINICAL FEATURES

Hemangiomas are common lesions that rarely ever reach a pathologist. Reported by Mirra and colleagues,[24] these tumors are found in approximately 10% of all autopsies and they are often seen by radiologists. They are usually asymptomatic. The vertebral bodies and the skull are most commonly affected (**Fig. 1**).[25] Kaleem and colleagues[26] analyzed all reported cases of hemangioma affecting the extremities in English literature through 2000 (n = 104) and found a mean age of 32 years and a slight preference for women (60%). When affecting the long bones, the diaphysis or metadiaphysis is the most common

Table 2
Differential diagnosis of vascular tumors of bone

Entity	Histologic and Molecular Findings	Immunohistochemistry
Hemangioma of bone	• Numerous smaller or larger blood-filled spaces, lined by flat endothelium • Reactive sclerosis of surrounding lamellar bone • *No specific genetic alterations*	CD31+ CD34+ ERG+
Epithelioid hemangioma of bone	• Lobular architecture (can be highlighted using actin immunohistochemistry) • Well-formed vessels lined by epithelioid endothelial cells • Eosinophilic infiltrate • No prominent nuclear atypia or atypical mitoses • Hemorrhagic and spindle cell areas can be prominent, especially in acral lesions • *Rearrangement of FOS*	CD31+ CD34+ ERG+
Atypical epithelioid hemangioma of bone	• Similar to epithelioid hemangioma, with more solid growth, increased cellularity, nuclear pleomorphism, and necrosis • *ZFP36-FOSB fusion*	Similar to epithelioid hemangioma
Pseudomyogenic (epithelioid sarcoma-like) hemangioendothelioma	• Sheets of spindled or epithelioid cells with abundant eosinophilic cytoplasm • Infiltrative growth • Neutrophilic infiltrate • Reactive woven bone and osteoclast-like giant cells can be present • *SERPINE-1-FOSB fusion*	ERG+ FLI1+ Keratin+ CD34− Desmin− Retention of INI1 FOSB+
Epithelioid hemangioendothelioma	• Epithelioid endothelial cells in strands and cords embedded in a hyaline or myxoid stroma • Intracytoplasmic vacuoles (blister cells) • No well-formed vessels • Infiltrative growth • Cytologic atypia and mitoses usually limited, but can be prominent • *WWTR1-CAMTA1 fusion*	CD31 100% CD34 85% FLI1 100% Keratin 25%–38% D2-40 54% Prox1 54% ERG 98% Claudin-1 88% CAMTA1 86%–88%
YAP1-TFE3 rearranged epithelioid hemangioendothelioma	• Focally well-formed vasoformative features in addition to solid areas • Voluminous deep eosinophilic or histiocytoid cytoplasm, sometimes feathery • Mild to moderate nuclear atypia • *YAP1-TFE3 fusion*	Same as EHE TFE3+
Angiosarcoma	• Vasoformative, with multilayering, or solid • In bone often epithelioid (>90%) • Inflammatory infiltrate • Nuclear atypia (with large nucleoli) • Brisk mitotic atypia, including atypical mitoses • *No specific genetic alterations*	CD31 95%–100% ERG 96% VWF 60%–75% CD34 39%–40% Actin 61% Keratin 69%–80% D2-40 31%
Intravascular papillary endothelial hyperplasia (Masson tumor)	• Can occur in a blood vessel, a hematoma or in a preexisting vascular lesion • Papillary structures containing fibrin or collagen, covered by a single layer of endothelial cells • No or limited cytologic atypia, no or limited mitotic activity, no multilayering	CD31+ CD34+ ERG+

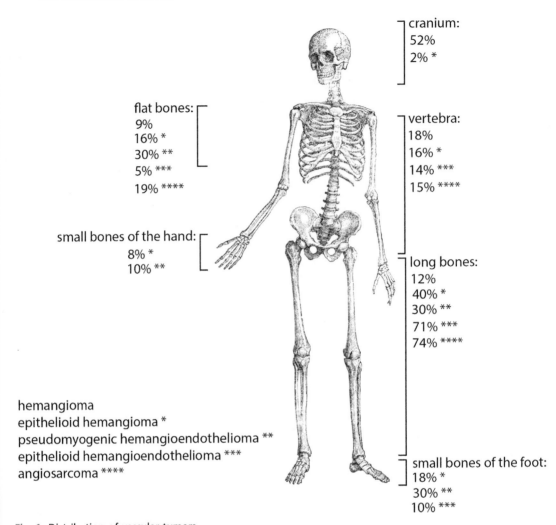

cranium:
52%
2% *

flat bones:
9%
16% *
30% **
5% ***
19% ****

vertebra:
18%
16% *
14% ***
15% ****

small bones of the hand:
8% *
10% **

long bones:
12%
40% *
30% **
71% ***
74% ****

hemangioma
epithelioid hemangioma *
pseudomyogenic hemangioendothelioma **
epithelioid hemangioendothelioma ***
angiosarcoma ****

small bones of the foot:
18% *
30% **
10% ***

Fig. 1. Distribution of vascular tumors.

location. Medullary origin is most frequent, but 45% of cases are either periosteal (33%) or intra-cortical (12%).[26] In the literature, 11 cases have been described with intracortical hemangioma of bone, 7 of which were located in the distal tibia.[27] Cavernous hemangioma is the most frequent type, although also (areas with) capillary hemangi-oma can be found. At imaging the lesions are radio-lucent due to the lack of bone and abundance of fat on radiologic images. Reportedly the tumors give a high MRI signal in T1 and T2 owing to their high fat presence.[5] No genetic aberrations have been described thus far.

HISTOLOGIC AND IMMUNOHISTOCHEMISTRY FEATURES

Macroscopically (Fig. 2A–C) the lesions show tra-beculated bone with a dark spongelike appearance. Histologically, the lesions show numerous blood-filled spaces, lined by a thin layer of flat endothelial cells, without atypia. The vascular spaces are sur-rounded by loose connective tissue and grow in-between the bone trabeculae that are often thick-ened (Fig. 2D).

EPITHELIOID HEMANGIOMA

DEFINITION, EPIDEMIOLOGY, AND CLINICAL FEATURES

Epithelioid hemangioma of bone is classified as an intermediate and locally aggressive but rarely metastasizing vascular tumor of bone.[8,9] On CT scans, a honeycomb pattern can be visible. Concise naming and classification of this tumor entity were only introduced recently by O'Connell and col-leagues.[28,29] Previously epithelioid hemangiomas of bone were reported as "hemangioendothelioma

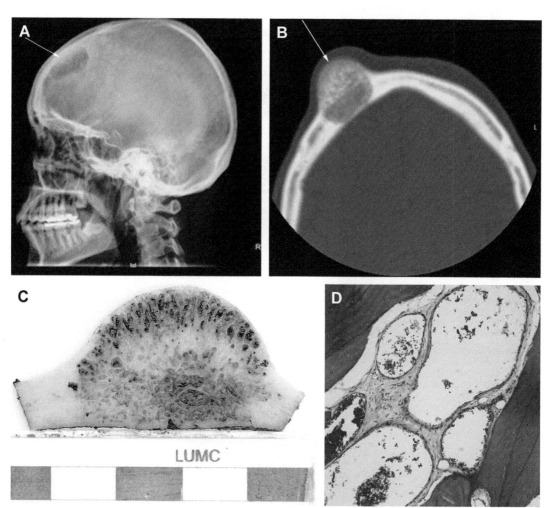

Fig. 2. Hemangioma of bone. (*A*) Radiograph of the skull with a sharply defined lytic lesion in the cranium. (*B*) Corresponding CT scan showing large protruding lytic lesion with calcifications (*arrows* point to tumors). Corresponding gross specimen shows trabeculations of the bone with spongelike appearance. (*D*) Microscopic image with large cavernous spaces lined by flat endothelium in between bony trabeculae (H&E).

of bone"[11] or "hemorrhagic epithelioid and spindle cell hemangioma."[11,30]

Nielsen and colleagues[11] revisited 50 epithelioid hemangiomas and described the age of occurrence as varying from 10 years to 75 years with a mean of 35 years and a slight preference for boys and men. Because epithelioid hemangioma is a rare entity, exact prevalence is difficult to determine.

Epithelioid hemangioma has been described as occurring in many different locations (see **Fig. 1**). Case reports and series of revisited cases seem to show there is a slight preference for the long tubular bones,[31] but the spine is also often affected.[32–35] Further reports include occurrences in the orbit.[36–41] Epithelioid hemangioma is also frequently reported to occur in the small tubular bones of the extremities.[42–45] Multifocal bone involvement occurs in approximately 18% of cases,[11] with 1 case involving 3 different bones.[46] Involvement of the draining lymph nodes has been described but is not often confirmed as metastatic,[47] although, as described by Nielsen and colleagues,[11] the lymph node can contains cells resembling epithelioid hemangioma.

HISTOLOGIC AND IMMUNOHISTOCHEMISTRY FEATURES

Epithelioid hemangioma is usually well defined, with a lobular architecture (**Fig. 3**C), but can extend into the soft tissue. The vessels are usually well formed and lined by epithelioid endothelial cells (**Fig. 3**D, E). The cells have an enlarged nuclei with open chromatin, without prominent nuclear atypia. The often loose stroma surrounding the

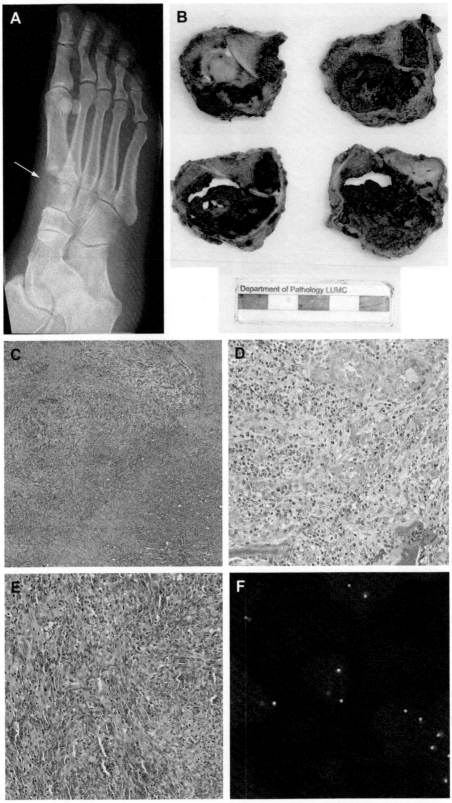

Fig. 3. Epithelioid hemangioma of bone. (*A*) Radiograph of the foot showing multiple sharply defined lesions (*arrow* points at the most prominent one). (*B*) Corresponding gross section. (*C*) Epithelioid hemangioma typically shows a lobular architecture (H&E). (*D*) Eosinophilic infiltrate surrounding the vessels lined by large epithelioid cells (H&E). (*E*) Hemorrhagic and spindled cell appearance can be prominent especially in acral lesions (H&E). (*F*) FISH with break-apart probes surrounding FOS shows a split signal.

vessels can be infiltrated with eosinophils (see **Fig. 3**E).

TUMORIGENESIS AND GENETICS

Previously it was believed that epithelioid hemangioma could be a reactive lesion. This was refuted with the detection of fusion genes involving FOS (see **Fig. 3**E) and FOSB with various fusion partners.[12–14] Discovery of specific fusion genes also showed that tumors with multiple foci are monoclonal suggesting multifocal regional spread instead of multiple primaries.[12] Overall, FOS rearrangements were found in 29% of epithelioid hemangiomas.[13] The frequency was higher in epithelioid hemangioma of bone compared with soft tissue (59%–71% vs 19%, respectively).[12,13] In the FOS translocated epithelioid hemangiomas, the fusion partners are at the C-terminal end of the protein and lead to a loss of the transactivating domain, regulating FOS turnover. It is speculated that this loss of the transactivation domain of FOS would lead to a reduced turnover, because FOS is normally rapidly degraded. Fusion genes involving FOSB are fused at the N-terminal end of the protein and are most likely activating promoter swap events. A specific subset of epithelioid hemangiomas was shown to harbor ZFP36-FOSB fusions.[14] This subset has atypical histologic features, including more solid growth, increased cellularity, nuclear pleomorphism, and necrosis.[14] These cases are predominantly located at the penis and in bone. Both FOS and FOSB are part of the AP-1 transcription factor complex.[48]

PSEUDOMYOGENIC (EPITHELIOID SARCOMA-LIKE) HEMANGIOENDOTHELIOMA

DEFINITION, EPIDEMIOLOGY, AND CLINICAL FEATURES

Most likely the first description in the literature of pseudomyogenic hemangioendothelioma was published in 1992 by Mirra and colleagues,[49] who reported a previously undescribed variant of epithelioid sarcoma. They reported 5 cases of epithelioid sarcoma displaying multicentric involvement of a single limb and osseous involvement, with bland diffuse fibrohistiocytic and rhabdoid cells. The first description as a distinct entity was in 2003 when Billings and colleagues[50] reported 7 histologically identical cases under the name epithelioid sarcoma-like hemangioendothelioma. In 2011, Hornick and Fletcher[16] presented a large patient series, including 29 cases; 24% of these had concurrent bone involvement. They proposed designating the tumors as pseudomyogenic

hemangioendothelioma. Most of the tumors arise in the extremities (see **Fig. 1**) with a male predominance (41 vs 9). Mean age was 31 years, ranging from 14 years to 80 years. Strikingly, 33 of 50 patients presented with multifocal disease in which multiple discontiguous nodules were found in different tissue planes. In 2016, Inyang and colleagues[17] published the largest series of pseudomyogenic hemangioendotheliomas of bone to date, describing 10 cases of a male predominance (9 male vs 1 female) and a mean age of 36 (range 12–74 years). They described the lesions as having intratumoral reactive woven bone and infiltration of osteoclast-like giant cells. The tumor is locally aggressive and rarely metastasizing, therefore of the intermediate category: 1 patient of 50 developed distant metastasis.[16] Reportedly the lesions are usually from 0.3 cm to 5.5 cm in size, with ill-defined margins (**Fig. 4**A).

HISTOLOGIC AND IMMUNOHISTOCHEMISTRY FEATURES

The tumor cells characteristically show an epithelioid sarcoma-like or rhabdomyoblast-like appearance, with abundant eosinophilic cytoplasm (**Fig. 4**B, C). The lesions can infiltrate in skeletal muscle. Infiltration with neutrophilic granulocytes can be prominent (see **Fig. 4**B). The tumor cells characteristically express keratin AE1AE3 (**Fig. 4**F), ERG, and FLI1 (**Fig. 3**E), whereas CD34 (**Fig. 3**D) and desmin are negative. CD31 is expressed in approximately 50% of the cases and INI1 is retained. FOSB was shown an excellent immunohistochemical marker for detecting the presence of the SERPINE1-FOSB fusion (discussed later), with 48 of 50 pseudomyogenic hemangioendothelioma cases showing positive nuclear staining.[51,52]

TUMORIGENESIS AND GENETICS

Trombetta and colleagues[53] published the first report of a balanced translocation between chromosomes 7 and 19 in pseudomyogenic hemangioendothelioma. The exact fusion partners were later identified as SERPINE1 and FOSB.[54] Fluorescence in situ hybridization (FISH) split probes for FOSB can be an excellent diagnostic marker (**Fig. 4**G). Most likely the SERPINE1-FOSB fusion leads to up-regulation of FOSB because FOSB is retained almost entirely (fused at exon 2) and gains the promoter of SERPINE1 (fusion occurs in intron 1). Up-regulation of FOSB could lead to activation of the AP-1 complex, which is a potent transcription factor leading to the tumorigenesis; thereby, the underlying molecular mechanism is very similar to epithelioid hemangioma in which

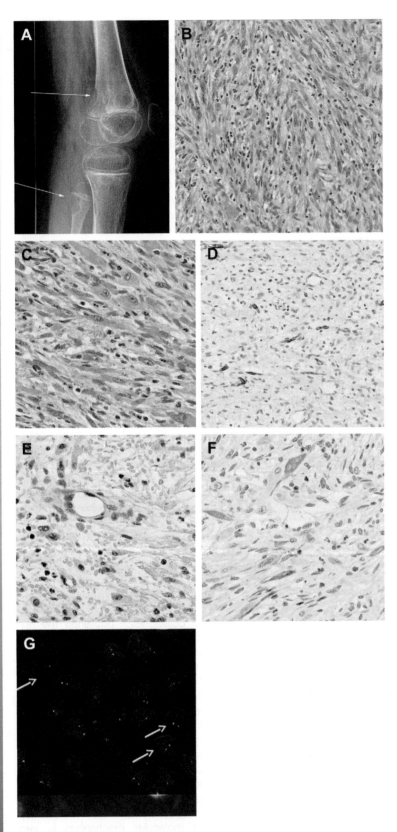

Fig. 4. Pseudomyogenic hemangioendothelioma of bone. (*A*) Radiograph shows a lesion in the left femur and fibula (*arrows*). (*B*) Spindle cells are seen admixed with neutrophils (H&E); (*C*) the cells display a rhabdomyoblast-like appearance (H&E). (*D*) CD34 is consistently negative. (*E*) FLI1 shows nuclear staining in the endothelial cells. (*F*) Keratin staining is positive in the tumor cells. (*G*) FISH demonstrating split apart (*arrows*) using a probe for FOSB indicative of FOSB rearrangement.

ZFP36-FOSB, as well as different types of FOS fusions, cause activation of the AP-1 complex.

EPITHELIOID HEMANGIOENDOTHELIOMA

DEFINITION, EPIDEMIOLOGY, AND CLINICAL FEATURES

Epithelioid hemangioendothelioma of bone is classified by the World Health Organization as a low-grade malignant vascular sarcoma.[8] Most are indolent, although 20% to 30% of the tumors metastasize and mortality is approximately 15%.[55] The first distinction of epithelioid hemangioendothelioma from angiosarcoma was made by Thomas in 1942,[56] who acknowledged that epithelioid hemangioendothelioma resembled epithelium in contrast to angiosarcoma. Moreover, he also described angiosarcoma as having a more malignant clinical course. The first comprehensive description of epithelioid hemangioendothelioma was formulated by Stout in 1943[57] who described 2 critical features. First, the formation of atypical endothelial cells in greater numbers than are required for the lining of blood vessels. Second, the formation of vascular tubes with a delicate framework of reticulin fibers.[57] Later the characteristic blister cells were added to the criteria for epithelioid hemangioendothelioma by Weiss and Enzinger.[58] The tumor could easily be mistaken for a carcinoma due to its epithelioid appearance and lack of vasoformation.

The combined literature shows that the age of occurrence is regularly distributed between 10 years and 60 years. There is a male predominance (68.9% of patients). The cases of reported metastasis showed that the preferred site for metastasis were the lungs followed by the skeleton, but it remains unclear whether these skeletal metastases should be considered true metastases or multifocal regional spread. Overall, epithelioid hemangioendothelioma of bone is polyostotic in greater than 50% of the cases.[59] It predominantly affects the lower extremity (approximately 81%) (see Fig. 1), and in up to 18% of the cases concurrent parenchymal tumors are found. Radiologically epithelioid hemangioendothelioma, like the other vascular tumors in bone, presents as a lytic lesion, without a sharp demarcation.

HISTOLOGIC AND IMMUNOHISTOCHEMISTRY FEATURES

Histologically, epithelioid hemangioendothelioma typically consists of epithelioid cells, with abundant eosinophilic cytoplasm, sometimes with intracytoplasmic vacuolization (so-called blister cells) (Fig. 5A, B). The cells are organized in short cords or strands and characteristically are embedded in hyalinized or myxoid stroma. The tumor has an infiltrative growth pattern and is lacking a lobular or vasoformative architecture. Marked nuclear atypia and/or necrosis is found in approximately 33% of the cases. Inflammatory cells are usually absent. Immunohistochemically, the tumor cells are positive for CD31 (100%) (Fig. 5C), CD34 (85%), FLI1 (100%), keratin (25%–38%), D2-40 (54%), Prox1 (47%), ERG (98%), and Claudin-1 (88%).[23,60,61] Recently, nuclear staining for CAMTA1 was shown a highly specific marker for epithelioid hemangioendothelioma, positive in 86% to 88% of the cases (Fig. 5D).[62,63] TFE3 immunohistochemistry can be used to identify the specific subset of epithelioid hemangioendotheliomas with YAP1-TFE3 fusions, although not all TFE3-positive cases carry the translocation (discussed later).[64] The clinical behavior of epithelioid hemangioendothelioma is highly variable and difficult to predict based on histologic features. Deyrup and colleagues[55] proposed a risk stratification scheme in which tumors larger than 3 cm, with more than 3 mitoses per 50 high-power fields (HPFs) have a 5-year survival rate of 59% and a metastatic rate of 32% compared with 100% 5-year survival for patients with tumors smaller than 3 cm with less than 3 mitoses per 50 HPFs. Whether this risk stratification scheme is also applicable to epithelioid hemangioendotheliomas with primary bone location remains to be established.

TUMORIGENESIS AND GENETICS

Two fusions have been described for epithelioid hemangioendothelioma, the most common is the WWTR1-CAMTA1 (Fig. 5E) fusion, which was concurrently described.[65,66] Reportedly almost all (89%–100%) epithelioid hemangioendothelioma with classic histologic features harbors this fusion. Using genetic analysis the monoclonal origin of multifocal epithelioid hemangioendothelioma has been established with WWTR1-CAMTA1 breakpoint analysis, indicating that multiple lesions arise from local or metastatic spread from a single primary as opposed to multiple independent primaries.[65]

In a distinct subset of epithelioid hemangioendotheliomas, which were negative for WWTR1-CAMTA1, a YAP1-TFE3 fusion has been described.[67] This specific subset affects predominantly young adults and has a distinct morphology, with vasoformative and vasoinvasive growth, combined with solid areas. The cytoplasm is

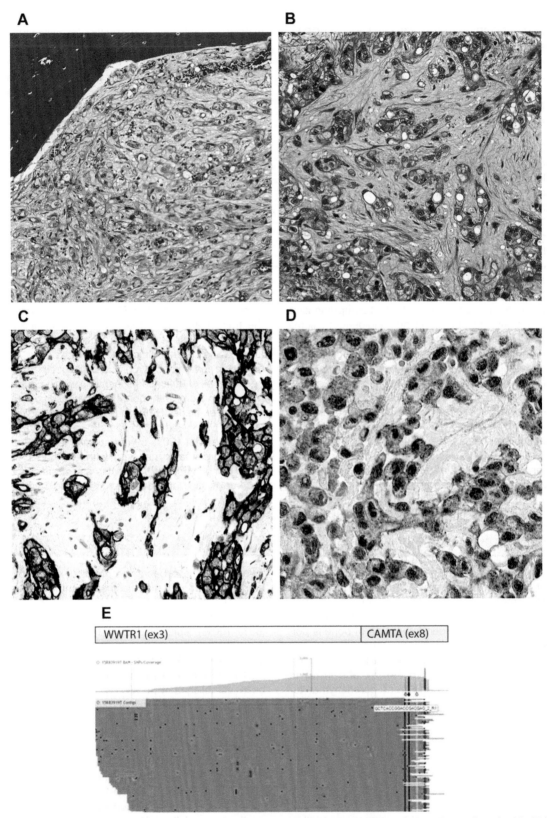

Fig. 5. Epithelioid hemangioendothelioma of bone. (*A*) Epithelioid tumor cells in cords and strands embedded in stroma (H&E). (*B*) Intracytoplasmic vacuoles can be seen (blister cells) (H&E). (*C*) CD31 confirms endothelial differentiation. (*D*) CAMTA1 shows positive nuclear staining. (*E*) The WWTR1-CAMTA1 fusion detected using next generation sequencing (Archer sarcoma fusion panel, Boulder, USA).

voluminous, deeply eosinophilic or histiocytoid, and sometimes feathery. The nuclei can be mild to moderately atypical. TFE3 FISH can be used to confirm the diagnosis.

The WWTR1-CAMTA1 fusion gene has been extensively studied. In contrast to what was speculated when the fusion was first described, the fusion is not a simple promoter swap where the WWTR1 promoter drives CAMTA1. The WWTR1-CAMTA1 fusion leads to activation of the Hippo signaling pathway, which is described as an important regulator of organ size. Because the chimeric protein contains the TEAD binding domain from WWTR1, it can activate the Hippo signaling pathway. The CAMTA1 part of the fusion protein leads to nuclear localization of the protein.[68] Although less well studied, it seems likely that the YAP1-TFE3 chimeric protein would also lead to activation of the Hippo signaling pathway.

ANGIOSARCOMA

DEFINITION, EPIDEMIOLOGY, AND CLINICAL FEATURES

Angiosarcomas are highly aggressive sarcomas affecting the cutis, deep soft tissue, bone, and viscera. Approximately 4% of all angiosarcomas arise primary in bone, Therefore, angiosarcoma of bone is rare. Angiosarcomas predominantly affect the long tubular bones (see Fig. 1) with a preference for the femur. In bone, 30% to 40% of angiosarcomas are multifocal.[21,69,70] Angiosarcomas are highly aggressive and predominantly occur in the seventh decade, with a male predominance. Angiosarcomas can be primary or arise secondary to radiation.[71] Angiosarcoma of bone should be treated with wide surgical resection, possibly with adjuvant radiation or chemotherapy. Virtually all patients die within a few years: the 1-year survival is 55% and the 5-year survival is 33%.[21,28] Radiologically, angiosarcoma presents as a well-defined, osteolytic lesion, with a geographic pattern of destruction.[70] Cortical destruction is found in 65% of cases. Because they are often multifocal, it is easily confused by radiologists with metastatic carcinoma. Macroscopically the tumors are hemorrhagic often with prominent necrosis.

HISTOLOGIC AND IMMUNOHISTOCHEMISTRY FEATURES

Microscopically ill-defined blood vessels lined by enlarged endothelial cells with hyperchromatic, pleomorphic nuclei are seen (Fig. 6A–C). In bone, greater than 90% of the angiosarcomas display epithelioid morphology.[20,21] In addition to the variable presence of vasoformative areas, often with multilayering, solid areas can be found. Mitoses are easily found, sometimes atypical forms.[6,21,28,72] Immunohistochemistry shows positivity for CD31 (95%–100%) (Fig. 6D), ERG (96%), VWF (60%–75%), CD34 (39%–40%), and smooth muscle actin (61%).[20,21,23,61] Keratin AE1AE3 is expressed in 69% to 80% of the angiosarcomas and in combination with a radiologic diagnosis of metastatic carcinoma and epithelioid morphology often causes misdiagnoses.[21] D2-40 is expressed in 31% of the angiosarcomas of bone and is associated with a worse outcome.[21] Likewise, loss of p16 is associated with a more aggressive clinical behavior.[73] In addition, the presence of a macronucleolus, 3 or more mitoses per 10 HPFs, and fewer than 5 eosinophilic granulocytes are associated with poor outcome.[21]

TUMORIGENESIS AND GENETICS

Many different genetic alterations have been described for the angiosarcomas. As reported by Verbeke and colleagues,[74] 2 groups of angiosarcomas could be identified: those with complex genetic profiles and a group with few gross genetic alterations. Inactivation of the p53 pathway is common in angiosarcoma. A study on angiosarcoma of the liver reported frequent events leading to inactivation of p53, where p14, p15 and p53 were analyzed for mutations and for methylation. In almost all cases, p53 was disabled due to promoter methylation or mutations in the aforementioned genes.[75,76] Antonescu and colleagues[77] described mutations in KDR in 7% restricted to breast angiosarcomas but later also reported a case in the lumbar spine. This mutation could lead to autophosphorylation, which would provide rationale for treatment with tyrosine kinase inhibitors. Furthermore, unsupervised clustering of gene expression profiles of angiosarcomas and other soft tissue sarcomas revealed that angiosarcomas cluster closely together, indicating they are a highly similar entity in their gene expression pattern even though the specific mutations per case can be different.[78] MYC amplifications are common events (55%–100%) in secondary angiosarcomas (after irradiation or chronic lymphedema).[79] Although MYC amplifications were first reported exclusively for secondary angiosarcomas, more recently they have been described in primary angiosarcoma cases as well as including angiosarcoma of bone.[74] Coamplification of FLT4 and additional mutations in PLCG1 and PTPRB can be found in secondary angiosarcoma.[71,80] Furthermore, Huang

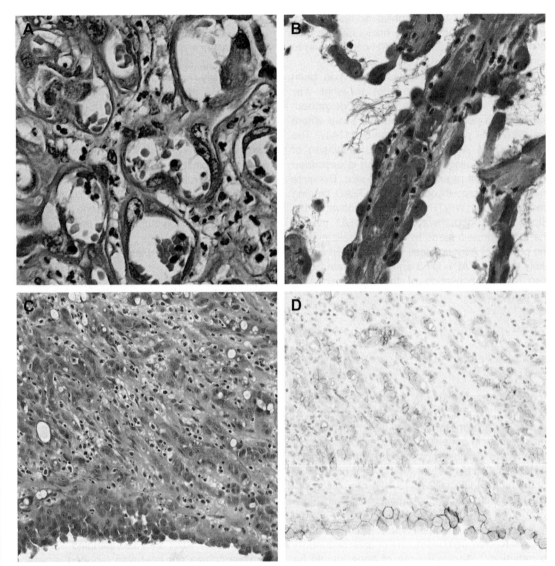

Fig. 6. Angiosarcoma of bone. (*A*) Angiosarcoma of bone showing high degree of nuclear atypia, often with prominent nucleoli (H&E). (*B*) Vessels are lined by epithelioid endothelial cells. Cells show nuclear atypia (H&E). (*C*) Diffuse growth can be seen and tumor cells can have cytoplasmic vacuoles (H&E). (*D*) Corresponding CD31 immunohistochemistry.

and colleagues[81] recently reported CIC abnormalities occurring in 9% of cases, affecting younger patients with primary angiosarcoma, with an inferior disease-free survival. Although alterations in these genes have not been described in angiosarcoma of bone, genetic information for angiosarcoma of bone is limited.

DISCUSSION

Vascular tumors consist of endothelial cells, often retaining the capacity to form vessels. Over time there has been much controversy surrounding the classification and naming of the various vascular tumors. But much of the confusion has been clarified with the discovery of a number of fusion genes and genetic alterations that point to distinct tumor entities.

Diagnosis of vascular tumors can be challenging because they are often similar in appearance but require different therapeutic approaches. Moreover, the epithelioid variants can show high keratin expression, leading to confusion with metastatic carcinoma.

Pitfalls

! Because radiologically vascular tumors in bone often present as multiple lytic lesions, raising suspicion of metastatic carcinoma or multiple myeloma, pathologists can easily misdiagnose a vascular tumor of bone for metastatic carcinoma, especially because most vascular lesions in bone are epithelioid and express keratin.

! Vascular tumors can include areas of hemorrhage with sometimes extensive intravascular papillary endothelial hyperplasia (Masson tumor), which can mimic angiosarcoma.

! The presence of intratumoral reactive woven bone and infiltration of osteoclast-like giant cells in pseudomyogenic hemangioendothelioma primary presenting in bone can cause confusion with osteoblastoma or giant cell tumor of bone

REFERENCES

1. Lamerato-Kozicki AR, Helm KM, Jubala CM, et al. Canine hemangiosarcoma originates from hematopoietic precursors with potential for endothelial differentiation. Exp Hematol 2006;34(7):870–8.
2. Kakiuchi-Kiyota S, Crabbs TA, Arnold LL, et al. Evaluation of expression profiles of hematopoietic stem cell, endothelial cell, and myeloid cell antigens in spontaneous and chemically induced hemangiosarcomas and hemangiomas in mice. Toxicol Pathol 2013;41(5):709–21.
3. Yoder MC, Ingram DA. Endothelial progenitor cell: ongoing controversy for defining these cells and their role in neoangiogenesis in the murine system. Curr Opin Hematol 2009;16(4):269–73.
4. Kovacic JC, Moore J, Herbert A, et al. Endothelial progenitor cells, angioblasts, and angiogenesis–old terms reconsidered from a current perspective. Trends Cardiovasc Med 2008;18(2):45–51.
5. Wenger DE, Wold LE. Benign vascular lesions of bone: radiologic and pathologic features. Skeletal Radiol 2000;29(2):63–74.
6. Wenger DE, Wold LE. Malignant vascular lesions of bone: radiologic and pathologic features. Skeletal Radiol 2000;29(11):619–31.
7. Bruder E, Perez-Atayde AR, Jundt G, et al. Vascular lesions of bone in children, adolescents, and young adults. A clinicopathologic reappraisal and application of the ISSVA classification. Virchows Arch 2009; 454(2):161–79.
8. Fletcher CDM, Bridge JA, Hogendoorn P, et al. Vascular tumours. Lyon (France): IARC; 2013.
9. Verbeke SLJ, Bovée JVMG. Primary vascular tumors of bone: a spectrum of entities? Int J Clin Exp Pathol 2011;4(6):541–51.
10. Volpe R, Mazabraud A. Hemangioendothelioma (angiosarcoma) of bone: a distinct pathologic entity with an unpredictable course? Cancer 1982;49(4): 727–36.
11. Nielsen GP, Srivastava A, Kattapuram S, et al. Epithelioid hemangioma of bone revisited: a study of 50 cases. Am J Surg Pathol 2009;33(2):270–7.
12. van IJzendoorn DGP, de Jong D, Romagosa C, et al. Fusion events lead to truncation of FOS in epithelioid hemangioma of bone. Genes Chromosomes Cancer 2015;54(9):565–74.
13. Huang SC, Zhang L, Sung YS, et al. Frequent FOS gene rearrangements in epithelioid hemangioma: a molecular study of 58 cases with morphologic reappraisal. Am J Surg Pathol 2015;39(10):1313–21.
14. Antonescu CR, Chen HW, Zhang L, et al. ZFP36-FOSB fusion defines a subset of epithelioid hemangioma with atypical features. Genes Chromosomes Cancer 2014;53(11):951–9.
15. Walter JW, North PE, Waner M, et al. Somatic mutation of vascular endothelial growth factor receptors in juvenile hemangioma. Genes Chromosomes Cancer 2002;33(3):295–303.
16. Hornick JL, Fletcher CDM. Pseudomyogenic hemangioendothelioma: a distinctive, often multicentric tumor with indolent behavior. Am J Surg Pathol 2011;35(2):190–201.
17. Inyang A, Mertens F, Puls F, et al. Primary pseudomyogenic hemangioendothelioma of bone. Am J Surg Pathol 2016;40(5):587–98.
18. Machado I, Mayordomo-Aranda E, Scotlandi K, et al. Immunoreactivity using anti-ERG monoclonal antibodies in sarcomas is influenced by clone selection. Pathol Res Pract 2014;210(8):508–13.
19. Perner S, Mosquera JM, Demichelis F, et al. TMPRSS2-ERG fusion prostate cancer: an early molecular event associated with invasion. Am J Surg Pathol 2007;31(6):882–8.
20. Deshpande V, Rosenberg AE, O'Connell JX, et al. Epithelioid angiosarcoma of the bone: a series of 10 cases. Am J Surg Pathol 2003;27(6):709–16.
21. Verbeke SLJ, Bertoni F, Bacchini P, et al. Distinct histological features characterize primary angiosarcoma of bone. Histopathology 2011;58(2):254–64.
22. Barak S, Wang Z, Miettinen M. Immunoreactivity for calretinin and keratins in desmoid fibromatosis and other myofibroblastic tumors: a diagnostic pitfall. Am J Surg Pathol 2012;36(9):1404–9.
23. Miettinen M, Wang ZF, Paetau A, et al. ERG transcription factor as an immunohistochemical marker for vascular endothelial tumors and prostatic carcinoma. Am J Surg Pathol 2011;35(3):432–41.

24. Mirra JM, Gold RH, Marcove RC. Bone tumors, diagnosis and treatment: diagnosis and treatment. Philadelphia: Lippincott Williams & Wilkins; 1980.

25. Picci P, Manfrini M, Fabbri N, et al. Atlas of musculoskeletal tumors and tumorlike lesions: the rizzoli case archive. Springer Science & Business Media; 2014.

26. Kaleem Z, Kyriakos M, Totty WG. Solitary skeletal hemangioma of the extremities. Skeletal Radiol 2000;29(9):502–13.

27. López-Barea F, Hardisson D, Rodríguez-Peralto JL, et al. Intracortical hemangioma of bone. Report of two cases and review of the literature. J Bone Joint Surg Am 1998;80(11):1673–8.

28. O'Connell JX, Nielsen GP, Rosenberg AE. Epithelioid vascular tumors of bone: a review and proposal of a classification scheme. Adv Anat Pathol 2001;8(2):74–82.

29. O'Connell JX, Kattapuram SV, Mankin HJ, et al. Epithelioid hemangioma of bone. A tumor often mistaken for low-grade angiosarcoma or malignant hemangioendothelioma. Am J Surg Pathol 1993;17(6):610–7.

30. Keel SB, Rosenberg AE. Hemorrhagic epithelioid and spindle cell hemangioma: a newly recognized, unique vascular tumor of bone. Cancer 1999;85(9):1966–72.

31. Mridha AR, Kinra P, Sable M, et al. Epithelioid hemangioma of distal femoral epiphysis in a patient with congenital talipes equinovarus. Malays J Pathol 2014;36(1):63–6.

32. Boyaci B, Hornicek FJ, Nielsen GP, et al. Epithelioid hemangioma of the spine: a case series of six patients and review of the literature. Spine J 2013;13(12):e7–13.

33. Calderaro J, Guedj N, Dauzac C, et al. A case of epithelioid hemangioma of the spine. Ann Pathol 2011;31(4):312–5, [in French].

34. Weaver SM, Kumar AB. Epithelioid hemangioma of the spine: an uncommon cause of spinal cord compression. Acta Neurol Belg 2015;115(4):843–5.

35. Akgun B, Ozturk S, Ucer O, et al. Epithelioid hemangioma of the thoracic spine. Neurol India 2015;63(4):610–1.

36. McEachren TM, Brownstein S, Jordan DR, et al. Epithelioid hemangioma of the orbit. Ophthalmology 2000;107(4):806–10.

37. Budimir I, Demirović A, Iveković R, et al. Epithelioid hemangioma of the orbit: case report. Acta Clin Croat 2015;54(1):92–5.

38. Sánchez-Orgaz M, Insausti-García A, Gregorio LY, et al. Epithelioid hemangioma of the orbit or angiolymphoid hyperplasia with eosinophilia. Ophthal Plast Reconstr Surg 2014;30(3):e70–2.

39. Alder B, Proia A, Liss J. Distinct, bilateral epithelioid hemangioma of the orbit. Orbit 2013;32(1):51–3.

40. Fernandes BF, Al-Mujaini A, Petrogiannis-Haliotis T, et al. Epithelioid hemangioma (angiolymphoid hyperplasia with eosinophilia) of the orbit: a case report. J Med Case Rep 2007;1:30.

41. Baili L, Cheour M, Hachicha F, et al. Orbital epithelioid hemangioma: a case report. J Fr Ophtalmol 2014;37(9):e133–6, [in French].

42. Svajdler M, Bohus P, Baumöhlová H, et al. Epithelioid hemangioma of the foot. Cesk Patol 2006;42(2):86–90, [in Slovak].

43. Luna JTP, DeGroot H 3rd. Five-year follow-up of structural allograft reconstruction for epithelioid hemangioma of the talus and navicular: a case report and review of the literature. Foot Ankle Int 2007;28(3):379–84.

44. Werhahn C, Lang M, Merkel KH, et al. Epithelioid hemangioma–a rare tumor of the hand. Handchir Mikrochir Plast Chir 1990;22(4):214–8, [in German].

45. El Harroudi T, Moumen M, Tijami F, et al. Giant epithelioid hemangioma of the hand. Chir Main 2008;27(5):240–2, [in French].

46. Sirikulchayanonta V, Jinawath A, Jaovisidha S. Epithelioid hemangioma involving three contiguous bones: a case report with a review of the literature. Korean J Radiol 2010;11(6):692–6.

47. Zhou Q, Lu L, Fu Y, et al. Epithelioid hemangioma of bone: a report of two special cases and a literature review. Skeletal Radiol 2016;45(12):1723–7.

48. Eferl R, Wagner EF. AP-1: a double-edged sword in tumorigenesis. Nat Rev Cancer 2003;3(11):859–68.

49. Mirra JM, Kessler S, Bhuta S, et al. The fibroma-like variant of epithelioid sarcoma. A fibrohistiocytic/myoid cell lesion often confused with benign and malignant spindle cell tumors. Cancer 1992;69(6):1382–95.

50. Billings SD, Folpe AL, Weiss SW. Epithelioid sarcoma-like hemangioendothelioma. Am J Surg Pathol 2003;27(1):48–57.

51. Hung YP, Fletcher CDM, Hornick JL. FOSB is a useful diagnostic marker for pseudomyogenic hemangioendothelioma. Am J Surg Pathol 2017;41(5):596–606.

52. Sugita S, Hirano H, Kikuchi N, et al. Diagnostic utility of FOSB immunohistochemistry in pseudomyogenic hemangioendothelioma and its histological mimics. Diagn Pathol 2016;11(1):75.

53. Trombetta D, Magnusson L, von Steyern FV, et al. Translocation t(7;19)(q22;q13)–a recurrent chromosome aberration in pseudomyogenic hemangioendothelioma? Cancer Genet 2011;204(4):211–5.

54. Walther C, Tayebwa J, Lilljebjörn H, et al. A novel SERPINE1-FOSB fusion gene results in transcriptional up-regulation of FOSB in pseudomyogenic haemangioendothelioma. J Pathol 2014;232(5):534–40.

55. Deyrup AT, Tighiouart M, Montag AG, et al. Epithelioid hemangioendothelioma of soft tissue: a proposal for risk stratification based on 49 cases. Am J Surg Pathol 2008;32(6):924–7.

56. Thomas A. Vascular tumors of bone: pathological and clinical study of 27 cases. Surg Gynec Obstet 1942;74:777–95.

57. Stout AP. Hemangio-endothelioma: a tumor of blood vessels featuring vascular endothelial cells. Ann Surg 1943;118(3):445–64.

58. Weiss SW, Enzinger FM. Epithelioid hemangioendothelioma: a vascular tumor often mistaken for a carcinoma. Cancer 1982;50(5):970–81.

59. Campanacci M, Boriani S, Giunti A. Hemangioendothelioma of bone: a study of 29 cases. Cancer 1980; 46(4):804–14.

60. Gill R, O'Donnell RJ, Horvai A. Utility of immunohistochemistry for endothelial markers in distinguishing epithelioid hemangioendothelioma from carcinoma metastatic to bone. Arch Pathol Lab Med 2009; 133(6):967–72.

61. Miettinen M, Rikala MS, Rys J, et al. Vascular endothelial growth factor receptor 2 as a marker for malignant vascular tumors and mesothelioma: an immunohistochemical study of 262 vascular endothelial and 1640 nonvascular tumors. Am J Surg Pathol 2012;36(4): 629–39.

62. Shibuya R, Matsuyama A, Shiba E, et al. CAMTA1 is a useful immunohistochemical marker for diagnosing epithelioid haemangioendothelioma. Histopathology 2015;67(6):827–35.

63. Doyle LA, Fletcher CDM, Hornick JL. Nuclear expression of CAMTA1 distinguishes epithelioid hemangioendothelioma from histologic mimics. Am J Surg Pathol 2016;40(1):94–102.

64. Flucke U, Vogels RJC, de Saint Aubain Somerhausen N, et al. Epithelioid Hemangioendothelioma: clinicopathologic, immunhistochemical, and molecular genetic analysis of 39 cases. Diagn Pathol 2014;9:131.

65. Errani C, Zhang L, Sung YS, et al. A novel WWTR1-CAMTA1 gene fusion is a consistent abnormality in epithelioid hemangioendothelioma of different anatomic sites. Genes Chromosomes Cancer 2011;50(8):644–53.

66. Tanas MR, Sboner A, Oliveira AM, et al. Identification of a disease-defining gene fusion in epithelioid hemangioendothelioma. Sci Transl Med 2011;3(98): 98ra82.

67. Antonescu CR, Le Loarer F, Mosquera JM, et al. Novel YAP1-TFE3 fusion defines a distinct subset of epithelioid hemangioendothelioma. Genes Chromosomes Cancer 2013;52(8):775–84.

68. Patel NR, Salim AA, Sayeed H, et al. Molecular characterization of epithelioid haemangioendotheliomas identifies novel WWTR1-CAMTA1 fusion variants. Histopathology 2015;67(5):699–708.

69. Young RJ, Brown NJ, Reed MW, et al. Angiosarcoma. Lancet Oncol 2010;11(10):983–91.

70. Vermaat M, Vanel D, Kroon HM, et al. Vascular tumors of bone: imaging findings. Eur J Radiol 2011; 77(1):13–8.

71. Mentzel T, Schildhaus HU, Palmedo G, et al. Postradiation cutaneous angiosarcoma after treatment of breast carcinoma is characterized by MYC amplification in contrast to atypical vascular lesions after radiotherapy and control cases: clinicopathological, immunohistochemical and molecular analysis of 66 cases. Mod Pathol 2012;25(1):75–85.

72. Evans HL, Raymond AK, Ayala AG. Vascular tumors of bone: a study of 17 cases other than ordinary hemangioma, with an evaluation of the relationship of hemangioendothelioma of bone to epithelioid hemangioma, epithelioid hemangioendothelioma, and high-grade angiosarcoma. Hum Pathol 2003; 34(7):680–9.

73. Verbeke SLJ, Bertoni F, Bacchini P, et al. Active TGF-β signaling and decreased expression of PTEN separates angiosarcoma of bone from its soft tissue counterpart. Mod Pathol 2013;26(9):1211–21.

74. Verbeke SLJ, de Jong D, Bertoni F, et al. Array CGH analysis identifies two distinct subgroups of primary angiosarcoma of bone. Genes Chromosomes Cancer 2015;54(2):72–81.

75. Weihrauch M, Markwarth A, Lehnert G, et al. Abnormalities of the ARF-p53 pathway in primary angiosarcomas of the liver. Hum Pathol 2002;33(9):884–92.

76. Garcia JM, Gonzalez R, Silva JM, et al. Mutational status of K-ras and TP53 genes in primary sarcomas of the heart. Br J Cancer 2000;82(6):1183–5.

77. Antonescu CR, Yoshida A, Guo T, et al. KDR activating mutations in human angiosarcomas are sensitive to specific kinase inhibitors. Cancer Res 2009;69(18):7175–9.

78. Segal NH, Pavlidis P, Antonescu CR, et al. Classification and subtype prediction of adult soft tissue sarcoma by functional genomics. Am J Pathol 2003;163(2):691–700.

79. Manner J, Radlwimmer B, Hohenberger P, et al. MYC high level gene amplification is a distinctive feature of angiosarcomas after irradiation or chronic lymphedema. Am J Pathol 2010;176(1):34–9.

80. Behjati S, Tarpey PS, Sheldon H, et al. Recurrent PTPRB and PLCG1 mutations in angiosarcoma. Nat Genet 2014;46(4):376–9.

81. Huang SC, Zhang L, Sung YS, et al. Recurrent CIC gene abnormalities in angiosarcomas: a molecular study of 120 cases with concurrent investigation of PLCG1, KDR, MYC, and FLT4 gene alterations. Am J Surg Pathol 2016;40(5):645–55.

Notochordal Tumors
An Update on Molecular Pathology with Therapeutic Implications

Takehiko Yamaguchi, MD, PhD[a],*, Hiroki Imada, MD[a],
Shun Iida, MD[a], Karoly Szuhai, MD, PhD[b]

KEYWORDS

- Notochordal tumor • Chordoma • Benign notochordal cell tumor (BNCT) • Molecular pathology
- Targeted therapy • Brachyury (T) • EGFR • PDGFR

Key points

- Benign notochordal cell tumor is a recently introduced benign counterpart of chordoma and may be a precursor of it. Their morphologic features overlap and it is sometimes difficult to differentiate them microscopically, particularly on small biopsies.

- From recent advances in molecular studies applied on chordoma samples it became clear that chordomas commonly express various receptor tyrosine kinases (RTKs) and activated signal transduction molecules and thereby may respond to RTK inhibitors.

- The transcription factor brachyury is essential in notochord differentiation and a germline duplication of the brachyury gene is often seen in familial chordoma.

- Chordomas often show epidermal growth factor receptor (EGFR) gene copy number variation and overexpression of EGFR activating downstream signaling pathways. EGFR is one of the major potential therapeutic targets of chordoma.

- Platelet-derivered growth factor-alpha (PDGFRA) and platelet-derivered growth factor-beta (PDGFRB) are highly expressed and phosphorylated in chordomas and this suggests the use of PDGFR inhibitors in chordoma.

ABSTRACT

Recent molecular investigations of chordoma show common expression of various receptor tyrosine kinases and activation of downstream signaling pathways contributing to tumor growth and progression. The transcription factor brachyury (also known as T) is important in notochord differentiation, and germline duplication of the gene is often found in familial chordomas. Nuclear expression of brachyury is consistent in chordoma and in benign notochordal cell tumor. Based on the molecular evidence, targeting of several kinds of molecular agents has been attempted for the treatment of uncontrolled chordomas and achieved partial response or stable condition in many cases.

OVERVIEW

The World Health Organization (WHO) classification of bone tumors published in 2013 introduced a new entity of benign notochordal cell tumor (BNCT), which is regarded as a benign counterpart of chordoma.[1] Nowadays, notochordal tumors consist of 2 entities: BNCT and chordoma. It has been shown that at least some of the BNCTs are precursors of chordoma[2–5] (**Fig. 1**), although many textbooks and articles still state that

---

Disclosure Statement: The authors have nothing to disclose.
[a] Department of Pathology, Koshigaya Hospital, Dokkyo Medical University, 2-1-50 Minami-Koshigaya, Koshigaya, Saitama 343-8555, Japan; [b] Department of Molecular Cell Biology, Leiden University Medical Center, PO Box: 9600, Post Zone: R-01-P, Leiden 2300 RC, The Netherlands
* Corresponding author.
E-mail address: takehiko@dokkyomed.ac.jp

Surgical Pathology 10 (2017) 637–656
http://dx.doi.org/10.1016/j.path.2017.04.008
1875-9181/17/© 2017 Elsevier Inc. All rights reserved.

surgpath.theclinics.com

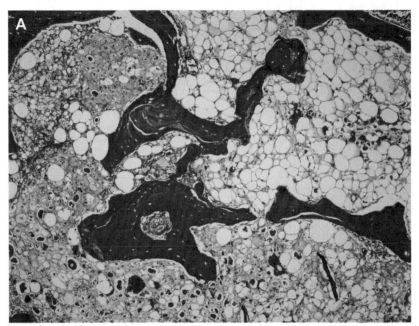

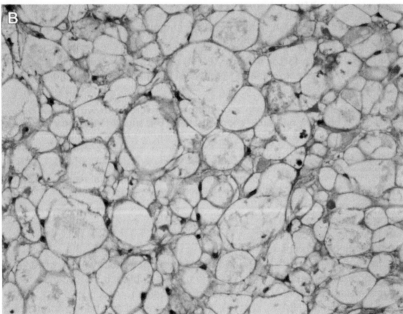

Fig. 1. BNCT. (A) BNCT consists of solid sheets of adipocytelike vacuolated and eosinophilic tumor cells without intercellular myxoid matrix. The affected bone trabeculae are preserved and show some appositional bone formation representing osteosclerosis (hematoxylin-eosin [H&E] staining, original magnification ×100). (B) Higher-power view reveals proliferation of adipocytelike vacuolated tumor cells with small bland nuclei. No intercellular myxoid matrix is evident (H&E staining, original magnification ×400).

chordoma develops in a notochordal rest. Jaffe[6] states that vertebral chordomas seem to occur in bone in spite of notochordal rests being much more frequently located within the intervertebral disk than in the vertebral body, so it is difficult to believe that chordoma arises in notochordal rests. Moreover, it is impossible to explain why chordoma periphericum develops in the extra-axial location based on the traditional theory.[7,8]

Therefore, it is reasonable that chordoma may develop through BNCT or directly (de novo) from stem cells with notochordal differentiation.[9] To compare genomic aberrations of chordoma and BNCT would be the best and easiest way to unravel the molecular mechanisms of malignant transformation from BNCT to chordoma. However, BNCT has not been investigated enough on a molecular basis because it is most often diagnosed purely based on radiological imaging without histology, and surgical treatment is not necessary.

BENIGN NOTOCHORDAL CELL TUMOR

BNCT was initially introduced in 2004[10,11] and subsequently recognized in the WHO classification of bone tumors in 2013.[1] It is a benign bone tumor composed of benign notochordal cells and may be a precursor of chordoma. Ecchordosis physaliphora spheno-occipitalis is another benign notochordal cell lesion. It is a polypoid lesion found on the clivus and is considered to be an extraosseous counterpart of BNCT.[1] BNCTs detected clinically are often found in the cervical and lumbar vertebrae; however, smaller lesions are also found in the sacrum, coccyx, and clivus at autopsy.[10,12] Most lesions are incidentally found on imaging examinations because they are usually asymptomatic.[12] Radiographs often fail to show any abnormality but occasionally reveal mild osteosclerosis. Computed tomography (CT) scan shows an intraosseous sclerotic lesion without extraosseous tumor extension. Magnetic resonance imaging (MRI) reveals homogeneously low signal intensity on T1-weighted imaging (T1-WI), homogeneously high signal intensity on T2-weighted imaging (T2-WI), and no contrast enhancement on gadolinium (Gd)-enhanced T1-WI.

GROSS FEATURES

The cut-surfaces of BNCT disclose an unencapsulated and well-demarcated tumor with a bright tan, glossy texture. No lobular structure is recognized.

MICROSCOPIC FEATURES

BNCTs are unencapsulated and consist of solid sheets of adipocytelike vacuolated and eosinophilic tumor cells with bland nuclei (see **Fig. 1**). Mitotic figures are rarely seen. The lesions lack intercellular myxoid matrix, although some cystic spaces filled with colloidlike material can be seen. The involved bone trabeculae are mildly, occasionally markedly, sclerotic. Bone marrow islands may be seen within the lesion. BNCTs never show a lobular configuration or formation of fibrous septa. The tumor cells are immunohistochemically positive for brachyury, epithelial markers, vimentin, and S-100 protein.

DIFFERENTIAL DIAGNOSIS

The radiological differential diagnosis includes sclerotic vertebral lesions, including enostosis (bone island), hemangioma, intraosseous hibernoma, and metastasis (**Table 1**).[13] The histologic differential diagnosis between BNCT and chordoma is important and is described later. The tumor cells might be overlooked as fatty bone marrow on biopsy examination because they are reminiscent of mature fat cells.

PROGNOSIS

Prognosis is excellent and the lesions do not require any surgical intervention because it is very indolent except for the risk of malignant transformation. It is necessary to follow up patients with BNCT with imaging, although the risk of malignant transformation to chordoma is considered to be extremely low.

CHORDOMA

Chordoma is a rare, slow-growing, malignant bone tumor showing notochordal differentiation. Usually, malignant mesenchymal tumors are called malignant XX-oma or XX-sarcoma; however, chordoma suggests malignancy with neither prefix nor postfix because a benign counterpart had not been recognized until BNCT was proposed as such in 2004. Most chordomas are conventional chordomas and there are 2 rare subtypes: chondroid and dedifferentiated chordomas. Conventional and chondroid chordomas are classified as grade II and dedifferentiated chordoma grade III in a 3-tier system.[14] Most of the chordomas develop after the fourth decade of life, with a peak incidence in the fifth decade, but rarely occur in children, young adults, and even in infants. Chordomas have a predilection for affecting the axial skeleton, particularly in the sacrum/coccyx and clivus, followed by mobile spine.[1,6,15] Very occasionally, chordomas develop on the surface of the vertebrae and in extraosseous locations.[8,16] Radiographs reveal osteolytic bone destruction. CT shows a destructive bone tumor with extraosseous tumor formation. MRI reveals low signal intensity on T1-WI, heterogeneously high signal intensity on T2-WI, and marginal or entire enhancement on Gd-enhanced T1-WI.

GROSS FEATURES

Almost all chordomas develop within bone and are associated with a huge extraosseous tumor mass. Chordomas with a smaller soft tissue mass more often have been found recently because of improved resolution of MRI. The tumor is well demarcated and encapsulated with a thin fibrous capsule. The cut surface shows a well-demarcated gelatinous tumor with lobular configuration. Dedifferentiated

Table 1
Differential diagnosis between spinal tumors showing osteosclerosis

	Bone Island	Hemangioma	BNCT	Hibernoma	Fibrous Dysplasia
Radiograph	Dense sclerosis with spokelike pattern	Osteolysis/sclerosis	Normal to mild osteosclerosis	Normal to mild osteosclerosis	Ground glass/osteolysis
CT Scan	Osteosclerosis	Polka dot sign	Osteosclerosis	Osteosclerosis	Ground glass
MRI T1-WI	Low	Intermediate/high	Low	Low	Low/intermediate
T2-WI	Low	High	High	High	Low/intermediate
Gd-enhanced T1-WI	–	+	–	+	+
Bone Scan/FDG-PET	Negative	Negative/positive	Negative	Positive	Positive
Histology	Compact bone with spokelike pattern	Proliferation of blood vessels with intervening fatty marrow Sclerotic trabecular bone	Solid sheets of adipocytelike and/or eosinophilic tumor cells Sclerotic trabecular bone	Solid sheets of multivacuolated brown fat cells Sclerotic trabecular bone	Irregular-shaped woven bone trabeculae within a bland fibrous background
Immunohistochemistry	NP	CD31, CD34	Brachyury, vimentin, epithelial markers, S-100 protein	UCP1	NP
Molecular	NDY	NDY	NDY	Breakpoint in 11q	GNAS gene mutation

Abbreviations: CD, cluster of differentiation; FDG, fluorodeoxyglucose; Gd, gadolinium; GNAS, guanine nucleotide binding protein (G protein), alpha stimulating activity polypeptide; NDY, not detected yet; NP, not specific; UCP, uncoupling protein; WI, weight imaging.

chordoma is associated with a nonmyxoid tumor component with a fairly sharp margin.

MICROSCOPIC FEATURES

Chordoma is an encapsulated lobular tumor composed of solid sheets and/or cords of epithelioid vacuolated tumor cells with a varying amount of intercellular myxoid matrix (Fig. 2A, B). Each lobule is separated by thin fibrous septum. The tumor cells show clear to eosinophilic cytoplasm. Nuclear atypia and pleomorphism vary from mild to severe between cases. The affected bone is usually destroyed and tumors may extend into the adjacent bone structure. Well-differentiated chordoma mimics BNCT (see Fig. 2C). Poorly differentiated chordoma looks like pleomorphic spindle cell sarcoma but the tumor cells show signs of notochordal differentiation (see Fig. 2D). Chondroid chordoma that has a predilection for the base of the skull shows chondrosarcoma-like components in addition to classic chordoma morphology. Dedifferentiated chordoma consists of 2 components: classic chordoma and

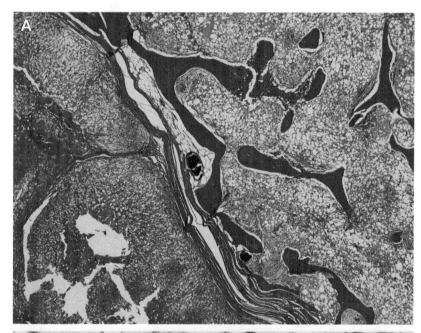
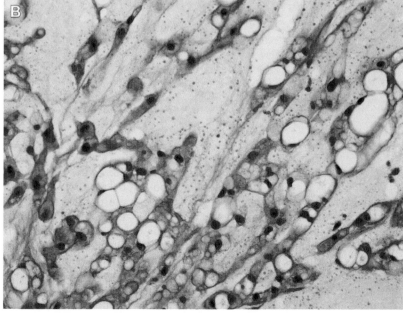

Fig. 2. Chordoma. (A) Chordoma consists of lobules of eosinophilic and/or clear tumor cells, separated by thin fibrous septa with vasculature (H&E staining, original magnification ×20). (B) Higher-power view reveals proliferation of eosinophilic, epithelioid tumor cells with intracytoplasmic vacuoles, forming solid sheets and/or cords, associated with a rich myxoid background (H&E staining, original magnification ×200).

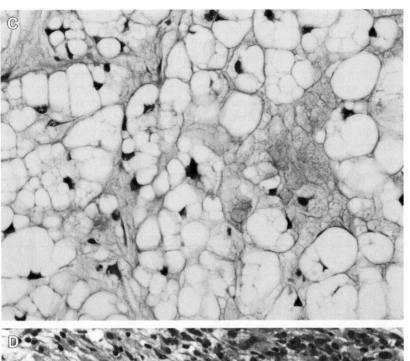

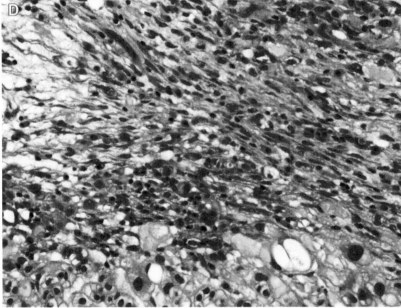

Fig. 2. (*continued*). (*C*) Well-differentiated chordoma consists of solid sheets of adipocytelike tumor cells, mimicking BNCT; however, myxoid matrix is present between tumor cells and nuclei are much more atypical (H&E staining, original magnification ×400). (*D*) Poorly differentiated chordoma shows proliferation of spindle-shaped tumor cells with pleomorphic nuclei, associated with occasional vacuolated tumor cells suggestive of notochordal differentiation (H&E staining, original magnification ×200).

high-grade sarcoma without notochordal differentiation (Fig. 3A). The border between 2 components is usually well demarcated. A recent study showed microskip metastasis, meaning that small tumor islands were seen around a mainly encapsulated tumor, which may reflect a higher recurrence rate (Akiyama T, Ogura K, Gokita T, et al. An analysis of the infiltrative features of chordoma: the relationship between micro-skip metastasis and postoperative outcomes, under submission). Immunohistochemically, the tumor cells of conventional and chondroid chordomas are positive for brachyury, vimentin, S-100 protein, and epithelial markers including pancytokeratins and epithelial membrane antigen (EMA). Dedifferentiated tumor cells in dedifferentiated chordoma may lack positive reaction for brachyury (see Fig. 3B). Careful observation of surgical specimens may detect a coexistent BNCT component adjacent to chordoma (Fig. 4).

Fig. 3. Dedifferentiated chordoma. (*A*) Dedifferentiated chordoma consists of classic chordoma and nonchordoma components. The former are composed of physaliferous cells and the latter show fascicular proliferation of undifferentiated spindle-shaped tumor cells (H&E staining, original magnification ×100). (*B*) Immunohistochemically, spindle-shaped tumor cells in the dedifferentiated component are negative for brachyury, whereas conventional chordoma cells show nuclear positivity for brachyury (En Vision: Agilent Technologies, Santa Clara, brachyury: SC-20109, Santa Cruz Biotechnology, Dallas, original magnification ×100).

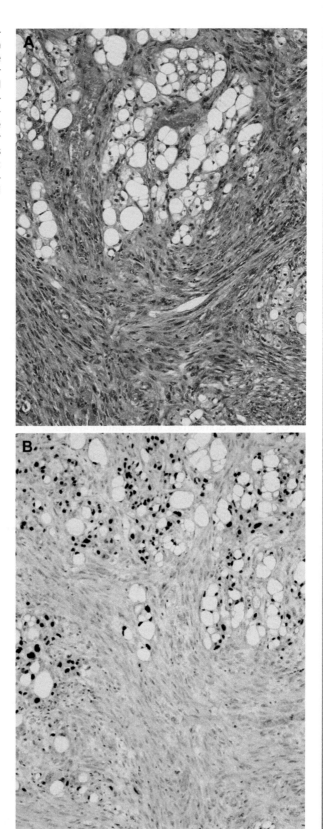

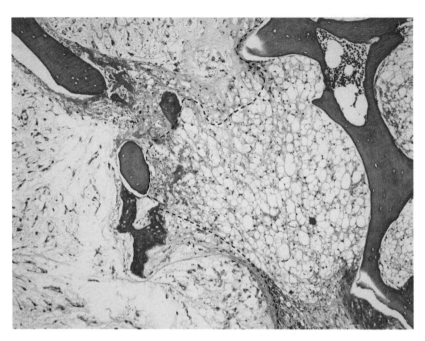

Fig. 4. Chordoma associated with BNCT. Histologic findings of chordooma (*left*) and coexistent BNCT (*right*). It is considered that chordoma can arise from BNCT. Blue dotted line indicates the interface between chordoma and BNCT (H&E staining, original magnification ×40).

DIFFERENTIAL DIAGNOSIS

The differential diagnosis between chordoma and BNCT is vital. Sometimes it is a daunting task, particularly on biopsy specimens, because histologic findings of well-differentiated chordoma are similar to those of BNCT, with an overlapping immunohistochemical profile (Table 2). Chordoma may show a histologic spectrum ranging from BNCT-like components to typical chordoma features. In addition, chordomas show fine fibrous capsules and/or septa with vasculature (see Fig. 2A, B), lobular configuration, intercellular myxoid matrix, and bone destruction. The border of chordoma to bone marrow cells of host bone seems very smooth because of a thin fibrous membrane existed (Fig. 5A). In contrast, the border of BNCT seems slightly zigzag along the contour of adjacent marrow adipocytes because of a lack of intervening fibrous membrane (see Fig. 5B).

The differential diagnosis also includes chondrosarcoma, myoepithelioma/myoepithelial carcinoma, chordoid meningioma, and metastatic carcinoma.[17,18] Distinguishing chordoma from chondrosarcoma is often difficult on small biopsies, particularly from the skull base. For the diagnosis of chondroid chordoma it is important to consider its morphologic mimicker, chondrosarcoma with myxoid matrix. Immunohistochemistry is helpful in differentiating them because chondrosarcomas are negative for epithelial markers and brachyury. Myoepithelial tumors, formerly called parachordoma, may mimic chordoma morphologically.[17] Immunohistochemically, myoepithelial tumors show a positive reaction for calponin, smooth muscle actin, GFAP, and p63, whereas they are consistently negative for brachyury. Cytogenetically, myoepithelial tumors developing outside the salivary glands commonly possess *EWSR1* gene rearrangement. Chordoid meningioma is one of the greatest differential diagnostic challenges for intracranial tumors. Chordoid meningioma often shows more typical meningioma histology in addition to chordoid components and is immunohistochemically negative for brachyury.[18] Metastatic mucinous adenocarcinoma, clear cell renal carcinoma, and hepatocellular carcinoma can mimic chordoma radiographically and/or microscopically. Immunohistochemical studies are helpful because carcinomas are negative for brachyury. In addition, mucinous adenocarcinoma may be positive for CDX2, whereas clear cell renal cell carcinoma is positive for CD10 and PAX8, and hepatocellular carcinoma is positive for AFP, HepPar1, and CEA, and negative for CK19 and EMA.

PROGNOSIS

Chordoma has been primarily managed by surgery for a long time. However, chordoma recurrence rate is high at locations where surgical excision with sufficient tumor-free margins is not possible, which directly affects the long-term survival rate of these patients. Next to local

Table 2
Clinicopathologic aspects of benign notochordal cell tumor and chordoma

	BNCT	Chordoma
Location	Cervical and lumbar spine (clinical cases)	Sacrum/coccyx and clivus >> cervical spine
Symptom	Asymptomatic or mild pain	Pain and neurologic deficits
Radiograph	Normal to mild osteosclerosis	Osteolysis/bone destruction
CT Scan	Osteosclerosis without extraosseous tumor extension	Bone destruction with extraosseous tumor formation
MRI	No extraosseous tumor mass T1-WI: homogeneously low signal T2-WI: homogeneously high signal Gd-enhanced T1-WI: not contrasted	Extraosseous tumor mass T1-WI: low signal T2-WI: heterogeneously high signal Gd-enhanced T1-WI: contrasted marginally or entirely
Bone Scan	Negative uptake	Positive uptake
Histology	No lobular configuration, no fibrous capsule Solid sheets of eosinophilic vacuolated tumor cells Bland nuclei, no mitotic figures No intercellular myxoid matrix Sclerotic reaction of involved bone trabeculae	Lobular configuration with thin fibrous capsule and septa Solid sheets or cords of clear to eosinophilic tumor cells with vacuolation Nuclear atypia in varying degree, mitotic figures Varying amounts of intercellular myxoid matrix Bone destruction
Immunohistochemistry	Brachyury, vimentin, epithelial markers, S-100 protein	Brachyury, vimentin, epithelial markers, S-100 protein
Treatment	Follow-up observation with MRI	Surgical excision, carbon ion, proton
Prognosis	Excellent, rare malignant transformation to chordoma	Poor, high local recurrent rate and distant metastasis in late clinical course

recurrence, metastasis to the lung, bone, lymph nodes, and skin occurs in 5% to 43% of patients.[15,19] The median overall survival is 4 to 7 years and the 10-year survival rate ranges from 40% to 60%. There is no significant difference in overall survival between patients with chondroid chordoma and conventional chordoma. Dedifferentiated chordoma is lethal, with systemic spread occurring in approximately 90% of cases. Traditional chemotherapy has not been effective so far, although adjuvant therapy is required. Instead of chemotherapy, proton therapy has been primarily applied in combination with surgery.[20] Carbon-ion radiation therapy has taken over from proton therapy to treat unresectable chordomas in some countries.[21–23] The 5-year local control, overall survival, and disease-free rates of carbon-ion radiation therapy are 77.2%, 81.1%, and 50.3%, respectively.[24] Despite the satisfying results, radiation therapy is not able to prevent distant metastasis even though it is effective in controlling local disease. As molecular analysis of chordoma has been

developed, potential new molecular targets have been discovered.

MOLECULAR PATHOLOGY AND THERAPEUTIC TARGETS OF CHORDOMA

Some reports of chordoma in children with tuberous sclerosis complex (TSC) suggested the possible involvement of receptor tyrosine kinases (RTKs) and their downstream pathways.[25–28] In TSC, mutations of TSC1 or TSC2 genes have been described, located on chromosomes 9q34 and 16p13, respectively. Inactivation of the wild-type allele in TSC-associated tumors by loss of heterozygosity have been shown, indicating a pivotal role of TSC-related pathways in chordoma development. TSC1 and TSC2 play important roles in the phosphatidylinositol 3 kinase (PI3K)/Ak strain transforming (Akt)/mammalian target of rapamycin (mTOR) pathway as being negative regulators of mTOR. Further investigation revealed that the PI3K/Akt/mTOR pathway is activated in

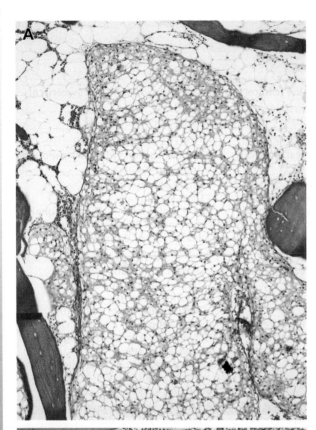

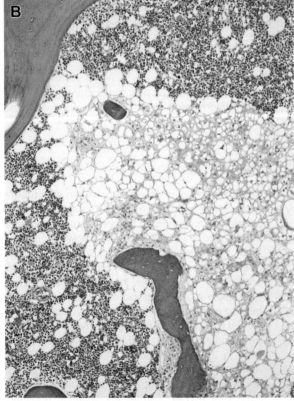

Fig. 5. Differential diagnosis between BNCT and chordoma. (A) Chordoma is encompassed by a thin fibrous membrane. The border of chordoma seems very smooth (H&E staining). (B) BNCT does not show any fibrous capsule formation. Therefore, the border of BNCT seems slightly zigzag along the contour of adjacent marrow adipocytes (H&E staining).

most chordomas and suggested that signaling through PI3K, Akt, and mTOR may be critical to chordoma pathogenesis.[29] Molecular cytogenetic studies have shown the gains of chromosomal material in chordomas, including familial cases, most prevalent at 7q, 12q, 17q, 20q, and 22q, whereas DNA sequence losses occurred mainly at 1p, 3p, 4q, 9p, 10q, and 13q[30–35] (Fig. 6). Detailed analysis of chordoma using whole-genome sequencing revealed that, in some cases, complex genomic changes mediated by massive genomic rearrangement acquired in a single catastrophic event, termed chromothripsis, could occur.[36] In the commonly deleted chromosomal loci, homozygous deletion or inactivation of tumor suppressor genes (cyclin-dependent kinase inhibitor 2A (CDKN2A), phosphatase and tensin homolog (PTEN), and SWI/SNF-related matrix-associated actin-dependent regulator of chromatin subfamily B member 1 (SMARCB1)) have been observed.[30,31,37] Some of these losses contribute to the loss of control in different RTK pathways; for example, PI3K, mTOR, and PTEN are located on chromosomes 3q26, 1p36.2, and 10q23, respectively. Molecular analysis of therapeutic targets for chordoma has progressed, particularly since the Chordoma Foundation was established in 2005, resulting in a coordinated effort to analyze this rare tumor entity and establish cell lines that are indispensable for functional analysis and testing of drugs for cancer treatment.[38] Consequently, several potentially targeted agents have been evaluated that inhibit specific molecules and their respective pathways that are known to be implicated in chordoma. The therapeutic molecular targets include epidermal growth factor receptor (EGFR), platelet-derived growth factor receptor (PDGFR), brachyury, PI3K/Akt/mTOR, mitogen-activated protein kinase (MAPK), wingless/int-1 (Wnt), signal transducer and activator of transcription (STAT), insulinlike growth factor-1 receptor (IGF1R), fibroblastic growth factor receptor (FGFR), transforming growth factor beta (TGFB), mesenchymal epithelial transition factor (c-MET), sonic hedgehog (SHH), nerve growth factor (NGF), programmed cell death protein 1 (PD1)-PD ligand 1 (PDL1), SMARCB1/integrase interactor 1 (INI1), methylthioadenosine phosphorylase, CDKN2A/CDKN2B (p16/p14), vascular endothelial growth factor (VEGF), and survivin.[39,40] Activated PI3K, Akt, and mTOR correlate inversely with outcome, in addition to inactivated TSC1 and TSC2.[41] From this list of potential targets a representative set is discussed in more detail later, including brachyury, EGFR, PDGFR, VEGF, IGF1R, PTEN, and SMARCB1.

BRACHYURY

Brachyury (official gene name is *T*) is an important transcription factor in notochord differentiation and a very specific marker of notochordal tumors.[42–45] The *T* gene is located on chromosome 6q27 and encodes a developmentally regulated transcription factor that is essential for notochordal development and formation of posterior mesodermal elements. Mature tissues do not express brachyury, whereas notochordal tumors, including chordoma and BNCT, show consistently positive immunoreaction for brachyury. Expression of brachyury is thought to be regulated by FGFRs through Ras/Raf/MEK and E26 transformation-specific 2

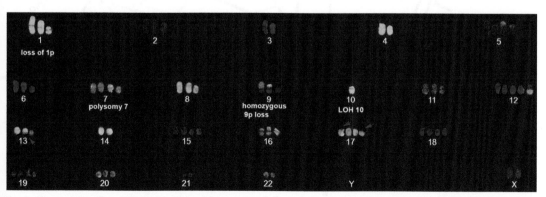

Fig. 6. Karyogram after COBRA (combined binary ratio) fluorescence in situ hybridization (FISH), multicolor FISH karyotyping, of a primary chordoma sample.[35] The tumor cell showed a 3n (69, XX, -X) karyotype with complex genomic changes involving several numerical and structural alterations. Genomic imbalances, loss of short arm of chromosome 1, and monosomy 10 leading to loss of heterozygosity and multiple copies of several chromosomes (4 or more copies) were present. Because of translocation, the short arm of hromosome 9 was lost, leading to a homozygous loss. Multiple fragments of chromosome 6 were involved in translocation, indicated by red arrows, leading to amplification of chromosome 6q segments.

(ETS2).[43] In genomic studies, no translocation was found to be associated with overexpression of brachyury that could be responsible for the dysregulated expression. Almost all chordomas do not show family history, but a cohort analyzing 4 familial chordoma sets identified recurrent germline duplication within chromosome 6q27.[44] Chordomas without family history show minor allelic gain of brachyury in only 4.5% of cases and genomic amplification in only 7% of cases.[46] Taken together, these data indicate that overexpression of brachyury is related to changes regulating expression control of the gene, most likely via epigenetic mechanisms. Enforced silencing of brachyury in the JHC7 and UCH-1 chordoma cell lines results in growth cessation, senescence, and differentiation. Thereby, inactivation of brachyury might serve as a potential target for treatment; however, so far no small molecules have been identified that could specifically block binding of a transcription factor to its target DNA sequence. Bypassing this problem, clinical trials are ongoing with patients with chordoma who are treated with a brachyury-specific vaccine, GI-6301, leading to tumor-specific target elimination because the expression of brachyury is limited in

other tissue compartments in adults, and in preclinical work it has been shown that avelumab, an anti-PD-L1 antibody, and vaccine treatment might have an enhanced effect.[47] Rarely, chordoma exist in a biphasic form that is composed of classic histologic features and high-grade undifferentiated sarcoma. Intriguingly, the dedifferentiated counterparts of these lesions lack expression of brachyury, warranting further investigation of dedifferentiated chordoma. As an alternative solution, because of the specific activation signature resulting from brachyury expression patterns, downstream activated genes could be targeted in chordoma; for example, the FGF/FGFR axis, or EGFR.

EPIDERMAL GROWTH FACTOR RECEPTOR

RTKs are key mediators of signal transductions induced from the extracellular compartments that in turn play important roles in cellular proliferation and differentiation.[48] EGFR is the cell surface receptor for members of the epidermal growth factor family of extracellular protein ligands and one of the most important cell-signaling pathways in cancer progression. The *EGFR* gene is located on

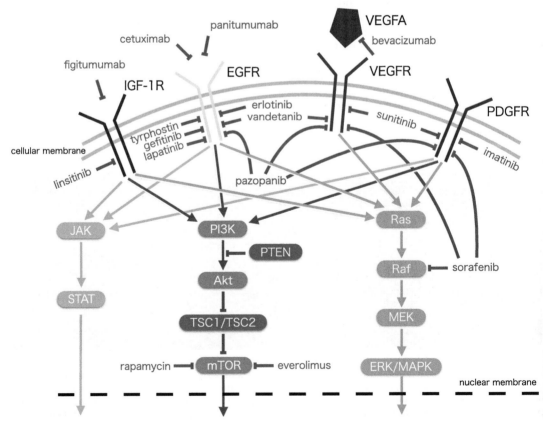

Fig. 7. Receptor tyrosine kinases and associated signaling pathways relevant to chordoma. Red terms indicate targeted molecular agents.

chromosome 7p12. Amplification as well as activating mutation and overexpression of EGFR have been described in several tumor types; for example, squamous cell carcinoma of the lung (COSMIC [Catalogue of Somatic Mutations in Cancer][49]). Activation of EGFR leads to the phosphorylation of signaling proteins involved in downstream pathways, including PI3K/Akt/mTOR and Ras/rapidly accelerated fibrosarcoma (Raf)/MEK (MAPK/ERK kinase)/extracellular signal-regulated kinase (ERK)/mitogen-activated protein kinase (MAPK) (Fig. 7). Both pathways are critical in regulating cellular apoptosis, proliferation, migration, and survival. Overexpression of EGFR, by disrupting the function of these pathways, can increase cellular proliferation and contribute to the aggressive nature of the tumor. Chordomas often show EGFR overexpression, which is associated with a more aggressive clinical behavior. Flanagan and colleagues[50,51] showed immunohistochemical EGFR expression in 69% of cases that they analyzed and high-level EGFR polysomy in 38%, high-level polysomy with focal amplification in 4%, low-level polysomy in 18%, and disomy in 39% of cases using fluorescence in situ hybridization. Activating mutations have not been found in chordoma. Copy number variation of chromosome 7 leading to EGFR gene copy number variation is one of the most common chromosomal aberrations found in chordomas.[52–56] Zhang and colleagues[57] revealed microRNA-608 (miR-608) to be a tumor-suppressive microRNA that regulates malignancy in chordoma, and that miR-608 expression inversely correlates with EGFR expression in chordoma cells. Based on this biological evidence, EGFR can be classified as a major potential therapeutic target for chordoma. It has been reported that a combination of cetuximab (EGFR antibody) and gefitinib, or erlotinib or lapatinib (EGFR-specific tyrosine-kinase inhibitors), in monotherapy or in combination with other small molecule inhibitors, resulted in treatment response both in patients with chordoma and in cell lines using in vivo and in vitro studies, respectively.[51,58,59]

PLATELET-DERIVED GROWTH FACTOR RECEPTOR

PDGFR is another RTK expressed in chordoma. There are 2 types of PDGFR: PDGFR-alpha (PDGFRA) and PDGFR-beta (PDGFRB), located on chromosomes 4q12 and 5q33, respectively. Activation of PDGFRA leads to the phosphorylation of signaling proteins involved in downstream pathways related to cell proliferation and growth, including PI3K/Akt/mTOR, ERK/MAPK, and STAT (see Fig. 7). Hyperactivation of PDGFRB and its

effects on downstream pathways can contribute to oncogenesis and tumor growth. PDGFRA was immunohistochemically positive in 75% of 72 analyzed patients with spinal chordoma.[60] Overexpression and activation of PDGFRB is fairly common in chordoma.[61,62] Both gains and losses of chromosome 5 (harboring the PDGFRB gene) have been observed and PDGFRA and/or PDGFRB are highly expressed and phosphorylated in chordomas.[41,61–64] The overexpression and activation of the PDGFR pathway may suggest the use of PDGFR inhibitors in chordoma. A well-studied PDGFR inhibitor, imatinib, could be used for this purpose. Furthermore, the use of sorafenib or sunitinib inhibits PDGFR in addition to VEGF receptor (VEGFR) and might be beneficial.

VASCULAR ENDOTHELIAL GROWTH FACTOR

VEGFA is one of the VEGF family. It is a signaling protein that stimulates vasculogenesis and angiogenesis, which contribute to tumor growth and metastasis. VEGF expression is mediated by hypoxia-inducible factor-1α (HIF-1α) expression under hypoxic conditions. VEGF may promote chordoma cell proliferation through activation of the Ras/ERK/MAPK pathway (see Fig. 7). The VEGFA locus is located on chromosome 6p12. Bayrakli and colleagues[65] found chromosome 6p12 aberration in only primary chordomas and suspected that the locus might be associated with chordoma pathogenesis. Most chordomas immunohistochemically express VEGFA in addition to hypoxia-inducible factor-1α (HIF-1α), matrix metalloproteinase-2 (MMP-2), and/or MMP-9.[66,67] Poor outcome is suggested in chordoma cases with high-level expression of VEGF.[68] Sorafenib potently inhibits VEGFR, PDGFR, and EGFR, serving as a good therapy option by attacking several of the RTKs in chordoma. Bevacizumab inhibits VEGFA and sunitinib, which inhibits downstream signaling of RTKs and potentially acts against VEGF-induced signaling.

INSULINLIKE GROWTH FACTOR-1 RECEPTOR

IGF1R is also one of the RTKs. IGF1R forms either a homodimer or heterodimer with insulin receptor A (IRA) or insulin receptor B (IRB). These IGF1R dimers are known to signal through the PI3K-Akt-mTOR, MAPK, and/or through Janus kinase (JAK)-STAT pathways (see Fig. 7) after binding of IGF1 or IGF2 as ligands. The IGF1R gene is located on chromosome 15 and no frequent alterations have been reported for this locus. IGF1R expression and signaling can play a role in

Table 3
Summary of clinically administrated molecular agents in chordomas

Inhibitors	Molecular Targets	N	Response	References
Cetuximab/gefitinib	EGFR	1	P/S (AWD for 9 mo)	Hof et al,[81] 2006
Cetuximab/gefitinib	EGFR	1	P/S (AWD for 4 mo)	Lindén et al,[82] 2009
Erlotinib	EGFR	1	P/S	Singhal et al,[83] 2009
1. Imatinib, followed by 2. Erlotinib	1. PDGFR 2. EGFR	1	1. PD 2. P/S (AWD for >12 mo)	Launay et al,[84] 2011
1. Imatinib, followed by 2. Erlotinib	1. PDGFR 2. EGFR	1	1. PD 2. P/S (AWD for >28 mo)	Houessinon et al,[85] 2015
Lapatinib	EGFR	18	13 out of 18: P/S (median PFS: 6 mo)	Stacchiotti et al,[86] 2013
1. Erlotinib + cetuximab, followed by 2. Erlotinib + bevacizumab	1. EGFR 2. EGFR + VEGFR	1	1. PD 2. P/S (AWD for 54 mo)	Asklund et al,[87] 2011; Asklund et al,[88] 2014
Erlotinib + bevacizumab	EGFR + VGEFR	1	P/S (AWD for 27 mo)	Asklund et al,[87] 2011
1. Erlotinib + cetuximab, followed by 2. Erlotinib + bevacizumab	1. EGFR 2. EGFR + VEGFR	1	1. PD 2. P/S (AWD for 24 mo)	Asklund et al,[87] 2011
Erlotinib + linsitinib	EGFR + IGF1R	1	P/S (AWD for >268 mo)	Macaulay et al,[71] 2016
Erlotinib + linsitinib	EGFR + IGF1R	1	P/S (AWD for >54 mo)	Aleksic et al,[72] 2016
Imatinib	PDGFR	6	4 out of 6: P/S	Casali et al,[89] 2004

Imatinib	PDGFR	18	11 out of 18: P/S (AWD for 14–70 mo)	Casali et al,[90] 2005
Imatinib	PDGFR	17	6 out of 11: P/S	Ferraresi et al,[91] 2010
Imatinib	PDGFR	56	36 out of 50: P/S	Stacchiotti et al,[92] 2012
Imatinib + Metronomic Cyclophosphamide	PDGFR	7	12-mo PFR: 3/7	Adenis et al,[93] 2013
Imatinib	PDGFR	50	34 out of 46: P/S (median PFS: 7 mo)	Hindi et al,[94] 2015
Sunitinib	VEGFR, PDGFR	9	2 out of 9: P/S at 6 mo	George et al,[95] 2009
Sorafenib	VEGFR, PDGFR	27	25 out of 27: P/S (9-mo PFR: 73.0%)	Bompas et al,[96] 2015
Sorafenib	VEGFR, PDGFR	26	9-mo PFR: 72.9%	Lebellec et al,[68] 2016
Pazopanib	VGEFR, PDGFR, EGFR	3	2 out of 3: P/S (AWD for 14 mo and 15 mo, respectively)	Lipplaa et al,[97] 2016
1. Imatinib, followed by 2. Pazopanib	1. PDGFR 2. VEDFR, PDGFR, EGFR	1	1. PD 2. PD	Lipplaa et al,[97] 2016
1. Imatinib, followed by 2. Sunitinib	1. EGFR 2. VEGFR, PDGFR	1	1. PD 2. P/S (AWD for 27 mo)	Lipplaa et al,[97] 2016
1. Imatinib, followed by 2. Rapamycin	1. PDGFR 2. mTOR	10	1. PD 2. 8 out of 10: P/S	Stacchiotti et al,[98] 2009
Rapamycin	mTOR	1	P/S (AWD for >10 mo)	Ricci-Vitiani et al,[99] 2013

Abbreviations: AWD, alive with disease; P/S, partial response or stable disease; PD, progressive disease; PFR, progression-free rate; PFS, progression-free survival.

transformation events and enhance cell survival, and overexpression of IGF1R has been linked to tumorigenesis and metastasis as well as to tumor resistance to cytotoxic therapies. Sommer and colleagues[69] reported that patients with phosphorylated isoforms of IGF1R (pIGF1R)-positive tumor showed significantly decreased median disease-free survival, whereas pIGF1R was absent in BNCT and fetal notochord. Another study indicated that IGF1R and its ligands, particularly IGF1, were consistently expressed in 76% of chordomas and that the IGF1R/IGF1 signaling pathway was activated in a subset of chordomas.[70] Based on these observations it was suggested that inhibition of IGF1R-signaling could serve as a potential target in chordomas. Linsitinib (OSI-906), an RTK inhibitor small molecule, and antibody targeting of IGF1R using, for instance, figitumumab (discontinued) were used in clinical trials for chordoma and/or several other tumor types.[71–73]

PTEN

PTEN plays a role in tumor suppression by negatively regulating the PI3K/Akt/mTOR signaling pathway (see Fig. 7). The *PTEN* gene is located on chromosome 10q23 and loss of heterozygosity of this locus was observed in ~25% of chordomas, associated with aggressive behavior, and correlated with an increased Ki-67 proliferative index.[74] Another study showed that expression of mTOR seems to correlate with the loss of PTEN expression in chordomas and suggested that PTEN and mTOR are prognostic predictors of poor prognosis.[75] These data suggest that a PDGFR inhibitor may disrupt growth and invasion of PTEN-deficient chordoma.

SMARCB1 (INTEGRASE INTERACTOR 1)

Lack of SMARCB1/INI-1 expression is characteristic of malignant rhabdoid tumor, atypical teratoid/rhabdoid tumor (AT/RT), and epithelioid sarcoma. The *SMARCB1/INI-1* gene is located on chromosome 22q11.2. It is a member of the ATP-dependent SWI/SNF chromatin-remodeling complex, is expressed in normal tissue, and is thought to function as a tumor suppressor gene. Recently, it was reported that tumor nuclei lack SMARCB1/INI-1 expression in pediatric chordomas immunohistochemically in addition to sporadic cases of malignant peripheral nerve sheath tumor, synovial sarcoma, extraskeletal myxoid chondrosarcoma, and myoepithelial carcinoma.[76–78] Deletions at the SMARCB1/INI-1 locus were observed in 3 of 8 cases of pediatric chordoma.[79] Poorly differentiated and pediatric chordomas tend to lose SMARCB1 expression, whereas most chordomas do express SMARCB1.[80] Lack of SMARCB1 expression may be a biomarker of chordoma with worse prognosis. c-Met expression in patients with spinal chordoma tends to correlate with younger patients and a favorable prognosis, like SMARCB1, although c-MET may contribute by a different molecular mechanism from SMARCB1.[60]

CLINICAL EVIDENCE OF TARGETED MOLECULAR AGENTS FOR CHORDOMA

Targeting of several kinds of molecular agents has been attempted to treat uncontrolled chordomas after surgery and/or radiotherapy.[68,71,72,81–99] Clinical evidence concerning targeted molecular agents is listed in Table 3. In many cases there was a partial response or stable disease, although cases with complete response are rarely reported in monotherapy. The combination of inhibitors against different RTKs might be necessary. Supporting this, chordoma cases were reported with partial but sustained response to erlotinib, pazopanib, sunitinib, or rapamycin after imatinib failure.[84,85,97,98]

RTK inhibitors have some hematopoietic and nonhematopoietic toxicity.[95,96,98,100] Major hematopoietic toxicity includes neutropenia, anemia, and thrombocytopenia. Nonhematopoietic toxicity consists of hand-foot syndrome, mucositis, weight loss, nausea, diarrhea, hypertension, infections, and thyroid dysfunction. However, no lethal side effects have been documented.

SUMMARY

From recent advances in molecular studies on chordoma it has become clear that chordomas commonly express various RTKs and thereby may respond to RTK inhibitors. At present, chordoma management is primarily based on surgical resection and, in combination with proton or carbon beam therapy, long-term cure can be achieved. However, in most cases tumor eradication is not possible, so additional treatment options should be explored. Chordoma management is still challenging; however, it is anticipated that further molecular investigations will yield new findings and contribute to the development of more effective molecular agents. From genetic studies on chordomas it has become clear that chordoma is a heterogeneous group of tumors comprising entities in which chromothripsis may occur, and tumors that (exceedingly rarely) arise in a hereditary background involving genomic changes of the T gene locus or the TSC. Secondary alterations, like gains or amplification of EGFR versus overexpression of EGFR or deletion of the CDKN2A/B locus or SMARCB1 locus, may act as secondary modifiers, resulting in different treatment outcomes. Next to the genetic heterogeneity, various expression levels of potential therapy-related target genes may add to the intratumor heterogeneity. These heterogeneous expression patterns might give a growth advantage to nonexpressing cells, consequently leading to the selection of the nonexpressing cell clones and resulting in therapy resistance. Correlating expression patterns in retrospective studies of responding and nonresponding patient samples with outcomes in different clinical trials might be used to identify predictive markers.

Stratification of rare tumor entities into subclasses is a daunting task for which a multi-institutional approach is needed. Active participation of patient organizations, like the Chordoma Foundation, might serve as a model for other rare disease entities, facilitating research and concentrating knowledge worldwide. In a joint effort, genetic and functional subclasses reacting differently to trial arms might then be identified, facilitating better identification of prognostic and/or predictive markers.

REFERENCES

1. Flanagan AM, Yamaguchi T. Notochordal tumours. In: Fletcher CDM, Bridge JA, Hogendoorn PCW, et al, editors. WHO classification of tumours of soft tissue and bone. 4th edition. Lyon (France): IARC; 2013. p. 325–9.
2. Yamaguchi T, Yamato M, Saotome K. First histologically confirmed case of a classic chordoma arising in a precursor benign notochordal lesion: differential diagnosis of benign and malignant notochordal lesions. Skeletal Radiol 2002;31:413–8.
3. Yamaguchi T, Watanabe-Ishiiwa H, Suzuki S, et al. Incipient chordoma: a report of two cases of early-stage chordoma arising from benign notochordal cell tumors. Mod Pathol 2005;18:1005–10.
4. Deshpande V, Nielsen GP, Rosenthal DI, et al. Intraosseous benign notochord cell tumors (BNCT)-further evidence supporting a relationship to chordoma. Am J Surg Pathol 2007;31:1573–7.
5. Nishiguchi T, Mochizuki K, Tsujio T, et al. Lumbar vertebral chordoma arising from an intraosseous benign notochordal cell tumour: radiological findings and histopathological description with a good clinical outcome. Br J Radiol 2010;83:e49–53.
6. Jaffe HL. Tumors and tumorous conditions of the bones and joints. Philadelphia: Lea & Febiger; 1958. p. 451–61.
7. Kikuchi Y, Yamaguchi T, Kishi H, et al. Pulmonary tumor with notochordal differentiation: report of two cases suggestive of benign notochordal cell tumor of extraosseous origin. Am J Surg Pathol 2011; 35:1158–64.
8. Suzuki H, Yamashiro K, Takeda H. Extra-axial soft tissue chordoma of wrist. Pathol Res Pract 2011; 15(207):327–31.
9. Yakkioui Y, van Overbeeke JJ, Santegoeds R, et al. Chordoma: the entity. Biochim Biophys Acta 2014; 1846:655–69.
10. Yamaguchi T, Suzuki S, Ishiiwa H, et al. Intraosseous benign notochordal cell tumors-overlooked precursors of classic chordomas? Histopathology 2004;44:597–602.
11. Yamaguchi T, Suzuki S, Ishiiwa H, et al. Benign notochordal cell tumors: a comparative histological study of benign notochordal cell tumors, classic chordomas, and notochordal vestiges of fetal intervertebral discs. Am J Surg Pathol 2004;28:756–61.
12. Yamaguchi T, Iwata J, Sugihara S, et al. Distinguishing benign notochordal cell tumor from vertebral chordoma. Skeletal Radiol 2008;37:291–9.
13. Bonar SF, Watson G, Gragnaniello C, et al. Intraosseous hibernoma: characterization of five cases and literature review. Skeletal Radiol 2014;43:939–46.
14. Grimer RJ, Hogendoorn PCW, Vanel D. Tumours of bone: introduction. In: Fletcher CDM, Bridge JA, Hogendoorn PCW, et al, editors. WHO classification of tumours of soft tissue and bone. 4th edition. Lyon (France): IARC; 2013. p. 243–7.
15. Czerniak B. Chordoma and related lesions. In: Czerniak B, editor. Dorfman and Czerniak's bone tumors. Philadelphia: Elsevier; 2016. p. 1174–216.
16. Matsubayashi J, Sato E, Nomura M, et al. A case of paravertebral mediastinal chordoma without bone destruction. Skeletal Radiol 2012;41:1641–4.
17. Fletcher CDM, Antonescu CR, Heim S, et al. Myoepithelioma/myoepithelial carcinoma/mixed tumour. In: Fletcher CDM, Bridge JA, Hogendoorn PCW, et al, editors. WHO classification of tumours of soft tissue and bone. Revised 4th edition. Lyon (France): IARC; 2013. p. 208–9.
18. Perry A, Louis DN, Budka H, et al. Meningiomas. In: Louis DN, Ohgaki H, Wrestler OD, et al, editors. WHO classification of tumours of the central nervous system. 4th edition. Lyon (France): IARC; 2016. p. 231–46.
19. Deshpande V, Nielsen GP, Rosenberg AE. Notochordal tumors. In: Nielsen GP, Rosenberg AE, Deshpande V, et al, editors. Diagnostic pathology: bone. Salt Lake City: Amirsys; 2013. p. 8-1–8-15.
20. Walcott BP, Nahed BV, Mohyeldin A, et al. Chordoma: current concepts, management, and future directions. Lancet Oncol 2012;13:e69–76.
21. Imai R, Kamada T, Sugahara S, et al. Carbon ion radiotherapy for sacral chordoma. Br J Radiol 2011;84:S48–54.

22. Matsumoto T, Imagama S, Ito Z, et al. Total spondylectomy following carbon ion radiotherapy to treat chordoma of the mobile spine. Bone Joint J 2013; 95-B:1392–5.

23. Nishida Y, Kamada T, Imai R, et al. Clinical outcome of sacral chordoma with carbon ion radiotherapy compared with surgery. Int J Radiat Oncol Biol Phys 2011;79:110–6.

24. Imai R, Kamada T, Araki N, Working Group for Bone and Soft Tissue Sarcomas. Carbon ion radiation therapy for unresectable sacral chordoma: an analysis of 188 cases. Int J Radiat Oncol Biol Phys 2016;95:322–7.

25. Schroeder BA, Wells RG, Starshak RJ, et al. Clivus chordoma in a child with tuberous sclerosis: CT and MR demonstration. J Comput Assist Tomogr 1987; 11:195–6.

26. Börgel J, Olschewski H, Reuter T, et al. Does the tuberous sclerosis complex include clivus chordoma? A case report. Eur J Pediatr 2001;160:138.

27. Lee-Jones L, Aligianis I, Davies PA, et al. Sacrococcygeal chordomas in patients with tuberous sclerosis complex show somatic loss of TSC1 or TSC2. Genes Chromosomes Cancer 2004;41:80–5.

28. McMaster ML, Goldstein AM, Parry DM. Clinical features distinguish childhood chordoma associated with tuberous sclerosis complex (TSC) from chordoma in the general paediatric population. J Med Genet 2011;48:444–9.

29. Presneau N, Shalaby A, Idowu B, et al. Potential therapeutic targets for chordoma: PI3K/AKT/TSC1/TSC2/mTOR pathway. Br J Cancer 2009;100:1406–14.

30. Hallor KH, Staaf J, Jönsson G, et al. Frequent deletion of the CDKN2A locus in chordoma: analysis of chromosomal imbalances using array comparative genomic hybridisation. Br J Cancer 2008;29(98): 434–42.

31. Le LP, Nielsen GP, Rosenberg AE, et al. Recurrent chromosomal copy number alterations in sporadic chordomas. PLoS One 2011;6:e18846.

32. Scheil-Bertram S, Kappler R, von Baer A, et al. Molecular profiling of chordoma. Int J Oncol 2014;44: 1041–55.

33. Miozzo M, Dalprà L, Riva P, et al. A tumor suppressor locus in familial and sporadic chordoma maps to 1p36. Int J Cancer 2000;87:68–72.

34. Kelley MJ, Korczak JF, Sheridan E, et al. Familial chordoma, a tumor of notochordal remnants, is linked to chromosome 7q33. Am J Hum Genet 2001;69:454–60.

35. Szuhai K, Tanke HJ. COBRA: combined binary ratio labeling of nucleic-acid probes for multi-color fluorescence in situ hybridization karyotyping. Nat Protoc 2006;1:264–75.

36. Stephens PJ, Greenman CD, Fu B, et al. Massive genomic rearrangement acquired in a single catastrophic event during cancer development. Cell 2011;144:27–40.

37. Choy E, MacConaill LE, Cote GM, et al. Genotyping cancer-associated genes in chordoma identifies mutations in oncogenes and areas of chromosomal loss involving CDKN2A, PTEN, and SMARCB1. PLoS One 2014;9:e101283.

38. Chordoma Foundation. Available at: https://www.chordomafoundation.org. Accessed December 15, 2016.

39. Therapeutic targets in chordoma. In: Chordoma Foundation. Available at: https://www.chordoma-foundation.org/targets/. Accessed December 15, 2016.

40. Tauziéde-Espariat A, Bresson D, Polivka M, et al. Prognostic and therapeutic markers in chordomas: a study of 287 tumors. J Neuropathol Exp Neurol 2016;75:111–20.

41. de Castro CV, Guimaraes G, Aguiar S Jr, et al. Tyrosine kinase receptor expression in chordomas: phosphorylated AKT correlates inversely with outcome. Hum Pathol 2013;44:1747–55.

42. Vujovic S, Henderson S, Presneau N, et al. Brachyury, a crucial regulator of notochordal development, is a novel biomarker for chordomas. J Pathol 2006;209:157–65.

43. Shalaby AA, Presneau N, Idowu BD, et al. Analysis of the fibroblastic growth factor receptor-RAS/RAF/MEK/ERK-ETS2/brachyury signalling pathway in chordomas. Mod Pathol 2009;22:996–1005.

44. Presneau N, Shalaby A, Ye H, et al. Role of the transcription factor T (brachyury) in the pathogenesis of sporadic chordoma: a genetic and functional-based study. J Pathol 2011;2(23):327–35.

45. Nibu Y, José-Edwards DS, Di Gregorio A. From notochord formation to hereditary chordoma: the many roles of Brachyury. Biomed Res Int 2013; 2013:826435.

46. Yang XR, Ng D, Alcorta DA, et al. T (brachyury) gene duplication confers major susceptibility to familial chordoma. Nat Genet 2009;41:1176–8.

47. Fujii R, Friedman ER, Richards J, et al. Enhanced killing of chordoma cells by antibody-dependent cell-mediated cytotoxicity employing the novel anti-PD-L1 antibody avelumab. Oncotarget 2016; 7:33498–511.

48. Di Maio S, Yip S, Al Zhrani GA, et al. Novel targeted therapies in chordoma: an update. Ther Clin Risk Manag 2015;11:873–83.

49. COSMIC. Available at: http://cancer.sanger.ac.uk/cosmic. Accessed January 04, 2017.

50. Shalaby A, Presneau N, Ye H, et al. The role of epidermal growth factor receptor in chordoma pathogenesis: a potential therapeutic target. J Pathol 2011;223:336–46.

51. Scheipl S, Barnard M, Cottone L, et al. EGFR inhibitors identified as a potential treatment for chordoma in a focused compound screen. J Pathol 2016;239:320–34.

52. Dewaele B, Maggiani F, Floris G, et al. Frequent activation of EGFR in advanced chordomas. Clin Sarcoma Res 2011;1:4.

53. Scheil S, Brüderlein S, Liehr T, et al. Genome-wide analysis of sixteen chordomas by comparative genomic hybridization and cytogenetics of the first human chordoma cell line, U-CH1. Genes Chromosomes Cancer 2001;32:203–11.

54. Brandal P, Bjerkehagen B, Danielsen H, et al. Chromosome 7 abnormalities are common in chordomas. Cancer Genet Cytogenet 2005;160:15–21.

55. Grabellus F, Konik MJ, Worm K, et al. MET overexpressing chordomas frequently exhibit polysomy of chromosome 7 but no MET activation through sarcoma-specific gene fusions. Tumour Biol 2010; 31:157–63.

56. Walter BA, Begnami M, Valera VA, et al. Gain of chromosome 7 by chromogenic in situ hybridization (CISH) in chordomas is correlated to c-MET expression. J Neurooncol 2011;101:199–206.

57. Zhang Y, Schiff D, Park D, et al. MicroRNA-608 and MicroRNA-34a regulate chordoma malignancy by targeting EGFR, Bcl-xL and MET. PLoS One 2014; 9:e91546.

58. Siu IM, Ruzevick J, Zhao Q, et al. Erlotinib inhibits growth of a patient-derived chordoma xenograft. PLoS One 2013;8:e78895.

59. Bozzi F, Manenti G, Conca E, et al. Development of transplantable human chordoma xenograft for preclinical assessment of novel therapeutic strategies. Neuro Oncol 2014;16:72–80.

60. Akhavan-Sigari R, Gaab MR, Rohde V, et al. Expression of PDGFR-α, EGFR and c-MET in spinal chordoma: a series of 52 patients. Anticancer Res 2014;34:623–30.

61. Tamborini E, Miselli F, Negri T, et al. Molecular and biochemical analyses of platelet-derived growth factor receptor (PDGFR) B, PDGFRA, and KIT receptors in chordomas. Clin Cancer Res 2006;12: 6920–8.

62. Tamborini E, Virdis E, Negri T, et al. Analysis of receptor tyrosine kinases (RTKs) and downstream pathways in chordomas. Neuro Oncol 2010;12: 776–89.

63. Orzan F, Terreni MR, Longoni M, et al. Expression study of the target receptor tyrosine kinase of imatinib mesylate in skull base chordomas. Oncol Rep 2007;18:249–52.

64. Akhavan-Sigari R, Abili M, Gaab MR, et al. Immunohistochemical expression of receptor tyrosine kinase PDGFR-α, c-Met, and EGFR in skull base chordoma. Neurosurg Rev 2015;38:89–98.

65. Bayrakli F, Guney I, Kilic T, et al. New candidate chromosomal regions for chordoma development. Surg Neurol 2007;68:425–30.

66. Chen KW, Yang HL, Lu J, et al. Expression of vascular endothelial growth factor and matrix metalloproteinase-9 in sacral chordoma. Neurooncol 2011;101:357–63.

67. Li X, Ji Z, Ma Y, et al. Expression of hypoxia-inducible factor-1α, vascular endothelial growth factor and matrix metalloproteinase-2 in sacral chordomas. Oncol Lett 2012;3:1268–74.

68. Lebellec L, Bertucci F, Tresch-Bruneel E, et al. Circulating vascular endothelial growth factor (VEGF) as predictive factor of progression-free survival in patients with advanced chordoma receiving sorafenib: an analysis from a phase II trial of the French Sarcoma Group (GSF/GETO). Oncotarget 2016;7:73984–94.

69. Sommer J, Itani DM, Homlar KC, et al. Methylthioadenosine phosphorylase and activated insulin-like growth factor-1 receptor/insulin receptor: potential therapeutic targets in chordoma. J Pathol 2010; 220:608–17.

70. Scheipl S, Froehlich EV, Leithner A, et al. Does insulin-like growth factor 1 receptor (IGF-1R) targeting provide new treatment options for chordomas? a retrospective clinical and immunohistochemical study. Histopathology 2012;60:999–1003.

71. Macaulay VM, Middleton MR, Eckhardt SG, et al. Phase I dose-escalation study of linsitinib (OSI-906) and erlotinib in patients with advanced solid tumors. Clin Cancer Res 2016;22:2897–907.

72. Aleksic T, Browning L, Woodward M, et al. Durable response of spinal chordoma to combined inhibition of IGF-1R and EGFR. Front Oncol 2016;6:96.

73. Scagliotti GV, Bondarenko I, Blackhall F, et al. Randomized, phase III trial of figitumumab in combination with erlotinib versus erlotinib alone in patients with nonadenocarcinoma nonsmall-cell lung cancer. Ann Oncol 2015;26:497–504.

74. Lee D-H, Zhang Y, Kassam AB, et al. Combined PDGFR and HDAC inhibition overcomes PTEN disruption in chordoma. PLoS One 2015;10:e0134426.

75. Chen K, Mo J, Zhou M, et al. Expression of PTEN and mTOR in sacral chordoma and association with poor prognosis. Med Oncol 2014;31:886.

76. Mobley BC, McKenney JK, Bangs CD, et al. Loss of SMARCB1/INI1 expression in poorly differentiated chordomas. Acta Neuropathol 2010;120:745–53.

77. Tirabosco R, Jacques T, Berisha F, et al. Assessment of integrase interactor 1 (INI-1) expression in primary tumours of bone. Histopathology 2012; 61:1245–7.

78. Mularz K, Harazin-Lechowska A, Ambicka A, et al. Specificity and sensitivity of INI-1 labeling in epithelioid sarcoma. Loss of INI1 expression as a frequent immunohistochemical event in synovial sarcoma. Pol J Pathol 2012;63:179–83.

79. Antonelli M, Raso A, Mascelli S, et al. SMARCB1/INI1 involvement in pediatric chordoma: a mutational and immunohistochemical analysis. Am J Surg Pathol 2017;41:56–61.

80. Yadav R, Sharma MC, Malgulwar PB, et al. Prognostic value of MIB-1, p53, epidermal growth factor receptor, and INI1 in childhood chordomas. Neuro Oncol 2014;16:372–8.

81. Hof H, Welzel T, Debus J. Effectiveness of cetuximab/gefitinib in the therapy of a sacral chordoma. Onkologie 2006;29:572–4.

82. Lindén O, Stenberg L, Kjellén E. Regression of cervical spinal cord compression in a patient with chordoma following treatment with cetuximab and gefitinib. Acta Oncol 2009;48:158–9.

83. Singhal N, Kotasek D, Parnis FX. Response to erlotinib in a patient with treatment refractory chordoma. Anticancer Drugs 2009;20:953–5.

84. Launay SG, Chetaille B, Medina F, et al. Efficacy of epidermal growth factor receptor targeting in advanced chordoma: case report and literature review. BMC Cancer 2011;11:423.

85. Houessinon A, Boone M, Constans J-M, et al. Sustained response of a clivus chordoma to erlotinib after imatinib failure. Case Rep Oncol 2015; 8:25–9.

86. Stacchiotti S, Tamborini E, Lo Vullo S, et al. Phase II study on lapatinib in advanced EGFR-positive chordoma. Ann Oncol 2013;24:1931–6.

87. Asklund T, Danfors T, Henriksson R. PET response and tumor stabilization under erlotinib and bevacizumab treatment of an intracranial lesion noninvasively diagnosed as likely chordoma. Clin Neuropathol 2011;30:242–6.

88. Asklund T, Sandström M, Shahidi S, et al. Durable stabilization of three chordoma cases by bevacizumab and erlotinib. Acta Oncol 2014;53:980–4.

89. Casali PG, Messina A, Stacchiotti S, et al. Imatinib mesylate in chordoma. Cancer 2004;101:2086–97.

90. Casali PG, Stacchiotti S, Messina A, et al. Imatinib mesylate in 18 advanced chordoma patients. J Clin Oncol 2005;23:9012.

91. Ferraresi V, Nuzzo C, Zoccali C, et al. Chordoma: clinical characteristics, management and prognosis of a case series of 25 patients. BMC Cancer 2010;10:22.

92. Stacchiotti S, Longhi A, Ferraresi V, et al. Phase II study of imatinib in advanced chordoma. J Clin Oncol 2012;20:914–20.

93. Adenis A, Ray-Coquard I, Italiano A, et al. A dose-escalating phase I of imatinib mesylate with fixed dose of metronomic cyclophosphamide in targeted solid tumours. Br J Cancer 2013;109:2574–8.

94. Hindi N, Casali PG, Morosi C, et al. Imatinib in advanced chordoma: a retrospective case series analysis. Eur J Cancer 2015;51:2609–14.

95. George S, Merriam P, Maki RG, et al. Multicenter phase II trial of sunitinib in the treatment of nongastrointestinal stromal tumor sarcomas. J Clin Oncol 2009;27:3154–60.

96. Bompas E, Le Cesne A, Tresch-Bruneel E, et al. Sorafenib in patients with locally advanced and metastatic chordomas: a phase II trial of the French Sarcoma Group (GSF/GETO). Ann Oncol 2015;26: 2168–73.

97. Lipplaa A, Dijkstra S, Gelderblom H. Efficacy of pazopanib and sunitinib in advanced axial chordoma: a single reference center case series. Clin Sarcoma Res 2016;6:19.

98. Stacchiotti S, Marrari A, Tamborini E, et al. Response to imatinib plus sirolimus in advanced chordoma. Ann Oncol 2009;20:1886–94.

99. Ricci-Vitiani L, Runci D, D'Alessandris QG, et al. Chemotherapy of skull base chordoma tailored on responsiveness of patient-derived tumor cells to rapamycin. Neoplasia 2013;15:773–82.

100. Eroukhmanoff J, Castinetti F, Penel N, et al. Autoimmune thyroid dysfunction induced by tyrosine kinase inhibitors in a patient with recurrent chordoma. BMC Cancer 2016;16:679.

Myoepithelial Tumors of Bone

 CrossMark

Wangzhao Song, MD[a], Uta Flucke, MD, PhD[b], Albert J.H. Suurmeijer, MD, PhD[a],*

KEYWORDS

- Myoepithelioma • Myoepithelial carcinoma • Bone • Pathology • Immunohistochemistry • EWSR1
- FUS • Fusion gene

ABSTRACT

Myoepithelial tumors (METs) of bone (BMETs) are a rare but distinct tumor entity. METs that are cytologically benign are termed myoepitheliomas; METs with malignant histologic features are called myoepithelial carcinomas. BMETs have a wide age range, may involve any part of the skeleton, and have a variable spindle cell and epithelioid morphology. Bone tumors to be considered in the differential diagnosis are discussed. Additional techniques are indispensable to correctly diagnose BMETs. By immunohistochemistry, BMETs often express cytokeratins and/or EMA together with S100, GFAP, or calponin. Half of BMETs harbor EWSR1 (or rare FUS) gene rearrangements with different gene partners.

OVERVIEW, HISTORICAL PERSPECTIVE

To the novice in musculoskeletal pathology who was taught in medical school that the most common bone tumors differentiate along mesenchymal or neuroectodermal lines, it may come as a surprise that some bone tumors show myoepithelial differentiation.

Myoepithelial tumors (METs) of bone (BMETs) are rare. To date, up to 30 cases have been described in the literature.[1–12] BMETs were recognized as a distinct clinicopathological entity only after their initial description in soft tissue.

In 1997, Kilpatrick and colleagues[13] first proposed the unifying concept that METs morphologically resembling myoepithelial counterparts presenting as skin adnexal or salivary gland tumors, may also occur in soft tissue. Hornick and Fletcher[14] described a series of 101 soft tissue METs in 2003, after which Gleason and Fletcher[15] reported a series of 29 soft tissue METs presenting in childhood in 2007. Soft tissue METs represent a wide histologic spectrum with cases showing benign and malignant histomorphology and clinical behavior. In the 2013 World Health Organization (WHO) classification of tumors of soft tissue and bone,[16] the terms myoepithelioma and mixed tumor are used for the benign variants and myoepithelial carcinoma is the proper name for the malignant phenotypes. Myoepithelioma is mainly composed of myoepithelial cells, whereas mixed tumor also shows clear-cut ductal differentiation. The older term parachordoma, which was still used as a synonym for myoepithelioma in the 2002 WHO classification,[16] reflects the morphologic resemblance of some METs to chordoma, but clearly chordoma is a completely different tumor entity, as shown by nuclear immunostaining for the T-box transcription factor brachyury.[17]

Only in the past decade have molecular pathologic studies revealed that the molecular genetic pathogenesis of METs of soft tissue and bone is different from those occurring in skin and salivary glands.

EPIDEMIOLOGY, SITES OF INVOLVEMENT, AND GROSS FEATURES

BMETs have a wide age distribution and show an almost equal sex distribution. Most patients are adults and adolescents, but BMETs also arise in teenagers. The elderly are seldom affected.

Disclosure statements: the authors have no commercial or financial conflicts of interest. W. Song receives funding from the China Scholarship Council (CSC) program (grant no: 201606940023).
[a] Department of Pathology and Medical Biology, University Medical Center Groningen, University of Groningen, PO Box 30.001, Groningen 9700RB, The Netherlands; [b] Department of Pathology, Nijmegen Medical Center, Radboud University, PO Box 9101, Nijmegen 6500HB, The Netherlands
* Corresponding author.
E-mail address: a.j.h.suurmeijer@umcg.nl

surgpath.theclinics.com

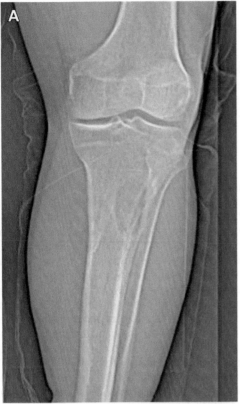

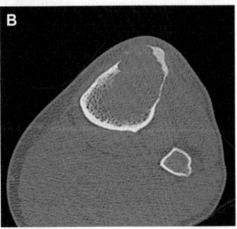

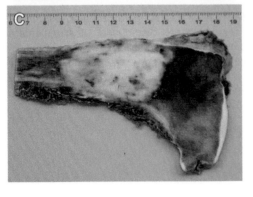

By location, BMETs have a variable distribution. The tumors most often present in long tubular bones (femur, tibia, fibula, humerus), but also occur in small tubular bones (phalanges), and axial skeleton (iliac bone, sacrum, vertebra, ribs, skull, and maxilla).

Although BMETs are usually intraosseous tumors, juxtacortical lesions also have been reported.[8]

By imaging studies (radiographs, computed tomography [CT], MRI) BMETs are well-demarcated, lytic tumors that may have aggressive features and show invasion of surrounding soft tissue (Fig. 1). By gross examination of surgical specimens, BMETs are solid, nodular tumors. Cortical destruction and extension in surrounding soft tissue may be present (see Fig. 1, Fig. 2).

Grossly, BMETs are well-demarcated, nodular, lobulated masses. On cut surface, color and consistency are proportionate to cellularity, collagenization, and myxoid change or hemorrhage. Commonly, BMETs are solid and gray-white, whereas myxochondroid areas are gelatinous and glistening.

MICROSCOPIC FEATURES AND DIAGNOSIS

The histology of benign BMETs (myoepitheliomas) is variable and resembles their salivary gland counterparts (Fig. 3). Microscopically, myoepithelial tumor cells can have different features,[18] with areas consisting of bland eosinophilic spindle cells, epithelioid cells, clear cells, squamous cells, or plasmacytoid cells (Figs. 4–7). Some tumors are predominantly composed of spindle cells arranged in bundles (Fig. 8), whereas other BMETs show foci with epithelioid cells and clear or vacuolated tumor cells that form cohesive cell nests and cords (Figs. 9 and 10). Myxoid areas with spindle or epithelioid cells can show a reticular architectural pattern (Fig. 11). These neoplastic myoepithelial cells are embedded in a variable amount of fibrous, hyaline fibrous, myxoid, or myxohyaline stroma (see Figs. 9–11, Fig. 12). Frank cartilaginous or osseous differentiation is rather rare.

Fig. 1. Myoepithelioma of the proximal tibia. (A) The plain radiograph and (B) MRI both show an intramedullary lytic lesion that is well demarcated, but destroys the cortical bone (arrows). (C) Gross examination of the cut surface of the resection specimen reveals a well-demarcated, solid, gray-white tumor that is located intramedullary but destroys cortical bone.

Fig. 2. Myoepithelioma of the scapula. This gross specimen shows a myoepithelioma that breaks through cortical bone and invades the surrounding soft tissue.

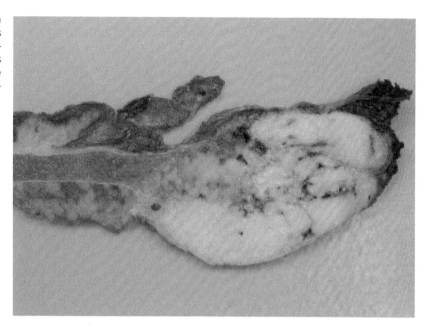

Malignant BMETs (myoepithelial carcinomas) show cytonuclear atypia, prominent nucleoli, increased mitotic activity, and areas of necrosis. Morphologic features that distinguish benign myoepitheliomas of bone from malignant variants are not well established.[7] In soft tissue locations, nuclear atypia and prominent nucleoli are currently considered to be the sole histologic features of (potential) malignant behavior. A subset of myoepithelial carcinomas is composed of solid sheets of round tumor cells with nuclear atypia with prominent nucleoli (**Fig. 13**).

The myoepithelial phenotype of BMETs can be demonstrated by immunohistochemistry (IHC) using an appropriate panel of antibodies (**Fig. 14**). The large majority of METs show combined expression of cytokeratins and/or epithelial membrane antigen (EMA) together with S100 and/or

Fig. 3. Myoepithelioma of bone. Hematoxylin and eosin (H&E, original magnification, ×50) microphotograph illustrating the variable histology of myoepithelioma with bundles of spindle cells (lower right) and cords of epithelioid cells embedded in hyalinized fibrous stroma (upper left and right).

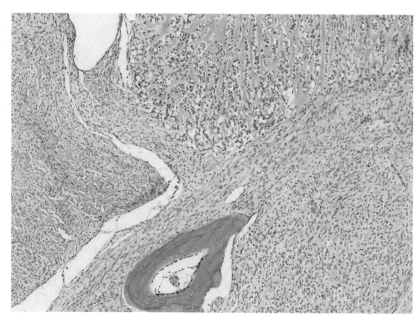

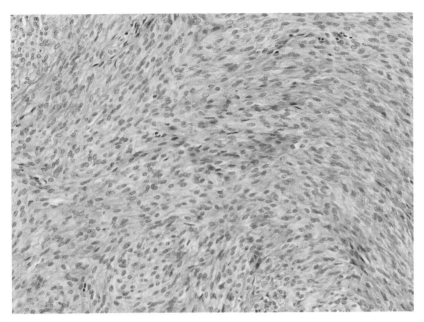

Fig. 4. Myoepithelioma of bone. H&E microphotograph showing an area of spindled tumor cells with monomorphic oval nuclei with fine chromatin and inconspicuous nucleoli. The tumor cells are surrounded by a small amount of fibrillary collagen (H&E, original magnification, ×200).

glial fibrillary acidic protein (GFAP), an immunophenotype required to make a confirmatory diagnosis (Fig. 15). Sox-10 is another useful marker for myoepithelial tumors.[19] Smooth muscle markers that have proven to be useful are calponin, smooth muscle actin (SMA), or smooth muscle myosin heavy chain (SMMS-1). A small percentage of myoepithelial carcinomas show loss of SMARCB1/INI1 in tumor cell nuclei.

Nearly half of the BMETs harbor recurrent EWSR1 (and rare FUS) gene fusions, that can be demonstrated using a break-apart fluorescence in situ hybridization (FISH) assay or, more specifically, by reverse-transcriptase polymerase chain reaction (RT-PCR) or next-generation sequencing (NGS). Several different fusion partners have been found in METs (Fig. 16). In BMETs, EWSR1 (or FUS) fusion partners described to date are

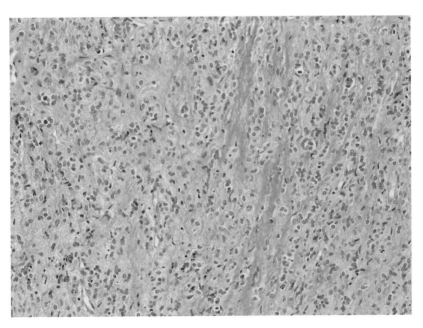

Fig. 5. Myoepithelioma of bone. H&E microphotograph showing an area in which the tumor is composed of epithelioid cells with monomorphic round nuclei with fine chromatin and inconspicuous nucleoli (H&E, original magnification, ×200).

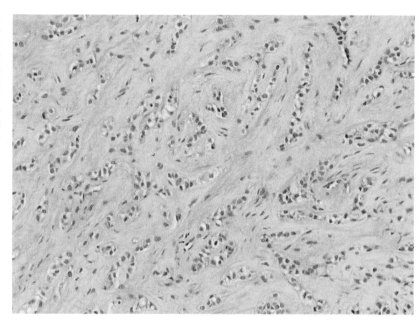

Fig. 6. Myoepithelioma of bone. H&E microphotograph showing an area in which the tumor is composed of clusters and cords of epithelioid tumor cells with clear and vacuolated cytoplasm. The tumor cells are embedded in myxohyaline stroma (H&E, original magnification, ×200).

POU5F1, PBX1, PBX3, and KLF17.[4,9,10,20] Additional fusion partners detected in soft tissue tumors are ZNF444 and ATF1.[10,21]

The molecular pathology of METs of bone and soft tissue is different from METs in salivary glands that lack EWSR1 fusion genes and often show PLAG1 rearrangements. Hence, despite morphologic overlap between these counterparts, METs in bone or soft tissue and salivary gland METs appear to be separate clinicopathological entities.

DIFFERENTIAL DIAGNOSIS

Given their rarity, occurrence in almost any bone, and variable histologic features, it is not surprising that the differential diagnosis of BMETs can be difficult and troubling. Moreover, in daily practice, needle bone biopsies taken for diagnostic histopathology of bone tumors may contain only a limited amount of tumor tissue. Therefore, IHC and molecular pathology are indispensable for an accurate diagnosis.

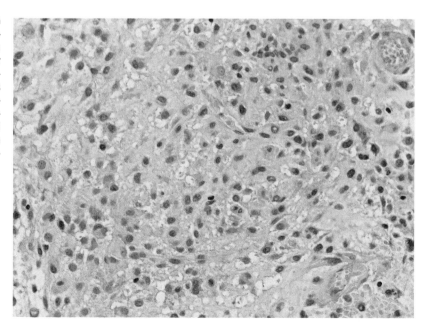

Fig. 7. Myoepithelioma of bone. H&E microphotograph showing an area in which the tumor is composed of plasmacytoid tumor cells with eccentric eosinophilic cytoplasm. The tumor cells are embedded in myxohyaline stroma (H&E, original magnification, ×200).

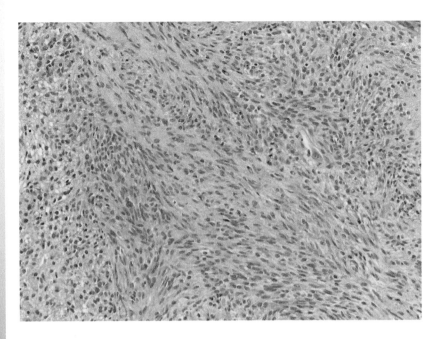

Fig. 8. Myoepithelioma of bone. H&E microphotograph illustrating that myoepithelioma may be predominantly composed of bundles of eosinophilic spindle cells, by which the tumor may be confused with a smooth muscle tumor (H&E, original magnification, ×200).

Herein, we focus on the differential diagnosis of METs presenting as bone tumors.

In the differential diagnosis, we consider the variable histologic appearance of BMETs and discuss bone tumors with relatively bland spindle cells and/or epithelioid cells that are embedded in a variable amount of fibrous, myxoid, or myxohyaline stroma.

Spindle cell bone tumors that enter the differential diagnosis of myoepithelioma are fibrous dysplasia, fibro-osseous dysplasia, desmoplastic fibroma, chondromyxoid fibroma, smooth muscle tumors, and myxoma of jawbones.

Fibrous dysplasia (FD) can present as a solitary nonaggressive and expansile bone lesion. FD often has a typical ground glass appearance on radiographs or CT images, whereas BMETs are lytic and radiolucent. Histologically, FD is easily discriminated from BMETs when areas of metaplastic woven bone are seen. However, needle

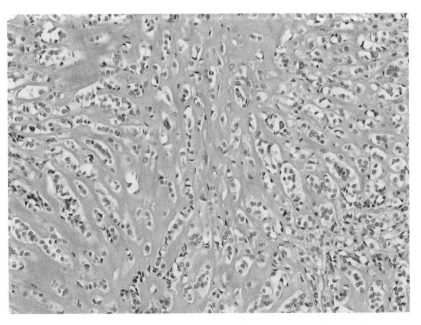

Fig. 9. Myoepithelioma of bone. H&E microphotograph showing an area in which the tumor is composed of hyaline stroma with radiating cords of cohesive tumor cells with eosinophilic and clear cytoplasm, by which the tumor may be confused with chordoma or extraskeletal myxoid chondrosarcoma (H&E, original magnification, ×200).

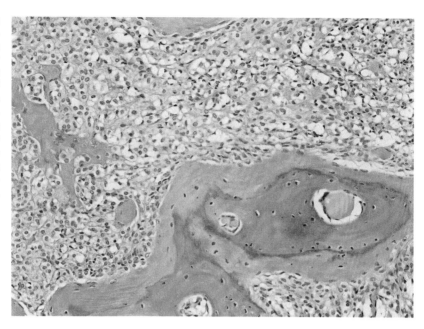

Fig. 10. Myoepithelioma of bone. H&E microphotograph showing an area in which the tumor invades bone marrow and is composed of tumor cells with eosinophilic and strongly vacuolated cytoplasm that is arranged in nests, by which the tumor may be confused with metastatic adenocarcinoma (H&E, original magnification, ×200).

biopsies may contain only the cellular component, woven bone being absent. The bland fibroblastic spindle cells in FD may be arranged in short storiform bundles, a growth pattern that is uncommon in BMETs. IHC expression of keratins and EMA does not occur in FD. Most FD lesions harbor GNAS1 gene mutations that may be detected by PCR, which is a very useful tool when confronted with diagnostically difficult cases.

Osteofibrous dysplasia (OFD) and the closely related OFD-like adamantinoma are bone tumors that predominantly occur in children. The typical location is the diaphysis of the tibia, with few cases presenting in the fibula. OFD and OFD-like

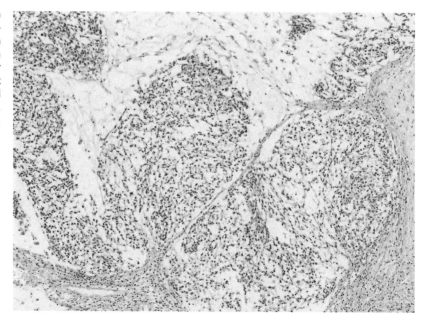

Fig. 11. Myoepithelioma of bone. H&E microphotograph, showing a myxoid area in which the tumor has a reticular architecture, reminiscent of extraskeletal myxoid chondrosarcoma (H&E, original magnification, ×100).

Fig. 12. Myoepithelioma of bone. H&E microphotograph showing an area in which the tumor has abundant fibrous stroma with spindle cells, by which the tumor may be confused with FD, fibro-osseous dysplasia, or DF (H&E, original magnification, ×50).

adamantinoma are intracortical lesions, clearly different from the intramedullary location of BMETs. Confusion may arise, however, because OFD and OFD-like adamantinoma contain single or grouped spindle cells that are positive for (basal type) cytokeratins and EMA. Importantly, IHC for S100, GFAP, and calponin is negative.

The clinical and radiologic presentation of desmoplastic fibroma (DF) and BMETs show much overlap, as both lesions may present as expansile, lytic lesions with cortical breakthrough. DF is most common in the mandible, but also may occur in other bones. Microscopically, DF is usually composed of bundles of fibroblastic spindle cells with tapering cytoplasm arranged in a collagenous stroma, by which the tumor resembles desmoid-type fibromatosis of soft tissue. Approximately half of DF cases show cytoplasmic staining for

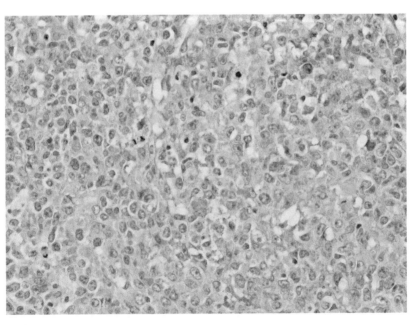

Fig. 13. Myoepithelial carcinoma. H&E microphotograph showing sheets of round tumor cells with hyperchromatic nuclei, prominent nucleoli, and mitotic activity (H&E, original magnification, ×200).

Fig. 14. Myoepithelioma of bone. IHC. Epithelioid areas are usually strongly positive for (*A*) cytokeratins and (*B*) EMA, whereas spindle cell areas show variable staining for (*C*) cytokeratins, (*D*) EMA, (*E*) S100, (*F*) calponin, and (*G*) SMA (H&E, original magnification, ×200).

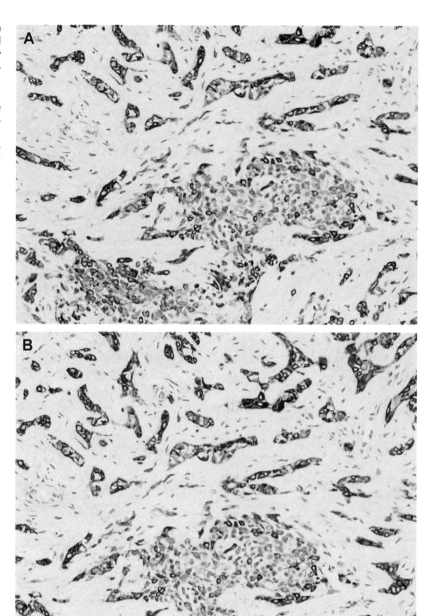

beta-catenin, whereas nuclear staining is seldom found. DF has no beta-catenin gene mutations. Moreover, DF lacks expression of the IHC markers and gene fusions typical of BMETs.

The clinical and radiologic presentation of chondromyxoid fibroma (CMF) and BMETs may mimic each other. Microscopically distinctive features of CMF are lobules of which central zones contain eosinophilic spindle and stellate cells in a myxoid background, whereas peripheral zones tend to be more cellular and harbor osteoclasts. CMF is often S100 positive, but lacks expression of cytokeratins, EMA, or GFAP.

The preferential sites of leiomyoma of bone are mandible and tibia. Well-differentiated leiomyosarcoma may present in the long tubular bones of the lower extremity but also in craniofacial bones. With imaging, leiomyoma and well-differentiated leiomyosarcoma are lytic lesions that may show cortical expansion. Microscopically, smooth

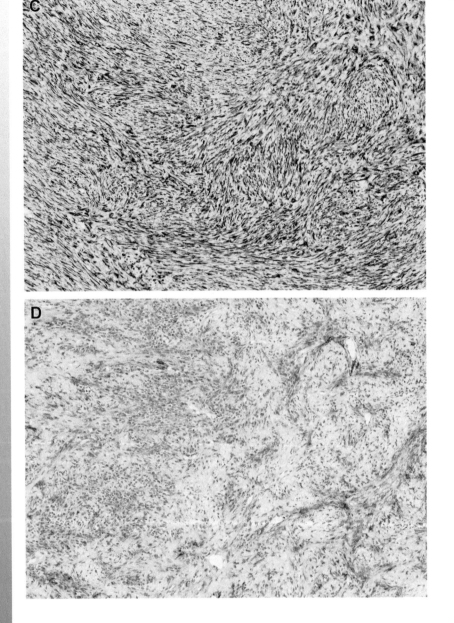

Fig. 14. (*continued*).

muscle tumors typically have interlacing bundles of eosinophilic spindle cells with elongated, hyperchromatic, cigar-shaped nuclei and well-defined eosinophilic cytoplasm. By IHC, smooth muscle tumors may express keratin, EMA, and calponin, but lack positivity for S100 or GFAP. Caldesmon and desmin are discriminatory markers of smooth muscle tumors. Given that primary smooth muscle tumors of bone are exceptionally rare, metastatic smooth muscle tumors should also be considered in the differential diagnosis. Metastatic gynecologic smooth muscle tumors show nuclear staining for hormone receptors.

Myxomas presenting in the mandible and maxilla, thought to be of odontogenic origin, are well-circumscribed lytic lesions and show a high T2-weighted signal by MRI. Histologically, myxomas of jawbones have abundant myxoid stroma containing bland stellate and spindle cells. BMETs may contain areas resembling myxoma, but

Fig. 14. (continued).

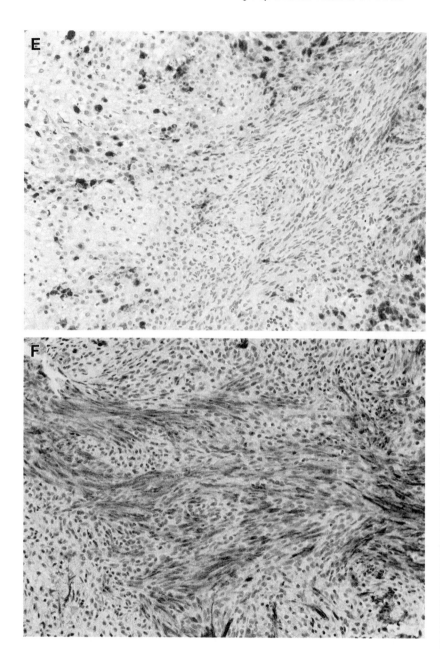

BMETs usually have a more variable histology and will stain for the IHC markers mentioned previously. Myxoma of jawbones does not have specific gene mutations or fusions (See Daniel Baumhoer's article, "Bone Related Lesions of the Jaws," in this issue).

Epithelioid tumors considered in the differential diagnosis of BMETs are chordoma, extraskeletal myxoid chondrosarcoma, sclerosing epithelioid fibrosarcoma, and epithelioid hemangioendothelioma.

Chordomas characteristically arise in the vertebral column, although rare extra-axial lesions also have been diagnosed.[17] Epithelioid areas in BMETs may show a striking resemblance to those seen in chordoma, hence the older term parachordoma for METs. However, usually, the tumor cells in chordomas are larger and more vacuolated than

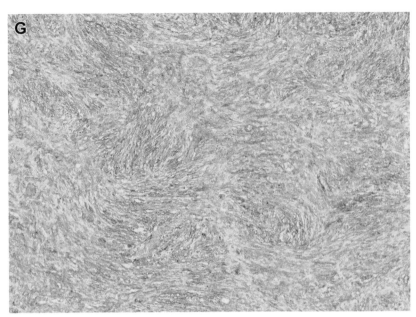

Fig. 14. (continued).

in BMETs. Both chordomas and BMETs express cytokeratins, EMA, and S100. Therefore, immunostaining for brachyury is required to diagnose chordoma (Fig. 17).[17]

Extraskeletal myxoid chondrosarcoma (EMC) is a distinct soft tissue sarcoma that may also show a striking resemblance to myoepithelioma. Although few cases have been described,[22] it is well appreciated that EMC also may present in bone. By IHC, EMC is often positive for S100 and EMA, but lacks cytokeratin expression. EMC often contains an NR4A3 fusion gene that allows a specific diagnosis. Importantly, EWSR1 is the most common fusion partner of NR4A3. Therefore, when using FISH, NR4A3 probes must be used instead of EWSR1 probes to distinguish between EMC and BMET.[23]

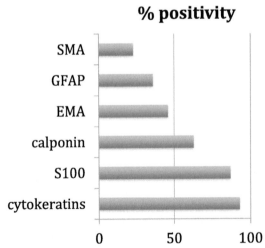

% positivity

Fig. 15. IHC markers for myoepithelial tumors. (*Data from* Hornick JL, Fletcher CD. Myoepithelial tumors of soft tissue: a clinicopathologic and immunohistochemical study of 101 cases with evaluation of prognostic parameters. Am J Surg Pathol 2003;27:1183–96.)

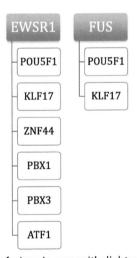

Fig. 16. Gene fusions in myoepithelial tumors.

Fig. 17. Extra-axial chordoma of the fifth metacarpal bone, originally diagnosed as parachordoma. (*A*) Plain radiograph showing a lytic and destructive tumor of the fifth metacarpal bone that invades surrounding soft tissue. (*B*) Gross specimen showing a glistening myxoid bone tumor that invades surrounding soft tissue.

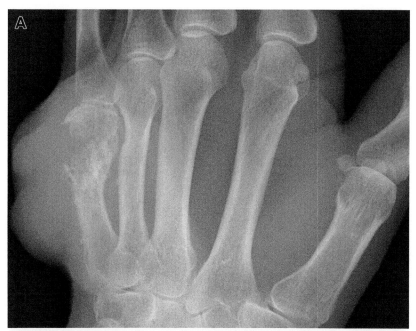

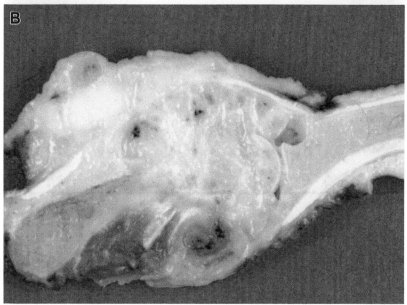

Sclerosing epithelioid fibrosarcoma (SEF) is a distinct soft tissue tumor that is related to low-grade fibromyxoid sarcoma (LGFMS). Rare cases of SEF have been described as primary bone tumors.[24] A case of SEF occurring in the distal femur is illustrated in Fig. 18. MUC4 immunostaining is very sensitive and specific for SEF and LGFMS. BMETs are negative for MUC4. SEF and LGFMS often have a gene fusion of either FUS or EWSR1

with CREBL1 or CREBL2. Thus, FISH for EWSR1 and FUS cannot be used to differentiate SEF from BMETs. RT-PCR or NGS can be applied for further confirmation of SEF by molecular pathology.

Epithelioid hemangioendothelioma (EHE) is an endothelial neoplasm composed of cords, nests, and strands of epithelioid endothelial cells arranged in myxohyaline stroma, by which it may

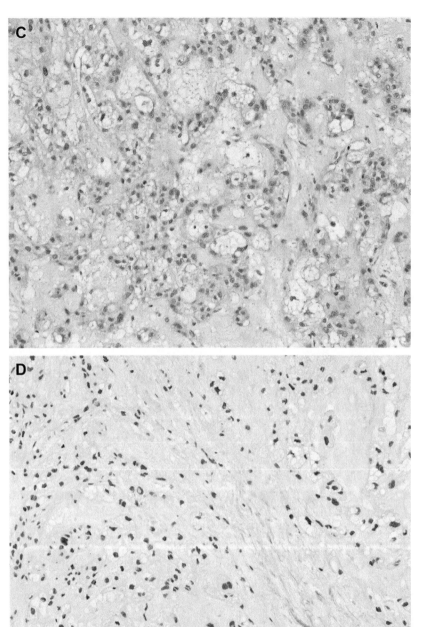

Fig. 17. (continued). (C) H and E microphotograph showing cords and nests with cohesive epithelioid tumor cells with strongly vacuolated (so-called physaliferous) cytoplasm. The tumor cells are embedded in myxohyaline stroma (H&E, original magnification, ×200). (D) IHC for brachyury showing nuclear staining of tumor cells (H&E, original magnification, ×200).

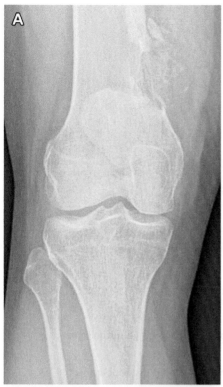

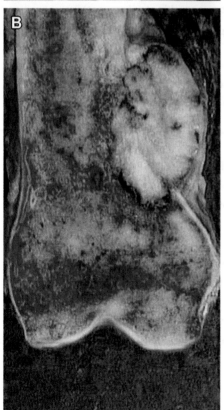

strongly resemble BMET. Bone locations of EHE include long and small tubular bones, vertebra, and jawbones.[25] The tumor cells of EHE often have vacuolated cytoplasm and may contain engulfed erythrocytes. EHE may express cytokeratins and EMA. However, IHC for endothelial markers (ERG, CD31, and CD34) will render a correct diagnosis. EHE has a consistent WWTR1-CAMTA1 fusion gene. An alternate YAP1-TFE3 fusion is present in a small subset of cases. For further details, see David G.P. van IJzendoorn and Judith V.M.G. Bovée's article, "Vascular Tumors of Bone: The Evolvement of a Classification Based on Molecular Developments," in this issue.

Understandably, myoepitheliomas with an epithelioid phenotype and cytoplasmic vacuolization or myoepithelial carcinomas showing clear-cut cytonuclear malignant features are easily confused with metastatic carcinoma. Hence, clinical evaluation and a panel of appropriate IHC markers for carcinomas that often metastasize to bone must be applied. Approximately 10% of myoepithelial carcinomas show loss of SMARCB1/INI1 in tumor cell nuclei by IHC.

Helpful distinguishing clinicopathological features of bone tumors mimicking BMETs are summarized in **Boxes 1** and **2**.

PROGNOSIS

Because of the rarity of METs in bone and limited follow-up of few published case series, it is as yet impossible to establish the prognostic value of cytologic features. It seems reasonable to adapt the criteria used for METs arising in soft tissue locations. Nuclear atypia and prominent nucleoli are currently considered to be the sole histologic features of (potential) malignant behavior. METs arising in soft tissue that show bland cytonuclear features usually have a good outcome, whereas METs with nuclear atypia and prominent nucleoli have metastatic potential.

Fig. 18. SEF of the distal femur. (*A*) Plain radiograph showing a lytic and destructive tumor of the distal femur that invades surrounding soft tissue. (*B*) Gross specimen showing a well-demarcated gray-white tumor that invades surrounding soft tissue. (*C*) H&E microphotograph showing cords of epithelioid tumor cells with clear cytoplasm surrounded by strands of hyalinized collagen (H&E, original magnification, ×100).

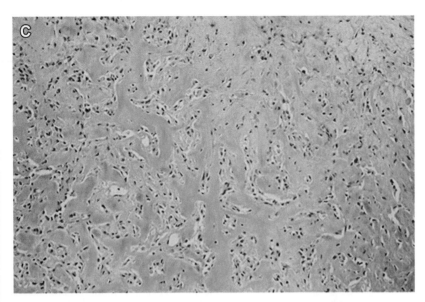

Fig. 18. (*continued*).

Box 1
Differential diagnosis of myoepithelioma

Helpful distinguishing features of spindle cell bone tumors resembling myoepithelioma

Fibrous dysplasia
- Imaging: nonaggressive, but often expansile lesion with ground glass appearance
- Histology: deposition of woven bone by spindle cells arranged in storiform pattern
- Immunohistochemistry (IHC): negative for keratins, epithelial membrane antigen (EMA), S100, glial fibrillary acidic protein (GFAP), and calponin
- Molecular pathology: 90% have GNAS1 mutations

Osteofibrous dysplasia (OFD) and OFD-like adamantinoma
- Epidemiology: predominantly presenting in children
- Imaging: cortical lesion in the diaphysis of the tibia
- Histology: deposition of woven bone by osteoblasts
- IHC: keratin/EMA-positive spindle cells are negative for S100, GFAP, and calponin

Desmoplastic fibroma
- Histology: collagen-rich bundles with fibroblasts, resembling desmoid fibromatosis
- IHC: negative for keratins, EMA, S100, and GFAP

Chondromyxoid fibroma
- Histology: lobular architecture with spindle and stellate cells in myxoid background
- IHC: S100 often positive, whereas keratins, EMA, and GFAP are negative

Leiomyoma and well-differentiated leiomyosarcoma
- Histology: interlacing bundles of smooth muscle cells with elongated nuclei
- IHC: caldesmon and desmin are positive in smooth muscle tumors, negative in bone myoepithelial tumors (BMETs)

Myxoma of jawbones
- Imaging: high T2-weighted signal on MRI
- Histology: abundant myxoid stroma with stellate tumor cells
- IHC: negative for keratins, EMA, S100, and GFAP

(*Continued*)

Box 1
Differential diagnosis of myoepithelioma (*continued*)

Helpful distinguishing features of epithelioid bone tumors resembling myoepithelioma

Chordoma

- Imaging: high T2-weighted signal on MRI
- Histology: large vacuolated (physaliferous) tumor cells
- IHC: chordoma is positive for the transcription factor brachyury

Extraskeletal myxoid chondrosarcoma

- IHC: EMC is keratin negative
- Molecular pathology: NR4A3 gene fusions (fluorescence in situ hybridization for EWSR1 does not help)

Sclerosing epithelioid fibrosarcoma

- IHC: MUC4 is a sensitive and specific marker
- Molecular pathology: FUS or EWSR1 gene fusions with CREBL1 or CREBL2

Epithelioid hemangioendothelioma

Histology: few vacuolated tumor cells have engulfed erythrocytes

IHC: tumor cells are positive for endothelial markers: ERG, CD31, and CD34

Molecular pathology: WWTR1-CAMTA1 fusion gene. A YAP1-TFE3 fusion is found in a small subset of epithelioid hemangioendothelioma cases

---

Box 2
Pathologic Key Features

Myoepithelioma of bone

- May arise in many different bones, including long and small tubular bones, the axial skeleton, and craniofacial bones
- Has a wide age range, but is rare in the elderly
- Has a variable histology, often with spindled and/or epithelioid cells in a variable amount of fibrous and myxohyaline stroma
- In addition to morphology, expression of cytokeratin/EMA with either S100 or GFAP, or calponin is required for an appropriate diagnosis
- Nearly half of the tumors harbor EWSR1 (or rare FUS) gene fusion with different partners
- Myoepithelial carcinoma shows cytonuclear atypia and prominent nucleoli and sometimes consists of sheets of undifferentiated round epithelioid cells

---

Key Features

- Myoepithelial tumors (METs) of bone (BMETs) are a rare but distinct tumor entity.
- METs that are cytologically benign are termed myoepitheliomas, whereas METs with malignant histologic features are called myoepithelial carcinomas.
- BMETs have a wide age range, may involve any part of the skeleton, and have a variable spindle cell and epithelioid morphology.

REFERENCES

1. Alberghini M, Pasquinelli G, Zanella L, et al. Primary malignant myoepithelioma of the distal femur. APMIS 2007;115:376–80.
2. Biradar P, Menon S, Patil A, et al. Primary myoepithelial carcinoma of rib bone: morphology, immunohistochemical evaluation and diagnostic dilemma in an unusual case. J Cancer Res Ther 2015;11:647.
3. Cuesta Gil M, Bucci T, Navarro Cuellar C, et al. Intraosseous myoepithelioma of the maxilla: clinicopathologic features and therapeutic considerations. J Oral Maxillofac Surg 2008;66:800–3.
4. Antonescu CR, Zhang L, Chang NE, et al. EWSR1-POU5F1 fusion in soft tissue myoepithelial tumours. A molecular analysis of sixty-six cases, including soft tissue, bone, and visceral lesions, showing common involvement of the EWSR1 gene. Genes Chromosomes Cancer 2010;49:1114–24.
5. Park JS, Ryu KN, Han CS, et al. Malignant myoepithelioma of the humerus with satellite lesion: a case report and literature review. Br J Radiol 2010; 83:161–4.
6. Rekhi B, Amare P, Gulia A, et al. Primary intraosseous myoepithelioma arising in the iliac bone and displaying trisomies of 11, 15, 17 with del (16q) and del (22q11)–a rare case report with review of literature. Pathol Res Pract 2011;207:780–5.
7. Kurzawa P, Kattapuram S, Hornicek FJ, et al. Primary myoepithelioma of bone: a report of 8 cases. Am J Surg Pathol 2013;37:960–8.
8. Franchi A, Palomba A, Roselli G, et al. Primary juxtacortical myoepithelioma/mixed tumour of the bone: a report of 3 cases with clinicopathologic, immunohistochemical, ultrastructural, and molecular characterization. Hum Pathol 2013;44:566–77.
9. Puls F, Arbajian E, Magnusson L, et al. Myoepithelioma of bone with a novel FUS-POU5F1 fusion gene. Histopathology 2014;65:917–22.
10. Huang SC, Chen HW, Zhang L, et al. Novel FUS-KLF17 and EWSR1-KLF17 fusions in myoepithelial tumors. Genes Chromosomes Cancer 2015;54:267–75.
11. Nambirajan A, Mridha AR, Sharma MC, et al. Primary intra-osseous myoepithelioma of phalanx mimicking an enchondroma. Skeletal Radiol 2016;4:1453–8.
12. Rekhi B, Joshi S, Panchwagh Y, et al. Clinicopathological features of five unusual cases of intraosseous myoepithelial carcinomas, mimicking conventional primary bone tumours, including EWSR1 rearrangement in one case. APMIS 2016;124:278–90.
13. Kilpatrick SE, Hitchcock MG, Kraus MD, et al. Mixed tumors and myoepitheliomas of soft tissue: a clinicopathologic study of 19 cases with a unifying concept. Am J Surg Pathol 1997;21:13–22.
14. Hornick JL, Fletcher CD. Myoepithelial tumours of soft tissue: a clinicopathologic and immunohistochemical study of 101 cases with evaluation of prognostic parameters. Am J Surg Pathol 2003;27:1183–96.
15. Gleason BC, Fletcher CD. Myoepithelial carcinoma of soft tissue in children: an aggressive neoplasm analyzed in a series of 29 cases. Am J Surg Pathol 2007;31:1813–24.
16. Kilpatrick SE, Limon J. Mixed tumor/myoepithelioma/parachordoma. In: Fletcher CDM, Unni K, Mertens F, editors. World Health Organization classification of tumours. Tumours of soft tissue and bone. Lyon (France): IARC; 2002. p. 198–9.
17. Tirabosco R, Mangham DC, Rosenberg AE, et al. Brachyury expression in extra-axial skeletal and soft tissue chordomas: a marker that distinguishes chordoma from mixed tumor/myoepithelioma/parachordoma in soft tissue. Am J Surg Pathol 2008;32:572–80.
18. Chitturi RT, Veeravarmal V, Nirmal RM, et al. Myoepithelial cells (MEC) of the salivary glands in health and tumours. J Clin Diagn Res 2015;9:14–8.
19. Miettinen M, McCue PA, Sarlomo-Rikala M, et al. Sox10-a marker for not only schwannian and melanocytic neoplasms but also myoepithelial cell tumors of soft tissue: a systematic analysis of 5134 tumors. Am J Surg Pathol 2015;39:826–35.
20. Agaram NP, Chen HW, Zhang L, et al. EWSR1-PBX3: a novel gene fusion in myoepithelial tumors. Genes Chromosomes Cancer 2015;54:63–71.
21. Flucke U, Mentzel T, Verdijk MA, et al. EWSR1-ATF1 chimeric transcript in a myoepithelial tumor of soft tissue: a case report. Hum Pathol 2012;43:764–8.
22. Demicco EG, Wang WL, Madewell JE, et al. Osseous myxochondroid sarcoma: a detailed study of 5 cases of extraskeletal myxoid chondrosarcoma of the bone. Am J Surg Pathol 2013;37:752–62.
23. Flucke U, Tops BB, Verdijk MA, et al. NR4A3 rearrangement reliably distinguishes between the clinicopathologically overlapping entities myoepithelial carcinoma of soft tissue and cellular extraskeletal myxoid chondrosarcoma. Virchows Arch 2012;460:621–8.
24. Wojcik JB, Bellizzi AM, Dal Cin P, et al. Primary sclerosing epithelioid fibrosarcoma of bone: analysis of a series. Am J Surg Pathol 2014;38:1538–44.
25. Flucke U, Vogels RJ, de Saint Aubain Somerhausen N, et al. Epithelioid hemangioendothelioma: clinicopathologic, immunohistochemical, and molecular genetic analysis of 39 cases. Diagn Pathol 2014;9:131.

Hematopoietic Tumors Primarily Presenting in Bone

Arjen H.G. Cleven, MD, PhD*,
Pancras C.W. Hogendoorn, MD, PhD

KEYWORDS

• Plasma cell myeloma • Lymphoma of bone • Langerhans cell histiocytosis

---

Key points

- Plasma cell myeloma cells typically secrete a monoclonal immunoglobulin.
- The clinical and pathologic features of primary lymphoma of bone overlap with osteomyelitis, Langerhans cell histiocytosis, and other malignant tumors.
- Diagnosing acute lymphoblastic leukemia/lymphoma requires the integration of aspirate and flow cytometry findings.
- *BRAF* mutations are a frequent finding in Langerhans cell histiocytosis.

ABSTRACT

Hematologic neoplasms that primarily present in bone are rare; this article describes the most common examples of hematologic tumors primarily presenting in bone, including plasma cell myeloma, solitary plasmacytoma of bone, primary non-Hodgkin lymphoma of bone, acute lymphoblastic leukemia/lymphoma, and Langerhans cell histiocytosis. The macroscopic and microscopic features, differential diagnosis, diagnostic workup, and prognosis of all these different entities are discussed, with special emphasis on common differential diagnosis.

may overlap between primary malignant hematologic tumors in bone and other malignant tumors as well as benign proliferations, a final diagnosis in bone lesions can be challenging. Therefore, in the diagnostic workup, it is important to correlate clinical features with morphology, immunohistochemistry, and sometimes additional molecular analysis for a definitive diagnosis. Most malignant hematopoietic tumors primarily presenting in the bone are treated with systemic chemotherapy, with a relatively good prognosis compared with their nodal counterparts in case of DLBCL.

OVERVIEW

Plasma cell myeloma is the most common primary malignant bone neoplasm and diffuse large B-cell lymphoma (DLBCL) is the most frequent type of non-Hodgkin lymphoma primarily presenting in bone. Because clinical and morphologic features

PLASMA CELL MYELOMA

Plasma cell myeloma is a plasma cell-based neoplasm composed of a clone of immunoglobulin-secreting, terminally differentiated B cells that typically secrete a monoclonal immunoglobulin.[1,2] Plasma cell myeloma is defined as a bone-marrow–based, multifocal plasma cell neoplasm associated with M protein in serum and or urine.[3]

Conflict of Interest: All authors declare that they have no conflict of interest.
Department of Pathology, Leiden University Medical Center, PO Box 9600, L1-Q, Leiden 2300 RC, The Netherlands
* Corresponding author.
E-mail address: a.h.g.cleven@lumc.nl

Surgical Pathology 10 (2017) 675–691
http://dx.doi.org/10.1016/j.path.2017.04.011

surgpath.theclinics.com

Plasma cell myeloma is the most common primary malignant bone neoplasm with a median age at diagnosis of 70 years and males being affected more frequently than females.[1,3] The thoracic vertebrae, ribs, skull, pelvis, femur, clavicle, and scapula are most commonly involved.[3] Most patients have pain or a pathologic fracture at first presentation.

Disease progression from normal plasma cell to plasma cell myeloma includes several steps of disease. Translocations in 14q32 and deletion of chromosomal 13 transform normal plasma cells into monoclonal neoplastic cells, which give rise to an early stage of disease, named 'monoclonal gammopathy of unknown significance' (MGUS). Additional oncogenic events such as N-RAS, K-RAS, and TP53 mutations, inactivation of p16 via methylation, MYC dysregulation by complex chromosomal abnormalities, and nuclear factor-kappa Beta pathway activating mutations result in further progression of the disease and manifestation of plasma cell myeloma.[4,5]

Key Features
PLASMA CELL MYELOMA

- Most common primary malignant neoplasm presenting in bone
- Neoplastic plasma cells secrete a monoclonal immunoglobulin
- CD138 positive

Pitfalls
PLASMA CELL MYELOMA

! Carcinomas are frequently confusingly positive by immunohistochemistry for the plasma cell marker CD138

! Plasma cell myeloma may be positive for epithelial membrane antigen

RADIOLOGIC AND GROSS FEATURES

Radiographic findings in plasma cell myeloma include lytic bone lesions centered in the bone marrow without identifiable matrix and approximately 44% show a multiloculated appearance (Fig. 1).[6] Plasma cell myeloma localizations in the long bones are usually well-circumscribed and may be encompassed by periosteal new bone formation, giving the appearance of expansion

and only rarely plasma cell myeloma generates sclerotic lesions.[6] In case of a pathologic fracture followed by surgery, gross specimen of the involved bone will show a friable, soft, and red appearance in which the underlying bone is eroded or fragile.[6]

MICROSCOPY

The morphology of plasma cell myeloma may vary from sheets of easily recognizable plasma cells to only scattered clusters of plasma cells to a highly pleomorphic malignant or blastoid type of morphology in which the plasma cell origin of the tumor cells is not recognized at first glance (Fig. 2A, C).

Mature-looking plasma cells show an eccentric nucleus with "spoke wheel" or "clock-face" chromatin without nucleoli and basophilic cytoplasm and perinuclear hof. The more immature plasmablasts-type of cells have a more dispersed nuclear chromatin, higher nuclear:cytoplasmic ratio, and often prominent nucleoli (see Fig. 2A). Nuclear immaturity and pleomorphism rarely occur in reactive plasma cells and are reliable indicators of neoplastic plasma cell myeloma (see Fig. 2C). Cytoplasmic Ig may produce a variety of morphologically distinctive findings like round eosinophilic bodies named Russell bodies in the cytoplasm or round eosinophilic bodies called Dutcher bodies in the nucleus (see Fig. 2C).

DIFFERENTIAL DIAGNOSIS

The most common differential diagnosis among plasma cell neoplasms is early myeloma versus monoclonal gammopathy of undetermined significance (MGUS) or reactive plasma cells in conditions such a chronic osteomyelitis. Normally, this differential diagnosis is not difficult for a pathologist, because clinical and pathologic findings such as lytic bone lesions and myeloma-related symptoms required for the diagnosis of plasma cell myeloma are lacking in MGUS or reactive plasma cell conditions.

Plasma cells of plasma cell myeloma can look like reactive plasma cells, which is a common finding in chronic osteomyelitis, but restriction for lambda or kappa light chain by performing immunohistochemistry is only observed in plasma cell myeloma and not in osteomyelitis. Furthermore, MGUS shows typical normal looking plasma cells in bone marrow with only a mild increase of clonal plasma cells of less than 10%.

Metastasis of poorly differentiated carcinoma to the bone can show overlapping morphologic features with the more pleomorphic type of plasma cell myeloma. Because both entities are CD138

Fig. 1. Plasma cell myeloma. Radiograph shows multiple osteolytic lesions in the ramus superior of the os pubis a large osteolytic lesion is present with cortical destruction (*black arrow*). Radiologic differential diagnosis includes plasma cell myeloma, lymphoma, or metastasis of unknown primary tumor.

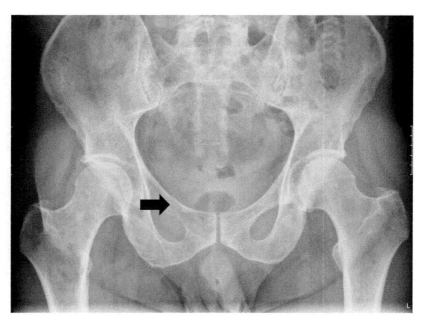

positive, additional pan-keratin stainings are mandatory to rule out poorly differentiated carcinoma. Additionally, poorly differentiated carcinomas do not show restriction for either kappa or lambda light chain immunohistochemistry. Epithelial membrane antigen may be positive in plasma cells and, thus, plasma cell myeloma as well.

In general, lymphoma primary of the bone (see also next paragraph) shows pleomorphic tumor cells mimicking the pleomorphic variant of plasma cell myeloma. CD20, PAX5 and CD79a (pan-B-lymphocyte markers) are strongly positive in B-cell lymphomas with negative staining for CD138

in contrast with strong positivity of CD138 in plasma cell myeloma. Plasma cell myeloma may show weak focal CD20 expression and strong CD79a expression, but PAX5 is generally not detected in plasma cell myeloma. Furthermore, plasma cell myeloma may be positive for CD56, MYC, and cyclin D1, which is also detectable in several other B-cell lymphomas.

Metastasis of melanoma can show overlapping morphology with the more blastoid or pleomorphic variants of plasma cell myeloma, but CD138 is negative and S100, Melan A, and HMB45 melanocytic markers are positive in most melanomas.

△△ Differential Diagnosis
OF PLASMA CELL MYELOMA

Plasma Cell Myeloma vs	Helpful Distinguishing Features
Chronic osteomyelitis	• Plasma cells in chronic osteomyelitis are polyclonal
MGUS	• Typical normal looking plasma cells
	• <10% clonal plasma cells
Poorly differentiated carcinoma	• Pan-keratin positive
	• No kappa or lambda light chain restriction
	• CD20 negative
Non-Hodgkin lymphoma	• Centroblastic or immunoblastic morphology
	• CD20$^+$, PAX5$^+$, CD138$^-$
	• BCL2/BCL6/MYC fluorescence in situ hybridization (FISH) dependent on lymphoma subtype may be positive
Melanoma	• S100$^+$, Melan A$^+$, HMB45$^+$, CD138$^-$

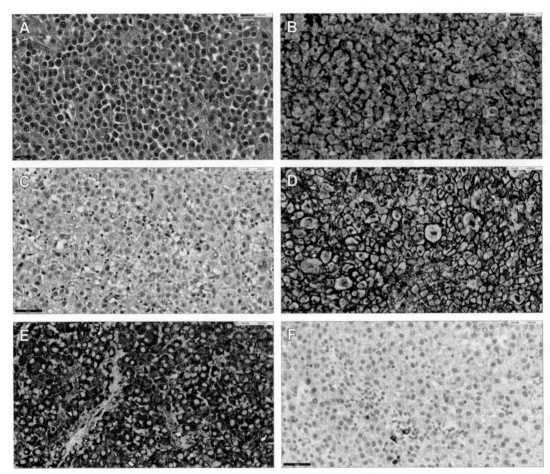

Fig. 2. Plasma cell myeloma in bone marrow biopsies. (*A*) Relatively uniform plasma cells with eccentrically located nuclei. Many nuclei contain a prominent centrally located brightly eosinophilic nucleolus. (*B*) Strong diffuse staining of CD138 in neoplastic plasma cells. (*C*) Neoplastic plasma cells with more pleomorphic morphology. (*D*) Strong diffuse staining of CD138 in pleomorphic plasma cells. (*E*) Restriction for kappa light chain in pleomorphic plasma cells. (*F*) Negative staining for lambda light chain in pleomorphic plasma cells. (*A, B, black bar* indicates 20 μm; *C–F, black bar* indicate 50 μm).

DIAGNOSIS

Plasma cells may be difficult to recognize and quantify in suboptimal biopsy material and when they are distributed interstitially in the bone marrow. Stains for plasma cell-associated antigens (CD138, CD38, CD79a, kappa, and lambda) usually stain plasma cells strongly on biopsy material, allowing an easy quantification for the pathologist (see *Fig.* 2B, D). Kappa and lambda light chain immunohistochemistry are useful in determining monoclonality in malignant plasma cell proliferations and differentiating them from reactive polyclonal plasma cells. Both plasma cells in reactive conditions as well as in plasma cell myeloma are rich in cytoplasmic immunoglobulin and stain strongly for antibodies to kappa or lambda light chains. In case of plasma cell myeloma, the neoplastic plasma cells express a monoclonal pattern of light chains reactivity (see *Fig.* 2E, F). In reactive plasma cells, there is a polyclonal pattern of reactivity, usually with a moderate predominance of kappa. CD138 is detected in 70% to 100% of plasma cell myeloma and seems to be specific for plasma cells; however, other B-cell disorders such as plasmablastic B-cell lymphoma may react with some CD138 antibodies. CD79a is positive in plasma cells and most cases of plasma cell myeloma, but is a pan-B-lymphocyte marker and therefore only useful to distinguish plasma cell myeloma from non–B-cell–type hematopoietic neoplasms and metastatic tumors. Furthermore, CD56 and cyclin D1 may be expressed in neoplastic plasma cells.

Molecular analyses are not part of the routine diagnostic workup for plasma cell myeloma, but both numerical and structural chromosomal abnormalities are common and chromosome translocations are observed in approximately 70% of cases involving the heavy chain locus on chromosome 14q32.[7] Furthermore, activating mutations are found in K-RAS and N-RAS in about 40% to 70% of cases.[7]

PROGNOSIS

Survival is closely related to the clinical stage of disease at the time of diagnosis. The most critical criterion for treating plasma cell myeloma is evidence of organ or tissue impairment manifested by anemia, hypercalcemia, lytic bone lesions, renal insufficiency, hyperviscosity, amyloidosis, or recurrent infection.

Plasma cell myeloma is incurable and treated with a combination of chemotherapy and radiation, with survival ranging from 6 months to more than 10 years. Standard chemotherapy regimens have improved median survival to approximately 30 to 36 months from diagnosis in patients with plasma cell myeloma. Thus, in most cases plasma cell myeloma is a progressive disease that infrequently enters complete remission, except after marrow transplantation.

Patients with karyotypic abnormalities on conventional cytogenetic studies have a significantly poorer prognosis than those without; deletion of chromosome 13, aneuploidy, or deletion of 17p13 are factors for an unfavorable prognosis.[6]

SOLITARY PLASMACYTOMA OF BONE

Solitary plasmacytoma of bone (SPB) is, similar to plasma cell myeloma, a plasma cell-based neoplasm composed of a clone of immunoglobulin-secreting, terminally differentiated B cells that typically secrete a monoclonal immunoglobulin.[1,2] SPB occurs in younger patients compared with plasma cell myeloma and is characterized by a single focus of bone destruction owing to clonal plasma cells and absence of systemic manifestations with little or no M-protein in serum or urine and no end-organ damage other than solitary osseous lesions.[3] The vertebra is the most frequent involved bone by SPB.

RADIOLOGY

Compared with plasma cell myeloma, which predominantly shows diffuse osteopenia with more ill-defined lytic lesions, SPB tends to be a more punched-out lytic lesion in a single bone.[6]

MICROSCOPY

The morphology of SPB is identical to plasma cell myeloma with typically easily recognizable plasma cells, although less often pleomorphic neoplastic plasma cells are seen (see Fig. 2A, C). Like plasma cell myeloma, within SPB the neoplastic plasma cells may harbor round eosinophilic bodies 'Russell bodies' in the cytoplasm or round eosinophilic bodies 'Dutcher bodies' in the nucleus that indicate the cell of origin.

DIFFERENTIAL DIAGNOSIS

The most important differential diagnosis of SPB is primary bone lymphoma and a combination of CD20, BCL6, CD138, kappa, and lambda easily differentiate between these entities, in which CD138+ with light chain restriction and a negative CD20 and BCL6 favors SPB. In case of a more polymorphic morphology, which occurs infrequently, the same workup should be followed as was outlined in the differential diagnosis of plasma cell myeloma.

DIAGNOSIS

For the diagnosis of SPB, in addition to the use of plasma cell-associated antigens (CD138, CD38, CD79a, kappa, and lambda), radiologic correlation is important to rule out systemic disease. Molecular analyses are not part of the routine diagnostic workup for SPB.

PROGNOSIS

SPB is treated with resection or radiation and one-third of patients remain disease free for more than 10 years. However, two-thirds eventually evolve to generalized myeloma that is incurable and treated with a combination of chemotherapy and radiation, with survival ranging from 6 months to more than 10 years.

PRIMARY NON-HODGKIN LYMPHOMA OF THE BONE

According to the World Health Organization (WHO), primary lymphoma of bone is defined as a neoplasm composed of malignant lymphoid cells, producing 1 or more masses within bone, without any supraregional lymph node involvement or other extranodal lesions.[3] Lymphoma primary of the bone is not a common disease, comprising approximately 7% of all malignant bone tumors, 5% of all extranodal lymphomas, and less than 1% of all non-Hodgkin lymphomas.[8] In contrast, primary nodal lymphomas frequently involve the skeletal system, with bone involvement seen in 16% to 20% of patients.[8] Approximately 50% of the patients with primary lymphoma of bone are older than 40 years, with only a minority arising in children.[8,9]

Primary bone lymphomas frequently occur in the femur followed by the pelvis, vertebrae, and humerus, usually arising in the metadiaphyseal region of the bone.[3] Approximately 10% to 40% of cases are multifocal, producing several lesions in 1 bone or involving multiple bones concurrently (polyostotic).[6]

The majority of primary bone lymphomas are DLBCL, only rarely follicular B-cell lymphoma, marginal zone B-cell lymphoma, Hodgkin lymphoma, anaplastic large T-cell lymphoma, or other T-cell lymphomas can originate primarily within the bone.[3]

At least one-half of the cases of DLBCL of bone exhibit a germinal center B-cell phenotype and a substantial number of cases a nongerminal center B-cell/activated B-cell phenotype,[10–12] in which the latter type of lymphoma harbors a poorer survival.[12] In primary lymphoma of the bone, gain of 1q and amplification of 2p16.1 and loss of 14q32.33 is frequently found,[10] proving that primary lymphoma of bone should be considered as a distinct entity from extranodal lymphomas.

RADIOLOGIC AND GROSS FEATURES

On radiologic imaging, primary lymphomas of bone show large, lytic, and destructive tumors that may erode the bone cortex or extend into the adjacent soft tissue (Fig. 3).[6] Bone margins are often "moth eaten" or permeative, and an onion skin periosteal reaction may be present.[6] In some cases, the tumor may elicit extensive medullary sclerosis. Occasionally, findings on plain radiography are minimal with abnormalities only recognized on bone scan, computed tomography or MRI. However, on MRI 31% of patient with primary lymphoma of bone showed an intraosseous tumor, with linear cortical signal abnormalities or even normal-appearing or thickened cortical bone without any soft tissue mass, reflecting a less-aggressive appearance.[13]

It is unusual to see gross specimens of primary bone lymphomas because the diagnosis is made on biopsy material and treatment consists of

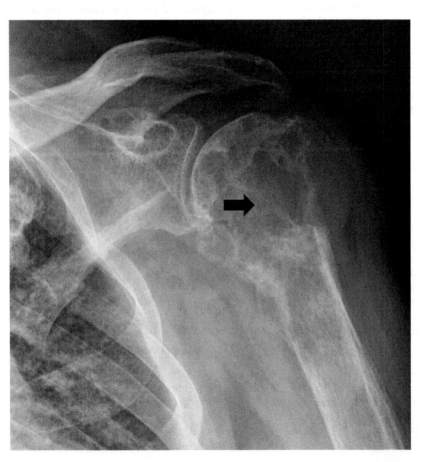

Fig. 3. Primary diffuse large B-cell lymphoma of bone. Radiograph shows a lytic destructive tumor in the proximal left humerus (black arrow) with cortical destruction and extension into the soft tissue. Radiologic differential diagnosis includes lymphoma, plasma cell myeloma or metastasis of unknown primary origin.

chemotherapy and radiotherapy without surgery. If available, macroscopy shows a gray-white and fleshy tumor in the bone, frequently with areas of necrosis.

MICROSCOPY

The histopathology of primary bone lymphomas exhibits the same features as nodal lymphomas, with DLBCL the most common type by far in both adults and children. In the majority of cases, the lymphoma shows a diffuse growth pattern with tumor cells infiltrating between the bone trabeculae and medullary fat. Most cases of DLBCL have a pleomorphic appearance (Fig. 4A) with prominent fibrosis and reactive osteoid (see Fig. 4B), with only a few cases showing an immunoblastic appearance. Pleomorphic B cells in DLBCL show large and irregular nuclei with a

cleaved, multilobulated appearance and prominent nucleoli (see Fig. 4A). Cytoplasm may be amphophilic, but is not abundantly present. Frequently, the tumor cells of DLBCL are crushed, which is a histologic finding that should raise the possibility of a lymphoma (see Fig. 4C).

In between the tumor cells, reticulin fibers are present that can give rise to thick fibrous bands and subsequently spindle cell changes in the tumor cells mimicking sarcoma (see Fig. 4D). An associated infiltrate of reactive, nonneoplastic lymphocytes can be a very prominent finding obscuring the malignant lesional cells.

Anaplastic large cell lymphoma in bone is very rare, but represents the most common primary T-cell lymphoma of bone. It has the characteristic features of its nodal counterpart including large cells with irregular nuclei and the hallmark cells with eccentric kidney-shaped nuclei.

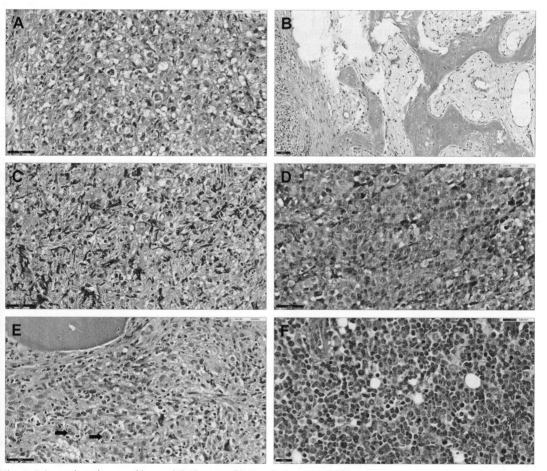

Fig. 4. Primary lymphoma of bone. (A) Pleomorphic B cells in case of diffuse large B-cell lymphoma (DLBCL) with large and irregular nuclei with a cleaved, multilobulated appearance and prominent nucleoli. (B) DLBCL with prominent fibrosis and reactive osteoid. (C) Frequently, tumor cells of DLBCL are crushed. (D) Spindle cell changes in the tumor cells of DLBCL. (E) Classical Reed Sternberg cells in Hodgkin lymphoma (*black arrow*). (F) Leukemic infiltrates in acute lymphoblastic leukemia. (A–F, *black bar*, 50 μm).

Classical Hodgkin lymphoma primarily arising in bone is very uncommon. If classical Reed Sternberg cells with a typical Hodgkin lymphoma immunophenotype (CD30$^+$, CD15$^+$, CD20$^-$) are present in the bone, this likely reflects extranodal localization of a primarily nodal Hodgkin lymphoma, because this can be seen in one-third of classical Hodgkin patients (see Fig. 4E).

DIFFERENTIAL DIAGNOSIS

The clinical and pathologic features of primary lymphoma of bone can overlap with reactive lesions like osteomyelitis or Langerhans cell histiocytosis (LCH), as well as other malignant tumors primary or secondary presenting in bone including osteosarcoma, Ewing sarcoma, carcinoma, or leukemia. By using a broad panel of immunohistochemical markers, a pathologist should not have great difficulties in most cases to differentiate between these entities. However, cases with poor representative biopsy material or abundant reactive lymphocytes, sclerosis, and spindle cell changes mimicking, for example, osteosarcoma or undifferentiated pleomorphic sarcoma, can be challenging.

When biopsy material is representative, and when immunohistochemistry for CD20 and PAX5 fails to demonstrate atypical large B cells, morphology with edematous stroma and a reactive infiltrate may indeed reflect chronic osteomyelitis. With these morphologic and immunohistochemical findings, a pathologist may favor chronic osteomyelitis, but only if clinical features (age, location) are appropriate. Likewise, LCH can be easily ruled out on representative biopsy material, by negative CD1a, Langerin, and S100 immunohistochemistry.

In contrast, the presence of large, atypical, pleomorphic cells or even monotonous large tumor cells may fit with the diagnosis of primary lymphoma of bone, metastasis, or other round cell tumors like Ewing sarcoma. When the patient is older than 50 years, metastasis from a primary carcinoma is a serious differential diagnosis, as is Ewing sarcoma in a young patient. Using an immunohistochemical panel including keratin AE1/AE3, CD20, PAX5, CD3, and CD4, a pathologist is able to differentiate between lymphoma or carcinoma. In case of a carcinoma (keratin positive, lymphoma markers negative), additional markers to determine the primary origin of carcinoma should be performed. In case of lymphoma, one should perform more markers to subclassify according to the WHO classification of lymphomas (see also Diagnosis). If this screening panel is negative, one should perform more keratin stainings to rule out poorly differentiated carcinoma, or stain for melanoma or other less frequent but malignant tumors than can present in bone such as rhabdomyosaroma (Desmin$^+$, MYF4$^+$) or germ cell tumors (PLAP$^+$, CD30$^+$).

Regarding the differential diagnosis of lymphoma with other primary malignant bone tumors such as osteosarcoma or Ewing sarcoma, by using an appropriate panel of immunohistochemical markers a pathologist should be able to distinguish these entities. Although primary lymphoma of bone can be accompanied with extensive sclerosis and spindle cell changes that reminds one of osteosarcoma, strong positive staining for CD20 and PAX5 rule out osteosarcoma. Important to be aware of is that Epstein-Barr virus–positive large B-cell lymphomas can be negative for

△△ **Differential Diagnosis**
OF PRIMARY LYMPHOMA OF BONE

PLB vs	Helpful Distinguishing Features
Chronic osteomyelitis	• No atypical large lymphoid cells
	• More T-cell than B-cell infiltrate
	• CD20 and PAX5 do not show sheets of atypical cells
LCH	• Intermixed with eosinophils
	• CD1A$^+$, Langerin$^+$, S100$^+$
	• BRAF V600 E
Carcinoma	• At least 1 pan keratin marker is positive, only focal weak CD20 or PAX5
Osteosarcoma	• Tumor osteoid produced by tumor cells
	• No strong staining for CD20 or PAX5
Ewing sarcoma	• *EWSR1* translocation in most Ewing sarcomas

CD20 but retain PAX5. For this reason it is mandatory to perform more than just 1 pan–B-cell marker.

Ewing sarcoma and lymphoma can share similar morphology and both are positive for CD99. However, Ewing sarcomas are unlikely to show expression of CD20, PAX5, BCL2, and BCL6, which is the most frequent profile found in large B-cell lymphomas. Demonstration of rearrangement of *EWSR1* is an additional tool to rule out lymphoma. Immunohistochemistry for FLI1 is not useful, because overexpression of *FLI1* can be detected in more than 20% of DLBCLs.[14] Of note, a minority of round cell sarcomas, so-called Ewing-like sarcomas show weaker heterogenous CD99 staining and rather than *EWSR1* involved translocation, harbor *BCOR, CIC,* or *NFATc2* involved translocations.[15–19] Furthermore some of the Ewing-like sarcomas, have profound reactive B-cell and T-cell infiltrate obscuring the neoplastic lesional cells.

Key Features
PRIMARY LYMPHOMA OF BONE

- 7% of all malignant bone tumors
- 50% of patients older than 40 years
- Frequently occurring in the femur
- Majority of primary bone lymphomas are DLBCLs

Pitfalls
PRIMARY LYMPHOMA OF BONE

! Spindle cell changes and sclerosis in malignant B cells may mimic sarcoma

! Associated infiltrate of reactive, nonneoplastic lymphocytes can be a very prominent finding obscuring the malignant B cells

DIAGNOSIS

The diagnostic workup for primary lymphomas of bone include a combination of microscopy with a broad panel of immunohistochemical lymphoma markers as well as molecular analysis such as FISH for BCL2/BCL6/MYC in case of DLBCL.

To accurately diagnose primary lymphoma of the bone, a pathologist should always correlate the morphology and immunohistochemical findings with the clinical and radiologic differential diagnosis. Most primary lymphomas of bone are mature B-cell lymphomas and stain with CD20, PAX5, and CD79a (Fig. 5A, B). Primary large B-cell lymphoma of bone can be further subdivided in germinal-center B-cell type and nongerminal center B-cell type by using BCL2, BCL6, CD10, and MUM1 (see Fig. 5C). CD10-, BCL2-, and BCL6-positive staining favors a germinal center B-cell type and MUM1 positive staining favors a nongerminal B-cell type that harbors a more inferior prognosis.[20]

In the case of DLBCL, performing BCL2/BCL6 and MYC FISH is recommend to identify a 'double hit' (MYC with BCL2 or BCL6 breakage) large B-cell lymphomas (see Fig. 5D), which are more aggressive lymphomas and, therefore, treated differently compared with their FISH-negative counterparts.[2,21] Recently, driver mutations were reported in genes like *MYD88, CD79a/b, CARD11,* and *TP53* that are linked with a more adverse prognosis and therapy resistance in DLBCL.[2,22,23] In parallel with the recommendation for performing triple (BCL2/BCL6/MYC) FISH on each DLBCL, in the near future it is likely that a targeted next generation sequencing approach will be part of the routine DLBCL diagnostics to better subclassify this heterogeneous group of DLBCLs and identify druggable targets.

Furthermore, if a patient is known to be in an immunosuppressive state, performing Epstein-Barr Virus (EBV) is necessary to classify a neoplastic large B-cell proliferation appropriate according to the WHO.

Anaplastic T-cell lymphomas are positive in at least 1 of these pan T-cell markers—CD3, CD2, CD4, or CD5—in combination with diffuse staining for CD30 and in case of an *ALK* translocation, expression of ALK protein is observed. Of note, depending on the amount of representative tissue material and clinical features, one should be cautious diagnosing anaplastic large T-cell lymphoma on biopsy material from bone, because many other T-cell lymphomas like peripheral T-cell lymphoma not otherwise specified or angioimmunoblastic T-cell lymphoma can be positive for CD30 and share morphologic findings with anaplastic T-cell lymphomas.

Immunoglobulin heavy and light chain genes are clonally rearranged in case of primary lymphoma of bone and can be tested for by polymerase chain reaction.[24] However, if there is no convincing morphologic or immunohistochemical substrate that raises suspicion for lymphoma, one should not test clonality because reactive conditions like osteomyelitis may show clonal immunoglobulin heavy and light chain gene rearrangements.[24,25]

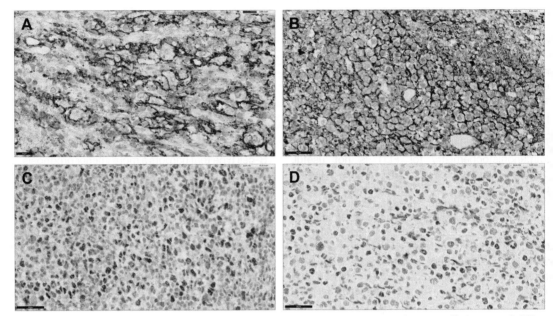

Fig. 5. Immunohistochemistry in primary lymphoma of bone. (*A*) Scattered neoplastic B-cells in case of diffuse large B-cell lymphoma (DLBCL) that stain for CD20. (*B*) Diffuse staining of CD20 in DLBCL. (*C*) Diffuse BCL6 positivity in DLBCL. (*D*) Strong MYC expression in more than 30% of neoplastic B cells, indicative for *MYC* involved translocation. (*A–D, black bar,* 50 μm).

PROGNOSIS

With current treatment protocols (combination of chemotherapy and radiotherapy), overall survival is excellent, in general reaching overall survival of more than 90%. Age is a significant factor associated with survival, with age less than 60 years indicative of a better survival. In nodal large B-cell lymphomas germinal center B-cell subtypes have an improved survival compared with non–germinal center B-cell type.[2]

In a small study cohort of 21 primary bone large B-cell lymphomas by Bhagavathi and colleagues,[26] 19% *BCL2*, 14% *BCL6*, and 9% of cases with a *MYC* involved rearrangements by FISH were detected, but no double hit lymphomas, which are known to harbor a more inferior survival in their nodal counterparts. Furthermore, within large B-cell lymphoma of bone the density of CD8+ T-cell infiltration and expression of BCL2 predict outcome and the PI3K/AKT/mTOR pathway seems to be an additional therapeutic target.[27]

ACUTE LYMPHOBLASTIC LEUKEMIA/LYMPHOMA

Acute lymphoblastic leukemia (ALL) and lymphoblastic lymphoma (LBL) are a continuum of neoplastic lymphoid disorders characterized by the proliferation of immature (blast) cells of precursor B-cell or precursor T-cell lineage. Patients with tissue involvement and less than 25% replacement of marrow cellularity by lymphoid blasts have been classified as acute LBL and patient with more than 25% bone marrow involvement have been classified as ALL.[1]

Most cases of LBL are of T-cell lineage and true B-cell lineage LBL is extremely rare. Both ALL and LBL can occur at any age, but the majority of cases arise in children. By definition, bone marrow is involved in all cases and liver, spleen, mediastinum, and lymph nodes are also frequently involved.

Key Features
ACUTE LYMPHOBLASTIC LEUKEMIA/LYMPHOBLASTIC LYMPHOMA

- Most cases of LBL are of T-cell lineage
- Diffuse growth with sheets of lymphoblasts
- Terminal deoxynucleotidyl transferase (TdT) positive

Pitfall
ACUTE LYMPHOBLASTIC LEUKEMIA/LYMPHOBLASTIC LYMPHOMA

! ALL/LBL share morphology and CD99 positivity with Ewing sarcoma

RADIOLOGY

Like other lymphomas in bone, radiologic imaging of ALL show lytic and destructive tumors and generalized osteoporosis.[6]

MICROSCOPY

Typically ALL and LBL show a diffuse growth pattern with sheets of lymphoblasts (Fig. 6A). The lymphoblasts may vary from small blasts with scant cytoplasm, condensed nuclear chromatin, and indistinct nucleoli to larger blasts with moderate amounts of cytoplasm and prominent nucleoli.

DIFFERENTIAL DIAGNOSIS

ALL and LBL must be distinguished from reactive conditions with expansion of precursor B-cells (hematogones), which may be seen in the bone marrow after prolonged infection, regeneration of hematopoiesis after chemotherapy, or bone marrow transplantation. Hematogones have a more heterogeneous aspect compared with the monotonous blasts found in ALL or LBL. Furthermore, hematogones have a distinct pattern of positive markers on flow cytometry and lack clonal immunoglobulin gene rearrangements.

The morphology of ALL and LBL may mimic Burkitt lymphoma/leukemia; however, the latter show a mature B-cell immunophenotype with strong CD20 and lack of TdT expression, which is a hallmark of ALL/LBL.

Compared with ALL and LBL, acute myeloid leukemia often shows a spectrum of morphologic differentiation in the addition of myeloid blasts with frequent dysplasia in other lineages of the hematopoiesis such as megakaryopoiesis. In addition, markers of the myeloid lineage (CD13+, CD33+) are positive in acute myeloid leukemia with negative TdT expression. Although leukemia with

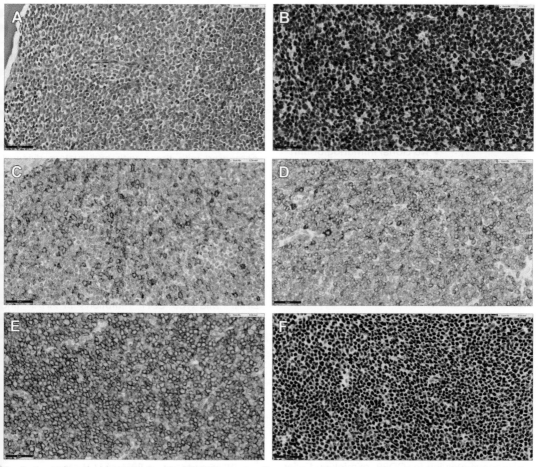

Fig. 6. Acute lymphoblastic leukemia. (A) Diffuse growth pattern with sheets of lymphoblasts. (B) Strong nuclear expression of TdT in lymphoblasts. (C) Heterogeneous expression for CD20 in lymphoblasts. (D) Strong homogenous expression for CD79a in lymphoblasts. (E) Strong homogenous expression of CD99 in lymphoblasts. (F) Strong FLI1 nuclear expression in lymphoblasts. (A–F, black bar, 50 μm).

ambiguous lineage exist, dependent on additional genetic aberrations, these groups of leukemias are further classified according to the WHO.

Significantly, small blue round cell tumors like Ewing sarcoma can closely mimic ALL, not only with respect to clinical presentation and radiologic findings but also with morphologic overlap. Important to realize is that CD45 may be negative in some cases of ALL and most LBLs are CD99 positive or FL1 positive (see Fig. 6E, F), which is also a characteristic finding in Ewing sarcoma. Therefore, beside performing a broad panel of immunohistochemical stainings to rule out other small blue round cell tumors, detection of *EWSR1* rearrangement is mandatory to rule out Ewing sarcoma in cases that do not harbor an immunohistochemical profile typical for ALL.

Differential Diagnosis
OF ACUTE LYMPHOBLASTIC LEUKEMIA/LYMPHOMA

ALL/LBL vs	Helpful Distinguishing Features
Hematogones	• Heterogeneous aspect of blasts
	• No sheets of blasts
	• Partial CD34 and CD20 expression
	• No clonal immunoglobulin gene rearrangements
Burkitt lymphoma	• Mature B-cell immunophenotype: strong CD20, TdT negative
Acute myeloid leukemia	• CD13$^+$, CD33$^+$, TdT$^-$
Ewing sarcoma	• TdT$^-$
	• *EWSR1* translocation in most Ewing sarcomas

DIAGNOSIS

Diagnosing ALL and LBL is a combination of integrating aspirate and flow cytometry findings of bone marrow with the morphology and immunohistochemical findings seen in the histology. ALL cells commonly do not express LCA and are positive for TdT, CD20 (weak), CD79a, and PAX5 (see Fig. 6B–D). Some cases of ALL show bright membranous staining for CD99, mimicking Ewing sarcoma (see Fig. 6E). Occasionally myeloperoxidase, a myeloid marker or a blast marker like CD34, can be positive in ALL. Cases of B-cell ALL lack immunoglobulin light chain restriction or surface immunoglobulins.

Furthermore, B-cell ALL is subclassified according to recurrent cytogenetic and molecular abnormalities into clinical important subgroups, including balanced translocations like *BCR-ABL1*, *MLL*, and *TEL-AML1*.[28] T-cell ALL is positive for CD2, CD4, CD10, CD34 and TdT on flow cytometry of the bone marrow as well as immunohistochemistry on most bone marrow biopsies.

PROGNOSIS

Almost 80% to 90% cure rate is achieved in children treated with extensive chemotherapy compared with a 5-year survival of 30% to 40% in adults treated with prolonged chemotherapy.[28]

LANGERHANS CELL HISTIOCYTOSIS

LCH is not a common disease, accounting for less than 1% of all bone tumors. Since the discovery of a recurrent activating mutation in *BRAF* in almost 80% of LCH cases, it is generally accepted to be a neoplastic disease rather than a reactive condition.[1,3,29,30] In approximately 40% of patients, skin involvement is seen and in less than 20% there is lymph node or lung localization.[31]

LCH is usually diagnosed during the first or third decade of life and can occur in any bone, but most commonly in skull and jaw.[3,32] Patients with monostotic disease have an excellent prognosis compared with those with multisystem disease. Treatment consists of curettage, or by direct intralesional injection of corticosteroids. Differences in telomerase expression and telomere length were found in Langerhans cells between monostotic disease versus multisystem disease.[33] Since the observation of frequent *BRAF* mutations in LCH, patients with more aggressive generalized disease (involving skin and bone) may benefit from *BRAF* inhibitors such as vemurafenib.[30,34] Recently in *BRAF* wild-type LCH, mutations in *ARAF* and *MAP1K1* are found that result in activation of the ERK pathway for which *MAP1K1* mutated tumors can be treated with MEK inhibitors.[35,36]

Key Features
LANGERHANS CELL HISTIOCYTOSIS

• Commonly in skull and jaw

• *BRAF* mutation in 80% of LCH cases

• Reactive eosinophilic granulocytes can be very prominent

Pitfalls
LANGERHANS CELL
HISTIOCYTOSIS

! Extensive sclerosis and reactive, nonneoplastic lymphocytes can be a very prominent finding obscuring the lesional Langerhans cells

! *BRAF* mutations also frequently found in tumors other than LCH

RADIOLOGIC AND GROSS FEATURES

LCH is a well-defined lytic lesion of 1 to 5 cm in diameter resembling osteomyelitis on radiologic imaging and cortical involvement may elicit a periosteal reaction (**Fig. 7**).[6] Healing of LCH is accompanied by progressive sclerosis of surrounding bone.[6] In line with other hematopoietic tumors in bone, it is unusual to see gross specimens of bone with localization of LCH.

MICROSCOPY

Langerhans cells are ovoid or round, histiocytic cells and are arranged in aggregates, sheets, or individually. The cells have eosinophilic cytoplasm and contain central ovoid coffee bean–shaped or deeply indented nuclei that have pale chromatin and linear grooves (**Fig. 8**A). Most Langerhans cells are mononuclear but some cells may contain multiple nuclei. Mitosis are seen but no atypical forms. Sclerosis and intermixing reactive eosinophilic granulocytes can be very prominent (see **Fig. 8**A), obscuring the lesional LCH cells. Other types of inflammatory cells like lymphocytes, plasma cells, macrophages, neutrophils, and osteoclast-type giant cells may be seen as well. Langerhans cells are able to recruit inflammatory cells like eosinophils and CD4[+] T cells via the production of chemokines and aberrant chemokine receptor expression.[37,38] Furthermore, osteoclast-like multinucleated giant cells seem to be intrinsic to LCH lesions and specific factors within the well-characterized chemokine production in LCH lesions are responsible for their formation.[39] The typical Birbeck granules of LCH cells are tubular pentalaminar membrane-bound cytoplasmic organelles and only observed with electron microscopy.

DIFFERENTIAL DIAGNOSIS

The imaging features of LCH may be indistinguishable from osteomyelitis, Ewing sarcoma, lymphoma, or other round cell malignancies. If biopsy material is representative, by using a broad panel of immunohistochemical markers, a pathologist should not have great difficulties in most cases to differentiate between these entities. However cases with poor representative biopsy material, sclerosis, or abundant reactive lymphocytes can be challenging for a pathologist.

Acute and chronic osteomyelitis may harbor many eosinophils and a mixed inflammatory infiltrate that may contain histiocytes, but no characteristic features of Langerhans cells are seen and CD1a, Langerin, and S100 immunohistochemistry is negative. Although imaging features are similar and the morphology may show overlapping features, clinical and laboratory findings are helpful in distinguishing LCH from osteomyelitis as well.

In contrast with LCH, malignant round cell tumors like Ewing sarcoma show morphology with

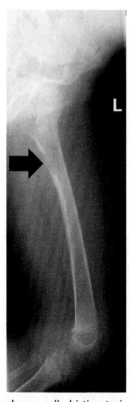

Fig. 7. Langerhans cell histiocytosis. Radiograph shows a lytic bone lesion in the proximal femur (*black arrow*) of a young patient with cortical destruction and a solid periosteal reaction. Radiologic differential diagnosis includes Langerhans cell histiocytosis, Ewing sarcoma, and osteomyelitis.

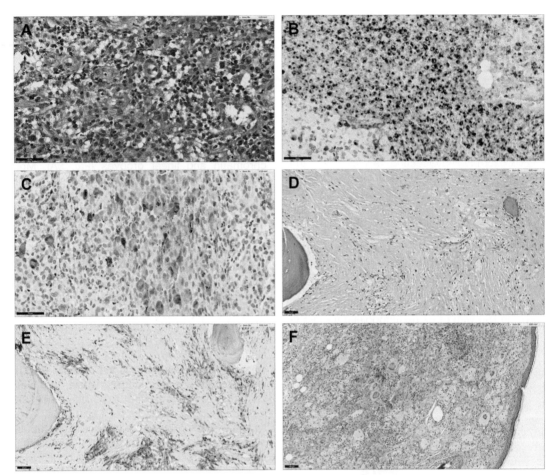

Fig. 8. Langerhans cell histiocytosis. (*A*) The cells have eosinophilic cytoplasm and contain central ovoid coffee bean–shaped or deeply indented nuclei that have pale chromatin and linear grooves. (*B*) Langerin-positive Langerhans cells. (*C*) S100-positive Langerhans cells. (*D*) Erdheim Chester disease with foamy macrophages and extensive sclerosis. (*E*) CD68 positivity in Erdheim Chester disease. (*F*) Concordant skin biopsy of patient with Erdheim Chester disease with dermal infiltrates of foamy macrophages. (*A–F, black bar,* 50 μm).

sheets of small uniform sized cells with hyperchromatic nuclei, but typical Langerhans cells of LCH or many eosinophils are not seen. Occasionally, biopsy material is poorly representative and malignant round cells are not identified easily. Performing immunohistochemistry is necessary in this differential diagnosis and in most cases of Ewing sarcoma will show bright membranous staining of CD99 without CD1a, Langerin, or S100 positivity. Because many other malignant round cell tumors, such as poorly differentiated synoviosarcoma or small cell carcinoma, can be strongly positive for CD99, detection of Ewing sarcoma specific translocations may be necessary.

The finding of *BRAF* mutations in approximately 80% of LCH cases can be used as an additional helpful tool for diagnosing LCH. However, Erdheim Chester disease may show overlapping histology with LCH and likewise harbors *BRAF* mutations in approximately 50% of cases.[40,41] Especially extensive sclerosis, which can occur in both LCH and Erdheim Chester disease (see **Fig. 8**D), can cause difficulties in differentiating between these disorders. Whether both entities are truly different diseases or a spectrum of the same disease still needs further investigation (see **Fig. 8**E and F).

LCH with multiple bone involvement may resemble Brown tumors of hyperparathyroidism but patient are much older in case of Brown tumor.[6] Furthermore, morphology of the latter shows many reactive stromal cells and multi-nucleated giant cells arranged in clusters which is not a feature seen in LCH.

△△ *Differential Diagnosis*
OF LANGERHANS CELL
HISTIOCYTOSIS

LCH vs	Helpful Distinguishing Features
Acute and chronic osteomyelitis	• No typical Langerhans cells • CD1a⁻, Langerin⁻, S100⁻
Ewing sarcomas	• No typical Langerhans cells • Sheets of small uniform sized cells with hyperchromatic nuclei • Strong uniform membranous CD99 staining • *EWSR1* translocation in most Ewing sarcomas

DIAGNOSIS

Diagnosing LCH for a pathologist encompasses a combination of representative morphology with the classical Langerhans cells in combination with positive immunohistochemistry for Langerin, CD1a and S100 protein (see **Fig. 8** B, C). Additional molecular analysis for *BRAF* mutations are not only diagnostically useful for LCH but may also have therapeutic implications for the use of *BRAF* inhibitors like vemurafenib in patients.[34,42–44]

PROGNOSIS

Prognosis in patients with LCH is generally good both in monostotic and limited polyostotic disease.[3] Although spontaneous healing in patients with LCH is observed frequently, recurrence is seen in approximately 10% of monostotic cases and up to 25% of polyostotic cases.[3] Patients with monostotic skeletal involvement have excellent prognosis, and usually remain disease free after adequate therapy; multifocal systemic disease has a guarded prognosis.

SUMMARY

Plasma cell myeloma and SPB are both characterized by neoplastic plasma cells that secrete monoclonal immunoglobulin. The fact that CD138, a plasma cell marker, can also be positive in carcinomas may be a caveat for the correct diagnosis. Primary bone lymphoma frequently occurs in the femur and needs to be distinguished from benign conditions like osteomyelitis or other malignant tumors like carcinoma, osteosarcoma, or Ewing sarcoma. By using a broad panel of immunohistochemical lymphoma markers, a pathologist should not have great difficulties in most cases. LCH is commonly located in the skull and jaw and frequently harbor ERK pathway activating mutations in *BRAF*, *MAP1K1*, and *ARAF*, which not only can be used as diagnostic tool but also have therapeutic implications.

REFERENCES

1. Swerdlow SH, Campo E, Harris NL, et al. WHO classification of Tumours of Haematopoietic and Lymphoid Tissues. In: Bosman TD, Jaffe ES, Lakhani SR, et al, editors. France: IARC; 2008. p. 202–8.
2. Swerdlow SH, Campo E, Pileri SA, et al. The 2016 revision of the World Health Organization classification of lymphoid neoplasms. Blood 2016;127(20): 2375–90.
3. Fletcher DM, Bridge JA, Hogendoorn PCW, et al. WHO classification of tumours of soft tissue and bone. France: IARC; 2013. p. 312–8.
4. Palumbo A, Anderson K. Multiple myeloma. N Engl J Med 2011;364(11):1046–60.
5. Kyle RA, Therneau TM, Rajkumar SV, et al. Prevalence of monoclonal gammopathy of undetermined significance. N Engl J Med 2006;354(13):1362–9.
6. Vigorita VJ, Ghelman B, Mintz D. Orthopaedic pathology. China: Lippincott Williams & Wilkins, a Wolters Kluwer Business; 2016.
7. Kuehl WM, Bergsagel PL. Molecular pathogenesis of multiple myeloma and its premalignant precursor. J Clin Invest 2012;122(10):3456–63.
8. Bhagavathi S, Fu K. Primary lymphoma of bone: a review. Semin Diagn Pathol 2014;31(1):48–52.
9. Heyning FH, Hogendoorn PC, Kramer MH, et al. Primary non-Hodgkin's lymphoma of bone: a clinicopathological investigation of 60 cases. Leukemia 1999;13(12):2094–8.
10. Heyning FH, Jansen PM, Hogendoorn PC, et al. Array-based comparative genomic hybridisation analysis reveals recurrent chromosomal alterations in primary diffuse large B cell lymphoma of bone. J Clin Pathol 2010;63(12):1095–100.
11. Koens L, Heyning FH, Szepesi A, et al. Nuclear factor-kappaB activation in primary lymphoma of bone. Virchows Arch 2013;462(3):349–54.
12. Heyning FH, Hogendoorn PC, Kramer MH, et al. Primary lymphoma of bone: extranodal lymphoma with favourable survival independent of germinal centre, post-germinal centre or indeterminate phenotype. J Clin Pathol 2009;62(9):820–4.
13. Heyning FH, Kroon HM, Hogendoorn PC, et al. MR imaging characteristics in primary lymphoma of bone with emphasis on non-aggressive appearance. Skeletal Radiol 2007;36(10):937–44.

14. Bonetti P, Testoni M, Scandurra M, et al. Deregulation of ETS1 and FLI1 contributes to the pathogenesis of diffuse large B-cell lymphoma. Blood 2013; 122(13):2233–41.

15. Specht K, Sung YS, Zhang L, et al. Distinct transcriptional signature and immunoprofile of CIC-DUX4 fusion-positive round cell tumors compared to EWSR1-rearranged Ewing sarcomas: further evidence toward distinct pathologic entities. Genes Chromosomes Cancer 2014;53(7):622–33.

16. Puls F, Niblett A, Marland G, et al. BCOR-CCNB3 (Ewing-like) sarcoma: a clinicopathologic analysis of 10 cases, in comparison with conventional Ewing sarcoma. Am J Surg Pathol 2014;38(10):1307–18.

17. Szuhai K, Ijszenga M, de Jong D, et al. The NFATc2 gene is involved in a novel cloned translocation in a Ewing sarcoma variant that couples its function in immunology to oncology. Clin Cancer Res 2009; 15(7):2259–68.

18. Szuhai K, IJszenga M, Tanke HJ, et al. Detection and molecular cytogenetic characterization of a novel ring chromosome in a histological variant of Ewing sarcoma. Cancer Genet Cytogenet 2007;172(1): 12–22.

19. Kajtar B, Tornoczky T, Kalman E, et al. CD99-positive undifferentiated round cell sarcoma diagnosed on fine needle aspiration cytology, later found to harbour a CIC-DUX4 translocation: a recently described entity. Cytopathology 2014;25(2):129–32.

20. Rosenwald A, Wright G, Chan WC, et al. The use of molecular profiling to predict survival after chemotherapy for diffuse large-B-cell lymphoma. N Engl J Med 2002;346(25):1937–47.

21. Sesques P, Johnson NA. Approach to the diagnosis and treatment of high-grade B cell lymphomas with MYC and BCL2 and/or BCL6 rearrangements. Blood 2016;129:280–8.

22. Pasqualucci L, Dalla-Favera R. The genetic landscape of diffuse large B-cell lymphoma. Semin Hematol 2015;52(2):67–76.

23. Dubois S, Viailly PJ, Bohers E, et al. Biological and clinical relevance of associated genomic alterations in MYD88 L265P and non-L265P-mutated diffuse large B-cell lymphoma: analysis of 361 cases. Clin Cancer Res 2017;23(9):2232–44.

24. Zamo A, Bertolaso A, van Raaij AW, et al. Application of microfluidic technology to the BIOMED-2 protocol for detection of B-cell clonality. J Mol Diagn 2012;14(1):30–7.

25. Langerak AW, Molina TJ, Lavender FL, et al. Polymerase chain reaction-based clonality testing in tissue samples with reactive lymphoproliferations: usefulness and pitfalls. A report of the BIOMED-2 Concerted Action BMH4-CT98-3936. Leukemia 2007;21(2):222–9.

26. Bhagavathi S, Micale MA, Les K, et al. Primary bone diffuse large B-cell lymphoma: clinicopathologic study of 21 cases and review of literature. Am J Surg Pathol 2009;33(10):1463–9.

27. Rajnai H, Heyning FH, Koens L, et al. The density of CD8+ T-cell infiltration and expression of BCL2 predicts outcome of primary diffuse large B-cell lymphoma of bone. Virchows Arch 2014;464(2):229–39.

28. Inaba H, Greaves M, Mullighan CG. Acute lymphoblastic leukaemia. Lancet 2013;381(9881):1943–55.

29. Chakraborty R, Burke TM, Hampton OA, et al. Alternative genetic mechanisms of BRAF activation in Langerhans cell histiocytosis. Blood 2016;128(21): 2533–7.

30. Emile JF, Abla O, Fraitag S, et al. Revised classification of histiocytoses and neoplasms of the macrophage-dendritic cell lineages. Blood 2016;127(22):2672–81.

31. Rigaud C, Barkaoui MA, Thomas C, et al. Langerhans cell histiocytosis: therapeutic strategy and outcome in a 30-year nationwide cohort of 1478 patients under 18 years of age. Br J Haematol 2016;174(6):887–98.

32. Egeler RM, van Halteren AG, Hogendoorn PC, et al. Langerhans cell histiocytosis: fascinating dynamics of the dendritic cell-macrophage lineage. Immunol Rev 2010;234(1):213–32.

33. da Costa CE, Egeler RM, Hoogeboom M, et al. Differences in telomerase expression by the CD1a+ cells in Langerhans cell histiocytosis reflect the diverse clinical presentation of the disease. J Pathol 2007;212(2):188–97.

34. Arceci RJ. Biological and therapeutic implications of the BRAF pathway in histiocytic disorders. Am Soc Clin Oncol Educ Book 2014;e441–5.

35. Nelson DS, van Halteren A, Quispel WT, et al. MAP2K1 and MAP3K1 mutations in Langerhans cell histiocytosis. Genes Chromosomes Cancer 2015;54(6):361–8.

36. Nelson DS, Quispel W, Badalian-Very G, et al. Somatic activating ARAF mutations in Langerhans cell histiocytosis. Blood 2014;123(20):3152–5.

37. Annels NE, Da Costa CE, Prins FA, et al. Aberrant chemokine receptor expression and chemokine production by Langerhans cells underlies the pathogenesis of Langerhans cell histiocytosis. J Exp Med 2003;197(10):1385–90.

38. Laman JD, Leenen PJ, Annels NE, et al. Langerhans-cell histiocytosis 'insight into DC biology'. Trends Immunol 2003;24(4):190–6.

39. da Costa CE, Annels NE, Faaij CM, et al. Presence of osteoclast-like multinucleated giant cells in the bone and nonostotic lesions of Langerhans cell histiocytosis. J Exp Med 2005;201(5):687–93.

40. Haroche J, Cohen-Aubart F, Charlotte F, et al. The histiocytosis Erdheim-Chester disease is an inflammatory myeloid neoplasm. Expert Rev Clin Immunol 2015;11(9):1033–42.

41. Parreau S, Haroche J, Pommepuy I, et al. Langerhans cell histiocytosis and Erdheim-Chester disease: a continuity? Rev Med Interne 2016;10:389–95.

42. Heritier S, Emile JF, Barkaoui MA, et al. BRAF mutation correlates with high-risk Langerhans cell histiocytosis and increased resistance to first-line therapy. J Clin Oncol 2016;34(25):3023–30.

43. Heritier S, Saffroy R, Radosevic-Robin N, et al. Common cancer-associated PIK3CA activating mutations rarely occur in Langerhans cell histiocytosis. Blood 2015;125(15):2448–9.

44. Schouten B, Egeler RM, Leenen PJ, et al. Expression of cell cycle-related gene products in Langerhans cell histiocytosis. J Pediatr Hematol Oncol 2002;24(9):727–32.

Bone-Related Lesions of the Jaws

Daniel Baumhoer, MD

KEYWORDS

- Osseous dysplasia • Ossifying fibroma • Fibrous dysplasia • Giant cell granuloma
- Aneurysmal bone cyst • Osteosarcoma

Key points

- Not all bone tumors or tumorlike lesions also occur in the jaws.
- Not all bone-related gnathic lesions occur in the peripheral skeleton.
- Some bone tumors behave differently when developing at this site.
- Radiologic and clinical correlations are mandatory for making adequate diagnoses.

ABSTRACT

The jaws combine several unique properties that mainly result from their distinct embryonic development and their role in providing anchorage for the teeth and their supporting structures. As a consequence, several bone-related lesions almost exclusively develop in the jaws (eg, osseous dysplasias, ossifying fibromas), have distinct clinical features (eg, osteosarcoma), or hardly ever occur at this location (eg, osteochondroma, enchondroma). The specific characteristics of these tumors and tumorlike lesions are outlined in this article.

OVERVIEW AND DEVELOPMENTAL CONSIDERATIONS

During early embryogenesis, the first pharyngeal arch develops a maxillary and a mandibular prominence. Intramembranous ossification inside the maxillary prominence forms the squamous temporal, maxillary, and zygomatic bones. The ventral parts of the first arch cartilage form a horseshoe-shaped primordium of the mandible, which later disappears after the mandible develops because of intramembranous ossification of the mandibular prominence–related mesenchyme. Only in the median plane of the chin and in the mandibular condyle is there also some enchondral ossification contributing to the normal development.[1]

Although it remains to be elucidated how and to what extent these developmental peculiarities influence the development of tumors and tumorlike lesions in this region, their contribution seems obvious. Enchondromas generally do not occur in the jaws and, despite well-documented cases of chondrosarcomas, no convincing studies have correlated morphology and IDH1/2 mutation status, which might be important to rule out osteosarcoma (OS) with a predominant chondroblastic differentiation. Giant cell tumor of bone is another example of a tumor that is common in the peripheral skeleton and virtually nonexistent in the jaws. Improvements in the molecular understanding of gnathic tumors will help to clarify the reasons for morphologic and clinical differences but are difficult to achieve because of the rarity of most lesions.

This article discusses bone-related lesions commonly occurring in the jaws, including fibro-osseous and giant cell–containing subtypes, and discusses their main differences and differential diagnoses. Furthermore, the distinct clinical behaviors of bone-forming tumors and particularly of

Disclosure Statement: Nothing to declare.
Bone Tumour Reference Centre at the Institute of Pathology, University Hospital Basel, University of Basel, Schoenbeinstrasse 40, Basel 4031, Switzerland
E-mail address: daniel.baumhoer@usb.ch

Surgical Pathology 10 (2017) 693–704
http://dx.doi.org/10.1016/j.path.2017.04.007
1875-9181/17/© 2017 Elsevier Inc. All rights reserved.

surgpath.theclinics.com

OSs are outlined and compared with lesions of the peripheral skeleton.

FIBRO-OSSEOUS LESIONS

This descriptively defined group of lesions comprises 3 distinct entities, of which some can be further divided into subtypes with characteristic clinical, radiologic, and histologic presentation:

1. Cemento-osseous dysplasia (COD), including periapical, focal, and florid subtypes
2. Cemento-ossifying fibroma (COF), including conventional, juvenile trabecular, and juvenile psammomatoid subtypes
3. Fibrous dysplasia (FD)

All lesions share a monomorphic fibroblastic stroma embedding various combinations of bone and cementumlike material (Table 1).

CEMENTO-OSSEOUS DYSPLASIA

COD constitutes the most common fibro-osseous lesion in the jaws and develops exclusively in the tooth-bearing areas of the gnathic bones. They are considered to derive from cells of the periodontal membrane and to represent nonneoplastic lesions of limited growth potential.[2] However, the molecular pathogenesis is largely unknown. In contrast with other fibro-osseous lesions, the matrix of COD matures into a dense mass over time, resulting in a characteristic radiologic and histologic appearance. There is a striking predilection for middle-aged (black) women.[2] Three distinct clinical variants can be distinguished:

1. Periapical COD: associated with a single or few mandibular incisors
2. Focal COD: single lesion not involving the anterior mandible, most prevalent in the posterior mandible
3. Florid COD: multifocal, generally present in multiple quadrants

Patients are usually asymptomatic and remain undiagnosed until routine dental radiographs are performed.[3] The radiology varies according to the stage of maturation. Early lesions appear as small periapical radiolucencies (Fig. 1A) that over time transform into heavily calcified and radio-opaque masses surrounded by a thin lytic rim. The periodontal ligament remains unaffected. Expansive growth and cortical thinning are not typical features of periapical and focal COD but can occur in the florid subtype.[4] Because classic COD does not require treatment and the clinical/radiographic constellation is highly characteristic, biopsy should not be required for the diagnosis. Surgical intervention is

even considered contraindicated because it can result in persistent infection that is difficult to treat.[5]

On histology, COD shows trabecular woven bone formation that typically fuses with the preexisting bone of the adjacent cortex. Osteoblastic rimming is not a prominent feature. In addition, a hypocellular or cell-free basophilic matrix can be observed that is generally regarded as cementum/cementicles[2] (see Fig. 1B). Because cementum is physiologically formed by cementoblasts after follicular ectomesenchymal cells have been stimulated by exposed dentin, some investigators questioned whether these globular deposits with concentric patterns of mineralization represent cementum and suggested to use "psammoma bodies" or at least "cementum-like material" as more descriptive terms. The World Health Organization (WHO) classification of head and neck tumors from 2005 omitted "Cemento-" in the definition of COD and COF, stating that the distinction between cementum and bone would be equivocal and without clinical relevance.[6] However the new edition of the WHO classification reintroduced the term, which seems reasonable because it underlines a highly characteristic histologic feature of those lesions irrespective of its true nature.[2] The matrix of COD is enclosed by a moderately cellular and monomorphic proliferation of fibroblastlike spindle cells without atypia and very low (if any) mitotic activity. Over time, the matrix mineralizes and coalesces to form calcified masses resembling ginger roots. Florid COD may be associated with pseudocystic changes that can resemble simple bone cysts. Malignant transformation does not occur.

CEMENTO-OSSIFYING FIBROMA

COFs comprise a group of benign fibro-osseous neoplasms of which 3 variants can be distinguished

1. Conventional cemento-ossifying fibroma (CCOF): a tumor of odontogenic origin exclusively developing in the tooth-bearing areas of the jaws, most frequently in the premolar/molar region of the mandible
2. Juvenile trabecular ossifying fibroma (JTOF): a rare bone tumor occurring most commonly in the maxilla but also in the mandible and rarely in extragnathic sites
3. Juvenile psammomatoid ossifying fibroma (JPOF): a rare tumor only infrequently affecting the jaws but more commonly developing in extragnathic sites, preferentially in the periorbital frontal and ethmoid bones

COF is rare and, similar to COD, primarily affects women in the third and fourth decades of life. JTOF and JPOF can occur at younger ages (8.5–12 years mean age for JTOF and 16–33 years for

Table 1
Fibro-osseous lesions

	Cemento-osseous Dysplasia	Cemento-osseous Fibroma	Fibrous Dysplasia
Age	Third–fourth decade	• COF: third–fourth decade • JTOF: first–second decade • JPOF: second–fourth decade	First–second decade
Gender predilection	Strong predilection for (black) women	• COF: female to male = 5:1 • JTOF: none • JPOF: none	None
Localization	• Periapical COD: apical areas of mandibular anterior teeth, solitary or multiple • Focal COD: apical areas of teeth other than those mentioned before, solitary • Florid COD: apical areas of teeth other than those mentioned before, multiple/multiquadrant	• COF: only tooth-bearing areas, mandible >maxilla, premolar and molar • JTOF: maxilla >mandible, extragnathic cases are rare • JPOF: extragnathic craniofacial bones (frontal and ethmoid bone) >gnathic bones	Maxilla >mandible, may involve adjacent bones, monostotic form 6–10× more common than polyostotic form
Symptoms	• Periapical and focal COD: nonspecific • Florid COD: nonspecific	Nonspecific	Nonspecific
Radiology	Well demarcated, primarily lytic but mineralizes increasingly over time, generally not expansive (except for florid COD)	Well demarcated with lytic rim, expansive, mixed radiolucent to radio-opaque, cortical thinning in advanced cases	Indistinct margins, expansive, ground-glass appearance
Histopathology	Moderately cellular and monomorphic fibroblastic stroma embedding Various proportions of woven bone trabeculae and cementumlike material, osteoblastic rimming is usually not prominent, matrix typically fuses with preexisting bone	Moderately cellular and monomorphic fibroblastic stroma embedding • COF: varying proportions of woven bone trabeculae with osteoblastic rimming and cementumlike material • JTOF: immature and slender bone trabeculae • JPOF: multiple psammoma body–like ossicles Matrix generally does not fuse with preexisting bone (separated by a slender rim of stroma)	Moderately cellular, monomorphic and loose fibroblastic stroma with varying numbers of irregularly shaped bone trabeculae, sometimes resembling Chinese script letters; generally no osteoblastic rimming, Sharpey fibers radiating from the trabeculae into the stroma, matrix typically fuses with preexisting bone
Genetics	Unknown	Unknown	Postzygotic missense mutations in the GNAS gene
Prognosis	Self-limited, no treatment required, no malignant transformation	Locally aggressive, recurrences rare after conservative surgery, no malignant transformation	Most cases stabilize with skeletal maturation; malignant transformation is exceedingly rare

Abbreviations: JPOF, juvenile psammomatoid ossifying fibroma; JTOF, juvenile trabecular ossifying fibroma.

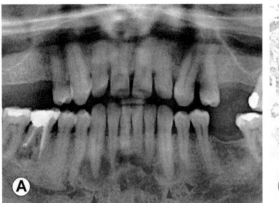
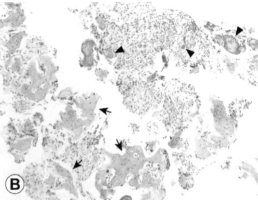

Fig. 1. (*A*) An orthopantomogram reveals several radiolucencies centered on the roots of the anterior mandibular incisors (*arrowheads*), highly characteristic of periapical cemento-osseous dysplasia (H&E, original magnification, ×25). (*B*) Morphologically, the lesion consists of a bland spindle cell stroma accompanied by the formation of woven bone (*arrows*) and cementumlike material (*arrowheads*) (H&E, original magnification, ×25).

JPOF) but the age distribution is broad and ranges up to the seventh decade.[8] The term "juvenile" has therefore been questioned by some investigators but has also been kept in the new WHO classification. With the exception of the exceedingly rare hyperparathyroidism jaw tumor syndrome and familial gigantiform cementoma (FGC), COFs present as single lesions.[5,9]

Patients typically notice a painless swelling of the affected bone, which can reach considerable and disfiguring dimensions if left untreated. Radiologically, early lesions appear purely lytic but show increasing matrix mineralization over time that is more unevenly distributed than in matured COD. Usually, a lytic rim remains encompassing the lesion. Although JTOF and JPOF can grow rapidly (and are therefore also called active or aggressive TOF/POF), COFs are generally well-circumscribed and expansile lesions that lead to cortical thinning (and potentially perforation). In case the mandible

is affected, a characteristic downward bowing of the inferior cortex can be observed. Wide destruction of cortical bone or aggressive periosteal reaction does not occur in COFs; they are furthermore not as intimately associated with teeth as COD. Infrequently, secondary aneurysmal bone cysts can develop, particularly in TPOF.[5]

On histology, COF is well defined and usually separated from the adjacent cortical bone by a thin rim of surrounding stroma (equivalent to the lytic rim seen on radiographs). Smaller lesions can therefore easily be enucleated, whereas COD (if erroneously excised) is usually retrieved in smaller fragments (see **Fig.** 1B). The matrix of COF consists of varying proportions of woven bone and cementumlike material in differing stages of maturation. Usually, bone trabeculae with prominent osteoblastic rimming can be found and are more consistently evident than in COD (**Fig.** 2A). Over time, lamellar maturation and

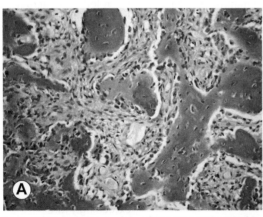
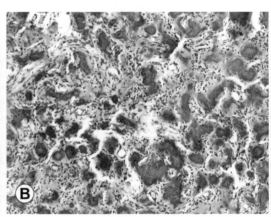

Fig. 2. (*A*) Trabecular new bone formation with osteoblastic rimming in a CCOF (H&E, original magnification, ×100). (*B*) Abundant psammoma body–like matrix deposits in a JPOF (H&E, original magnification, ×50).

mineralization increase and the matrix coalesces into more complex structures. JTOFs can infiltrate into the surrounding bone and typically show slender strands of woven bone that lack evidence of maturation. JPOFs contain spherical and pauci-cellular matrix deposits reminiscent of psammoma bodies/cementumlike material (see Fig. 2B). Over time, these basophilic cementicles can coalesce and induce new bone formation. The matrix of COF is embedded in a moderately cellular and monomorphic fibroblastlike stroma without significant atypia. Spindle cells can show storiform whorls and feature hyperchromatic nuclei; mitoses are usually difficult to find. Frequently, multinucleated giant cells are observed, particularly in JTOF and JPOF.[5,7]

COF is a slowly growing neoplasm that generally can be managed by surgical excision; only in very large lesions might en bloc resection be required. Recurrences are rare in CCOF and more common in JTOF and JPOF, and malignant transformation has not been documented so far for any COF. In recent publications, juvenile ossifying fibromas have been suggested as potential precursors of osteogenic sarcoma because of an increased amount of MDM2 and RASAL1 templates identified by quantitative polymerase chain reaction, which the investigators interpreted as evidence for gene amplification.[10,11] Although polysomy of the long arm of chromosome 12 (comprising both MDM2 and RASAL1) is probably the more appropriate term for the described and nevertheless interesting finding, it is clearly distinct from the MDM2 amplifications that can be found in a small subset of low-grade central OSs (discussed later) and is not sufficient to infer a relationship between these clearly distinct entities.[12]

A very rare and usually multifocal/multiquadrant subtype of COF is FGC, which exclusively affects the jaws and can result in severe facial deformity. It is still unclear whether FGC should be regarded as a subtype of COF or COD; however, the kind of matrix mineralization forming large calcified masses resembles that observed in COD.[5,13,14]

FIBROUS DYSPLASIA

FD is a skeletal anomaly caused by a postzygotic missense mutation of the GNAS gene encoding the activating alpha subunit of the stimulatory G protein. It may involve single (monostotic) or multiple (polyostotic) bones and can occur along with a range of endocrinopathies and skin lesions (Café-au-lait pigmentation) as McCune-Albright syndrome or together with intramuscular myxoma as Mazabraud syndrome. The mutation leads to a proliferation of undifferentiated, bone marrow–related stem cells that replace the hematopoietic marrow with a loose fibrous stroma and develop into functionally impaired bone-forming osteoprogenitors. In the craniofacial bones, FD typically affects multiple adjacent bones, which is still considered as monostotic involvement and should be designated as craniofacial FD.[15–17]

Active FD is a disease of the growing skeleton and most frequently involves the femur and the craniofacial bones. Eighty percent of cases are diagnosed in the first and second decades of life.[18] The monostotic form is 6 to 10 times more common than polyostotic FD; in principle, any bone can be affected.[19] In the jaws, the maxilla is most frequently involved and lesions can involve multiple adjacent bones. Patients usually recognize a painless swelling that can lead to facial asymmetry and/or teeth displacement/malocclusion caused by significant expansion of the affected bones. Radiologically, early FD is primarily lytic but over time develops a homogeneous ground-glass appearance that is highly characteristic. The margins are indistinct and blend into the surrounding normal bone (Fig. 3A); in the jaws, narrowing of the periodontal ligament and blurring of the dura surrounding the teeth can be observed. In most cases, the diagnosis can be made without requiring histologic proof.[20]

Morphologically, FD shows a bland and uniform fibroblastlike spindle cell stroma without atypia or increased mitotic activity. The stroma appears immature and shows loosely arranged collagen fibers. Directly evolving from the spindle cells, varying amounts of a usually delicate woven bone formation can be observed that typically lacks osteoblastic rimming. The trabeculae can resemble Chinese script letters, but cases with only scarce matrix deposits do occur (see Fig. 3B). Using special stains (eg, van Gieson), a typical pattern of Sharpey fibers that radiate perpendicularly from the trabeculae into the surrounding stroma is usually present.[21,22] Over time, the woven bone matures slowly into lamellar bone and the lesional cells carrying the causative mutation get progressively thinned out by apoptosis.[23] As a consequence, the stroma becomes increasingly hypocellular and the lesional matrix can resemble reactive osteosclerosis. For the same reason, it can become increasingly difficult to detect GNAS mutations because the amount of mutant gene copies can decrease below the detection threshold of the diagnostic method used.[24] Despite a presentation that is still radiologically and clinically typical, the histologic appearance therefore shifts into more nonspecific findings that can be difficult to interpret,

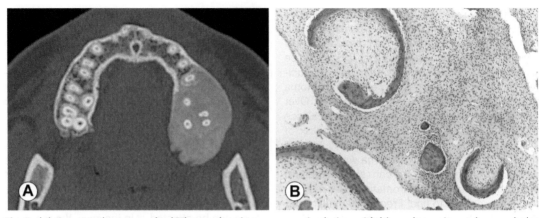

Fig. 3. (*A*) Computed tomography (CT) scan showing an expansive lesion with blurred margins and ground-glass appearance, typical for FD. (*B*) On histology, immature new bone formation surrounded by a moderately cellular and monomorphic fibroblastlike stroma are typical hallmarks (H&E, original magnification, ×50).

particularly without clinical and radiologic correlation and a negative GNAS mutation analysis.

FD usually stabilizes with skeletal maturation, which is why surgical intervention should be delayed as long as possible. Simple contouring of the affected bone is required in some cases. Malignant transformation, mostly into high-grade OS, is very rare.[25]

GIANT CELL–CONTAINING LESIONS

In contrast with the peripheral skeleton, conventional giant cell tumors of bone generally do not occur in the jaws, probably with the exception of very rare cases affecting the condylar process. Most lesions with giant cells represent central giant cell granuloma (CGCG) and aneurysmal bone cyst (ABC), particularly the solid variant (**Table 2**).

CENTRAL GIANT CELL GRANULOMA

CGCGs are localized but locally aggressive lesions of the jaws that most commonly affect the anterior mandible. They occur most frequently in women and usually develop before the age of 20 years. Most lesions grow slowly and remain asymptomatic except for painless swellings; however one-third of cases follow a more aggressive clinical course and can cause pain, resorption, and displacement of teeth, erosion, or even destruction of bone and soft tissue infiltration.[26] CGCGs are usually solitary lesions but can occur multifocally, particularly when related to neurofibromatosis 1 or Noonan-/LEOPARD syndrome.[27,28]

Radiologically, CGCGs appear lytic and multilobulated. They can reach considerable dimensions with marked expansion of the affected bone and cortical thinning (**Fig. 4**A). Aggressive permeative growth or periosteal reaction are generally absent. Because of metaplastic bone formation, the lesions can develop sclerotic areas but never become as extensively calcified as the aforementioned fibro-osseous lesions. In the differential diagnosis to ameloblastoma, which can radiographically also present as polylobulated and expansile osteolysis, these sclerotic parts can nevertheless be of diagnostic help because they are typically missing in ameloblastoma.[27,28]

On histology, CGCGs show a lobular proliferation of mononuclear cells that appear spindle shaped or polygonal and can be arranged in a storiform pattern. Intermingled, varying numbers of small multinucleated giant cells are found (<15 nuclei per section) that typically cluster around vascular spaces and hemosiderin deposits but are not as homogeneously distributed or may even dominate the histology as in conventional giant cell tumor of bone (see **Fig. 4**B). The nuclei of the mononuclear and multinucleated components are both inconspicuous and strikingly similar without significant anisomorphy or atypia. Mitoses are easily identified in the mononuclear cells but are not atypical. The lobules of tumor cells are usually incompletely separated by fibrous septae or metaplastic new bone formation, which is present to some extent in most cases.

Because hyperparathyroidism-related brown tumors can appear identical to CGCG on histology, laboratory testing should be complemented to rule out this differential diagnosis. The giant cell lesions occurring as part of the syndromes mentioned earlier are also virtually identical to classic CGCG, although in some the spindle cell morphology of the mononuclear cells is more

Table 2
Giant cell–containing lesions

	Central Giant Cell Granuloma	Aneurysmal Bone Cyst	Cherubism
Age	First–second decade	First–second decade	First decade
Gender predilection	Female >male	None	None
Localization	Anterior: mandible >maxilla	Posterior: mandible >maxilla	All 4 quadrants
Symptoms	Nonspecific	Nonspecific	Swelling of all 4 quadrants, which can lead to facial deformity
Radiology	Well demarcated, expansive, primarily lytic with limited central matrix mineralization, cortical thinning in advanced cases	Well demarcated, expansive, primarily lytic, can contain bony septae, cortical thinning in advanced cases, fluid-fluid levels on MRI	Well demarcated, largely expansive, usually contains bony septae, cortical thinning
Histopathology	Lobules of monomorphic spindle cells with scattered (small) multinuclear giant cells, fibrous septae with metaplastic woven bone formation	Pseudocysts lined by mononuclear polygonal cells, (small) multinuclear giant cells and siderophages, metaplastic new bone formation can appear bluish (so-called blue bone); more solid forms can occur	Identical to CGCG
Genetics	Unknown except for syndrome-related lesions	USP6 rearrangements in ~70% of primary ABC	SH3BP2 germline mutation
Prognosis	Recurrences may occur following curettage, no malignant transformation	Recurrences may occur following curettage, no malignant transformation	Most cases regress after puberty, no malignant transformation

pronounced and the numbers of giant cells tend to be reduced.[26,28] Another differential diagnosis with a strikingly similar morphology is cherubism, which has a characteristic clinical/radiographic presentation and should not lead to diagnostic difficulties (discussed later).

Molecular studies have not yielded any hints to the underlying pathogenesis of CGCG but clearly

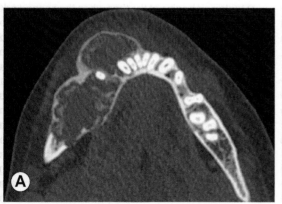
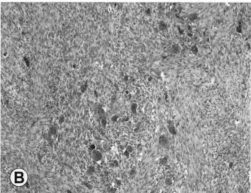

Fig. 4. (*A*) CGCG presenting as a polylobulated and expansile osteolysis of the right mandible. (*B*) Histology shows storiform spindle cells and foci of clustered multinucleated giant cells (H&E, original magnification, ×50).

excluded a relationship to giant cell tumor of bone and to solid variants of ABC. Conventional giant cell tumors have been shown to harbor point mutations in the H3F3A gene in up to 95% of cases, and these have not been detected in larger sets of CGCG.[29] The same holds true for the USP6 rearrangements that can be found in roughly 70% of (primary) ABC but not in CGCG. In contrast, the giant cell lesions of the small tubular bones of the hand and feet that histologically also resemble CGCG were found to show USP6 alterations and therefore to represent solid variants of ABC in at least a subset of cases.[30]

Most CGCG can be sufficiently treated by curettage, although recurrences do occur, particularly in aggressive and syndrome-related types. The role of adjuvants such as RANK (receptor activator of nuclear factor kappa-B) ligand inhibitors or bisphosphonates should be considered in lesions that are difficult to treat by surgery only.[31]

There is also a soft tissue correlate of CGCG that has been designated peripheral giant cell granuloma and that typically develops in the gingiva or alveolar mucosa. It probably develops as a result of chronic irritation and is also known as giant cell epulis. Clinically, it presents as a sessile or pedunculated mass that has a fleshy appearance and is histologically identical to CGCG except for being less lobulated. Excision is usually sufficient but should include the periosteum to avoid recurrences.[32]

ANEURYSMAL BONE CYST

ABC is a pseudocystic lesion of bone that shows an expansile and commonly eccentric growth. It usually contains spaces filled with fluid or blood but also occurs in a more solid variant that histologically can mimic CGCG. ABC typically develops in the first 2 decades of life (80%), although all age groups can be affected; in the jaws, the posterior mandible is the most commonly involved site.[33,34]

Patients complain of expansile swellings that can be painful and reach large dimensions. Teeth remain vital but can become displaced or mobile, and root resorption can also be observed. Radiographically, ABC typically presents as single or multilobulated lytic lesion that can contain bony septae; in MRI scans, fluid-fluid levels are highly characteristic.

On histology, the pseudocystic septae contain polygonal mononuclear cells and multinucleated giant cells to varying degrees. The giant cells are again small (<15 nuclei per section) and participate in lining the pseudocystic walls. Frequently, there are also hemosiderin deposits, siderophages, foam cells, and reactive new bone formation that typically appears basophilic and is known as blue bone. Mitoses can occur and are sometimes frequent; significant atypia or atypical mitoses are generally absent (if not, consider telangiectatic OS).[33,34]

ABC-like areas can be observed in a variety of bone tumors and tumorlike lesions, including juvenile ossifying fibroma, FD, and osteoblastoma, a phenomenon designated as secondary ABC. These lesions, as well as telangiectatic osteosarcoma, have not been reported to show USP6 rearrangements so far that can be identified in 70% of primary ABC. Importantly, only the mononuclear component of ABC represents the true lesional cell and harbors the molecular aberration, so it is vital to evaluate only those cells for molecular confirmation. In areas with abundant reactive cells this can be particularly difficult and can result in false-negative testing. USP6 rearrangements comprise gene fusions with a variety of different genes (CDH11, COL1A1, OMD, TRAP150, ZNF9) but consistently seem to result in upregulation of USP6. The exact role of USP6 in ABC formation is still largely unknown.[35]

Curettage is usually sufficient to treat ABC, although larger lesions might require en bloc resection. Recurrences can occur but malignant transformation has not convincingly been described so far.

CHERUBISM

Cherubism is a rare genetic disorder generally caused by germline mutations of the SH3BP2 gene with variable penetrance and expression levels. Patients present with marked expansion usually of all 4 quadrants of the jaws during childhood, and this can reach disfiguring dimensions. Because of an autosomal dominant inheritance, patients commonly have a known family history of the disease; however, spontaneous mutations occur in up to 50% of cases.[36,37]

The disease is linked to the normal development of teeth and begins at the time when the second primary molar erupts and the second and third permanent molars start to mineralize (between 2 and 3 years of age).[38,39] In early stages as well as in milder forms, the bone defects may only be detected radiographically. However, over time, most patients develop bilateral swellings that lead to facial deformity and can result in the retraction of the facial skin, including the eyelids, and the typical Putti-like phenotype (incorrectly referred to as cherubs). The posterior aspects of all quadrants appear polylobulated and lytic with cortical thinning and irregular bony septae inside. Depending on the extent of bone expansion, patients can develop tooth displacement, altered tooth eruption, or loosening of teeth, and rarely upper airway obstruction or obliteration occurs. During adolescence, most patients experience spontaneous regression so surgery should be reserved only for severe cases with an expected functional benefit.[40]

On histology, cherubism resembles CGCG, which can be misleading in cases in which the clinical context is not known. In early phases, osteoclastic giant cells can be very prominent and contain up to 100 nuclei; in later phases, the osteoclasts generally decrease in number and size. Malignant transformation has not been reported.

BONE-FORMING TUMORS

OSTEOMA

Osteoma is a benign tumor composed of mature bone that has a predilection for the craniofacial bones. It can occur at the surface of compact bone or arise in the medullary cavity, also known as enostosis or bone island.[41,42] Both forms are more common in the mandible and appear as well-circumscribed radio-opaque masses, usually measuring less than 2 cm. On histology, osteomas are predominantly composed of lamellar bone and can be divided into compact, spongious, and mixed subtypes. If cancellous areas occur, the bone can show osteoblastic rimming and a well-vascularized and moderately cellular fibrous stroma. Multiple osteomas can be a manifestation of the autosomal dominantly inherited Gardner syndrome, a variant of familial adenomatous polyposis. Usually, osteomas of the jaws do not require treatment and follow an indolent clinical course.[43]

OSTEOID OSTEOMA AND OSTEOBLASTOMA

Both osteoid osteoma (OO) and osteoblastoma (OB) are benign bone-forming tumors that only rarely occur in the craniofacial bones.[44–47] OO is characterized by a self-limiting growth potential (<2 cm) and nocturnal pain that typically responds to nonsteroidal antiinflammatory drugs (NSAIDs), although this phenomenon might be less obvious in jaw tumors. Radiographically, OO presents with a lytic nidus and perifocal sclerosis that can be extensive and potentially obscure the nidus. OB differs from OO by size (>2 cm) as well as progressive growth and usually does not respond to NSAIDs. In the literature, 10% of all OBs are reported to occur in the craniofacial bones, particularly in the posterior mandible, but this figure might be overrated because of the inclusion of cementoblastomas (morphologically similar lesions intimately associated with the roots of teeth and characterized by calcified cementumlike matrix deposition) in some studies. The radiologic presentation is predominantly lytic but can contain areas of calcification caused by mineralization of bone. On histology, OO and OB are virtually indistinguishable and show haphazardly arranged trabeculae of woven bone rimmed by activated osteoblasts with perinuclear halos (prominent Golgi apparatus). The matrix formation is embedded in a well-vascularized fibrous stroma that can contain scattered osteoclasts (Fig. 5). Infiltrative growth into the surrounding bone, high-grade atypia, atypical mitoses, or areas of tumor cell proliferation without bone formation are generally absent and should lead to the consideration of (osteoblastomalike) OS. Surgical excision or curettage is usually curative.

OSTEOSARCOMA

OS is the most common primary malignant tumor of bone and typically affects the metaphyses of long bones during skeletal growth.[48,49] Most

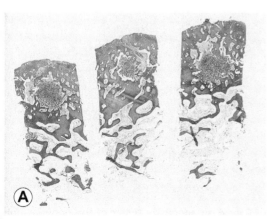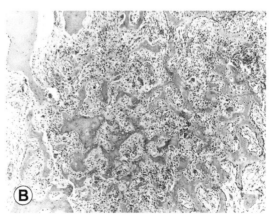

Fig. 5. (A) A small cortical nidus of an OO embedded in sclerotic bone (H&E, original magnification, ×10). (B) Greater magnification highlights the trabecular new bone formation surrounded by a highly vascularized stroma containing activated osteoblasts (H&E, original magnification, ×50).

cases develop around the knee and in the proximal humerus but the jawbones are the fourth most prevalent site, accounting for about 6% of cases. OS in this location tends to occur after skeletal maturity and 1 to 2 decades later than its peripheral counterparts. Men and women are equally affected, and there is a slight predilection for the mandible.[49–52] As in the rest of the skeleton, 2% to 8% of all OSs represent low-grade and intermediate-grade tumors, whereas almost all are conventional high-grade tumors.

Symptoms are nonspecific and can include pain, swelling, and loosening of teeth. Radiographically, OS presents as mixed radiolucencies reflecting the extent of matrix formation and mineralization. Aggressive features such as cortical permeation and periosteal reaction are generally present in high-grade tumors (Fig. 6A, B). On histology, gnathic OSs are identical to peripheral tumors and consist of pleomorphic tumor cells producing bone. The degree of atypia, mitotic activity, and necrosis varies but is usually less pronounced than in the peripheral skeleton (see Fig. 6C, D). A chondroblastic component is common and can mimic chondrosarcoma.[50] It should therefore be kept in mind that chondrosarcoma is exceedingly rare in the jawbones and cannot be diagnosed with certainty in core needle biopsies, except for tumors harboring IDH1/2 mutations. From another perspective, OS should always be considered if cartilage is present in a gnathic biopsy and a fracture with callus formation can be ruled out.

Immunohistochemistry with antibodies against SATB2, procollagen I, and osterix can help to confirm an osteoblastic lineage but is usually not required. There are no molecular markers available so far, with the exception of MDM2/CDK4 amplification in about 79% of parosteal OS and 29% of central low-grade OS. Immunohistochemistry against MDM2 can be used as a surrogate but needs confirmation using fluorescence in situ

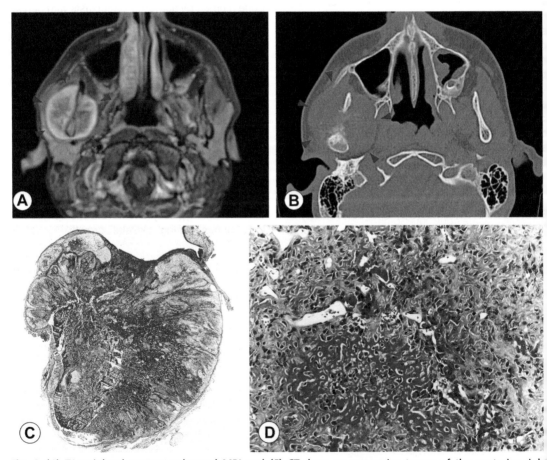

Fig. 6. (A) T1-weighted contrast-enhanced MRI and (B) CT show an aggressive tumor of the posterior right mandible (*arrowheads*) with bone destruction, periosteal reaction, and bony matrix mineralization. (C) Overview of a gnathic OS permeating through the preexisting alveolar bone (H&E, original magnification, ×10). (D) Higher magnification shows atypical tumor cells producing lacelike tumor osteoid (H&E, original magnification, ×100).

hybridization. In conventional high-grade OS, MDM2 amplification is rare (<10%), implying that only a positive result can help in the differential diagnosis.[12]

Gnathic OSs metastasize far less frequently (6%–21%) and later in the course of the disease compared with their peripheral counterparts, which is why resection with clear margins can be curative and results in 10-year survival rates greater than 80%. The role of additional chemotherapy is therefore still controversial. Notably, this favorable prognostic impact is restricted to OS of the jaws, whereas tumors of the skull or facial bones behave similar to peripheral tumors.[49,50]

REFERENCES

1. Moore KL, Persaud TVN. The developing human: clinically oriented embryology. 7th edition. Philadelphia: Saunders; 2003.
2. El-Mofty SK, Nelson B, Toyosawa S, et al. Cemento-osseous dysplasia. In: El-Naggar AK, Chan JKC, Grandis JR, et al, editors. WHO classification of head and neck tumours. Lyon (France): IARC Press; 2017. p. 254–5.
3. Owosho AA, Potluri A, Bilodeau EA. Osseous dysplasia (cemento-osseous dysplasia) of the jaw bones in western Pennsylvania patients: analysis of 35 cases. Pa Dent J (Harrisb) 2013;80(6):25–9.
4. Das BK, Das SN, Gupta A, et al. Florid cemento-osseous dysplasia. J Oral Maxillofac Pathol 2013; 17(1):150.
5. El-Mofty SK. Fibro-osseous lesions of the craniofacial skeleton: an update. Head Neck Pathol 2014; 8(4):432–44.
6. Slootweg PJ, El-Mofty SK. Ossifying fibroma. In: Barnes L, Eveson JW, Reichart P, et al, editors. World Health Organization classification of tumours. Pathology and genetics of head and neck tumours. Lyon (France): IARC Press; 2005. p. 319–20.
7. El-Mofty SK, Nelson B, Toyosawa S. Ossifying fibroma. In: El-Naggar AK, Chan JKC, Grandis JR, et al, editors. WHO classification of head and neck tumours. Lyon (France): IARC Press; 2017. p. 251–2.
8. El-Mofty S. Psammomatoid and trabecular juvenile ossifying fibroma of the craniofacial skeleton: two distinct clinicopathologic entities. Oral Surg Oral Med Oral Pathol Oral Radiol Endod 2002;93(3):296–304.
9. Carpten JD, Robbins CM, Villablanca A, et al. HRPT2, encoding parafibromin, is mutated in hyperparathyroidism-jaw tumor syndrome. Nat Genet 2002;32(4):676–80.
10. Guerin M, Thariat J, Ouali M, et al. A new subtype of high-grade mandibular osteosarcoma with RASAL1/MDM2 amplification. Hum Pathol 2016;50:70–8.
11. Tabareau-Delalande F, Collin C, Gomez-Brouchet A, et al. Chromosome 12 long arm rearrangement covering MDM2 and RASAL1 is associated with aggressive craniofacial juvenile ossifying fibroma and extracranial psammomatoid fibro-osseous lesions. Mod Pathol 2015;28(1):48–56.
12. Salinas-Souza C, De Andrea C, Bihl M, et al. GNAS mutations are not detected in parosteal and low-grade central osteosarcomas. Mod Pathol 2015; 28(10):1336–42.
13. Raubenheimer EJ, Noffke CE, Boy SC. Osseous dysplasia with gross jaw expansion: a review of 18 lesions. Head Neck Pathol 2016;10(4):437–43.
14. Kumar VV, Ebenezer S, Narayan TV, et al. Clinico-pathologic conference: multiquadrant expansile fibro-osseous lesion in a juvenile. Oral Surg Oral Med Oral Pathol Oral Radiol 2012;113(3):286–92.
15. Bianco P, Riminucci M, Majolagbe A, et al. Mutations of the GNAS1 gene, stromal cell dysfunction, and osteomalacic changes in non-McCune-Albright fibrous dysplasia of bone. J Bone Miner Res 2000; 15(1):120–8.
16. Weinstein LS, Shenker A, Gejman PV, et al. Activating mutations of the stimulatory G protein in the McCune-Albright syndrome. N Engl J Med 1991; 325(24):1688–95.
17. El-Mofty SK, Nelson B, Toyosawa S. Fibrous dysplasia. In: El-Naggar AK, Chan JKC, Grandis JR, et al, editors. WHO classification of head and neck tumours. Lyon (France): IARC Press; 2017. p. 253–4.
18. Waldron CA. Fibro-osseous lesions of the jaws. J Oral Maxillofac Surg 1993;51(8):828–35.
19. Siegal GP, Bianco P, Dal Cin P. Fibrous dysplasia. In: Fletcher CDM, Bridge JA, Hogendoorn PCW, et al, editors. WHO classification of tumours of soft tissue and bone. Lyon (France): IARC Press; 2013. p. 352–3.
20. MacDonald-Jankowski DS. Fibro-osseous lesions of the face and jaws. Clin Radiol 2004;59(1):11–25.
21. Alawi F. Benign fibro-osseous diseases of the maxillofacial bones. A review and differential diagnosis. Am J Clin Pathol 2002;118(Suppl):S50–70.
22. Slootweg PJ. Maxillofacial fibro-osseous lesions: classification and differential diagnosis. Semin Diagn Pathol 1996;13(2):104–12.
23. Riminucci M, Robey PG, Saggio I, et al. Skeletal progenitors and the GNAS gene: fibrous dysplasia of bone read through stem cells. J Mol Endocrinol 2010;45(6):355–64.
24. Liang Q, Wei M, Hodge L, et al. Quantitative analysis of activating alpha subunit of the G protein (Gsα) mutation by pyrosequencing in fibrous dysplasia and other bone lesions. J Mol Diagn 2011;13(2): 137–42.
25. Ruggieri P, Sim FH, Bond JR, et al. Malignancies in fibrous dysplasia. Cancer 1994;73(5):1411–24.
26. Raubenheimer E, Jordan RC. Central giant cell granuloma. In: El-Naggar AK, Chan JKC, Grandis JR, et al, editors. WHO classification of head and neck tumours. Lyon (France): IARC Press; 2017. p. 256–7.

27. Vered M, Buchner A, Dayan D. Central giant cell granuloma of the jawbones–new insights into molecular biology with clinical implications on treatment approaches. Histol Histopathol 2008;23(9):1151–60.

28. Flanagan AM, Speight PM. Giant cell lesions of the craniofacial bones. Head Neck Pathol 2014;8(4): 445–53.

29. Presneau N, Baumhoer D, Behjati S, et al. Diagnostic value of H3F3A mutations in giant cell tumour of bone compared to osteoclast-rich mimics. J Pathol Clin Res 2015;1(2):113–23.

30. Agaram NP, LeLoarer FV, Zhang L, et al. USP6 gene rearrangements occur preferentially in giant cell reparative granulomas of the hands and feet but not in gnathic location. Hum Pathol 2014;45(6):1147–52.

31. Gupta B, Stanton N, Coleman H, et al. A novel approach to the management of a central giant cell granuloma with denosumab: A case report and review of current treatments. J Craniomaxillofac Surg 2015;43(7):1127–32.

32. Shadman N, Ebrahimi SF, Jafari S, et al. Peripheral giant cell granuloma: a review of 123 cases. Dent Res J (Isfahan) 2009;6(1):47–50.

33. Motamedi MH, Behroozian A, Azizi T, et al. Assessment of 120 maxillofacial aneurysmal bone cysts: a nationwide quest to understand this enigma. J Oral Maxillofac Surg 2014;72(8):1523–30.

34. Jordan RC, Koutlas I, Raubenheimer E. Aneurysmal bone cyst. In: El-Naggar AK, Chan JKC, Grandis JR, et al, editors. WHO classification of head and neck tumours. Lyon (France): IARC Press; 2017. p. 258–9.

35. Oliveira AM, Perez-Atayde AR, Inwards CY, et al. USP6 and CDH11 oncogenes identify the neoplastic cell in primary aneurysmal bone cysts and are absent in so-called secondary aneurysmal bone cysts. Am J Pathol 2004;165(5):1773–80.

36. Papadaki ME, Lietman SA, Levine MA, et al. Cherubism: best clinical practice. Orphanet J Rare Dis 2012;7(Suppl 1):S6.

37. Jordan RC, Raubenheimer E. Cherubism. In: El-Naggar AK, Chan JKC, Grandis JR, et al, editors. WHO classification of head and neck tumours. Lyon (France): IARC Press; 2017. p. 257–8.

38. Hyckel P, Berndt A, Schleier P, et al. Cherubism - new hypotheses on pathogenesis and therapeutic consequences. J Craniomaxillofac Surg 2005; 33(1):61–8.

39. Yoshitaka T, Mukai T, Kittaka M, et al. Enhanced TLR-MYD88 signaling stimulates autoinflammation in SH3BP2 cherubism mice and defines the etiology of cherubism. Cell Rep 2014;8(6):1752–66.

40. Prescott T, Redfors M, Rustad CF, et al. Characterization of a Norwegian cherubism cohort; molecular genetic findings, oral manifestations and quality of life. Eur J Med Genet 2013;56(3):131–7.

41. Baumhoer D, Bras J. Osteoma. In: Fletcher CDM, Bridge JA, Hogendoorn PCW, et al, editors. WHO classification of tumours of soft tissue and bone. Lyon (France): IARC Press; 2013. p. 276.

42. Toner M, Allen CM, Castle J. Osteoma. In: El-Naggar AK, Chan JKC, Grandis JR, et al, editors. WHO classification of head and neck tumours. Lyon (France): IARC Press; 2017. p. 246.

43. Kaplan I, Nicolaou Z, Hatuel D, et al. Solitary central osteoma of the jaws: a diagnostic dilemma. Oral Surg Oral Med Oral Pathol Oral Radiol Endod 2008;106(3):e22–9.

44. Horvai A, Klein M. Osteoid osteoma. In: Fletcher CDM Bridge JA, Hogendoorn PCW, et al, editors. WHO classification of tumours of soft tissue and bone. Lyon (France): IARC Press; 2013. p. 277–8.

45. de Andrea CE, Bridge JA, Schiller A. Osteoblastoma. In: Fletcher CDM, Bridge JA, Hogendoorn PCW, et al editors. WHO classification of tumours of soft tissue and bone. Lyon (France): IARC Press; 2013. p. 279–80.

46. Toner M, Allen CM, Castle J. Osteoblastoma. In: El-Naggar AK, Chan JKC, Grandis JR, et al, editors. WHO classification of head and neck tumours. Lyon (France): IARC Press; 2017. p. 249.

47. Toner M, Allen CM, Castle J. Osteoid osteoma. In: El-Naggar AK, Chan JKC, Grandis JR, et al, editors. WHO classification of head and neck tumours. Lyon (France): IARC Press; 2017. p. 249.

48. Rosenberg AE, Cleton-Jansen A-M, de Pinieux G et al. Conventional osteosarcoma. In: Fletcher C Bridge J, Hogendoorn P, et al, editors. WHO classification of tumours of soft tissue and bone. Lyon (France): IARC Press; 2013. p. 282–8.

49. Baumhoer D, Lopes M, Raubenheimer E. Osteosarcoma. In: El-Naggar AK, Chan JKC, Grandis JR et al, editors. WHO classification of head and neck tumours. Lyon (France): IARC Press; 2017. p. 244–6.

50. Baumhoer D, Brunner P, Eppenberger-Castori S et al. Osteosarcomas of the jaws differ from their peripheral counterparts and require a distinct treatment approach. Experiences from the DOESAK Registry. Oral Oncol 2014;50(2):147–53.

51. Lee RJ, Arshi A, Schwartz HC, et al. Characteristics and prognostic factors of osteosarcoma of the jaws a retrospective cohort study. JAMA Otolaryngol Head Neck Surg 2015;141(5):470–7.

52. Thariat J, Julieron M, Brouchet A, et al. Osteosarcomas of the mandible: are they different from other tumor sites? Crit Rev Oncol Hematol 2012;82(3): 280–95.

Soft Tissue Tumors Rarely Presenting Primary in Bone; Diagnostic Pitfalls

Marta Sbaraglia, MD[a], Alberto Righi, MD[b],
Marco Gambarotti, MD[b], Daniel Vanel, MD[b],
Piero Picci, MD[b], Angelo P. Dei Tos, MD[a,c,*]

KEYWORDS

- Primary sarcoma of bone • Malignant fibrous histiocytoma • Hemangiopericytoma
- Leiomyosarcoma of bone • Synovial sarcoma of bone

Key points

- Primary bone sarcomas (nonosteosarcoma, nonchondrosarcoma, and non-Ewing sarcoma) rank among the rarest malignancies and represent a major diagnostic challenge.
- The reappraisal of now obsolete entities, such as malignant fibrous histiocytoma (MFH) and hemangiopericytoma (HPC), has led to recognition of specific tumor entities.
- Leiomyosarcoma (LMS) represents the most common lesion; however, a broader variety of soft tissue sarcomas may rarely occur in bone.
- Diagnosis relies on integration of clinical, radiologic, immunomorphologic, and molecular findings, ideally in context of expert centers.

ABSTRACT

Primary bone sarcomas represent extremely rare entities. The use of now abolished labels, such as malignant fibrous histiocytoma and hemangiopericytoma, has significantly hampered the chance of identifying specific entities. It is now accepted that a broad variety of mesenchymal malignancies most often arising on the soft tissue may actually present as primary bone lesions. A more accurate morphologic partition is justified based on availability of distinct therapeutic options. An integrated diagnostic approach represents the only way to achieve a correct classification. In consideration of the significant complexity, primary bone sarcomas should ideally be handled in the context of expert centers.

OVERVIEW

When dealing with primary bone malignant mesenchymal tumors, pathologists are offered a limited number of diagnostic options, including mainly osteosarcoma, Ewing sarcoma, and chondrosarcoma. Aside from the intrinsic diagnostic challenges that these entities generate, a broader variety of lesions that arise predominantly in the soft tissues may present as a primary bone malignancy. In the past, most of these cases have been lumped within 2 main categories; MFH and

Disclosure Statement: No disclosures.
[a] Department of Pathology, Azienda ULSS2 Marca Trevigiana, Treviso, Italy; [b] Department of Pathology, Istituto Ortopedico Rizzoli, Bologna, Italy; [c] Department of Medicine, University of Padua School of Medicine, Padua, Italy
* Corresponding author. Department of Pathology, Azienda ULSS2 Marca Trevigiana, Piazza Ospedale, 1, Treviso 31100, Italy.
E-mail address: angelo.deitos@unipd.it

Surgical Pathology 10 (2017) 705–730
http://dx.doi.org/10.1016/j.path.2017.04.013

fibrosarcoma. In the past 2 decades both MFH and fibrosarcoma underwent a profound conceptual reappraisal. The latest *WHO Classification of Tumours of Soft Bone and Soft Tissue Tumours*[1] has ultimately denied to MFH the dignity of a specific entity. This decision has been taken based on MFH at best representing a collection of unrelated pleomorphic sarcomas (ie, pleomorphic variants of rhabdomyosarcoma [RMS], LMS, and liposarcoma), even including nonmesenchymal lesions, such as metastatic sarcomatoid melanoma and carcinoma. The term, MFH, is currently replaced by the label, undifferentiated pleomorphic sarcoma (UPS), to designate those rare pleomorphic sarcomas in which no specific line of differentiation can be demonstrated. Fibrosarcoma, as defined by the presence of a spindle cell malignancy featuring a herringbone pattern of growth, in the current view corresponds to the fibrosarcomatous variant of dermatofibrosarcoma protuberans. There exist, however, a variety of fibroblastic sarcomas that includes distinctive entities, such as infantile fibrosarcoma, low-grade fibromyxoid sarcoma (LGFMS), sclerosing epithelioid fibrosarcoma (SEF), and myxoinflammatory fibroblastic sarcoma, that have also contributed to replacing fibrosarcoma as a defined clinicopathologic entity.

The process of reclassification was mostly generated within the soft tissue sarcoma community but, unavoidably, has also contaminated the bone sarcoma one. As a consequence, both MFH and fibrosarcoma in bone have also disappeared, replaced by morphologically distinct tumor entities.[2–5]

Sarcomas in general are known to represent one of the most challenging areas of surgical pathology; however, the situation in which a rare tumor arises in an exceptional location like bone generates even greater difficulty. This review is aimed at discussing the main clinicopathologic features of a selected group of malignant and locally aggressive and/or rarely metastasizing soft tissue lesions that can rarely occur primarily in the bone. Together they do not represent more than 5% of all primary bone malignancies.

LEIOMYOSARCOMA

Primary LMS of bone accounts for a majority of primary bone (nonosteogenic/chondrogenic and non-Ewing) sarcomas. They tend to occur in adult or elderly patients and the vast majority occurs in the long bones.[6–8] The femur is the most frequently affected site followed by the tibia and the pelvic bones.

Radiologically, LMS most often presents as a large, mostly lytic lesion, almost always breaking the cortex and extending into the surrounding soft tissue (Fig. 1).

Macroscopically, LMS exhibits a gray to white cut surface, associated in most cases with foci of necrosis and hemorrhage (Fig. 2). The lesion tends to be well demarcated, most often featuring extension in the soft tissues.

The microscopic features of LMS, similarly to its soft tissue counterpart, vary according to the degree of differentiation. Well-differentiated lesions are characterized by fascicles composed of spindle cells containing oval, blunt-ended nuclei and distinctive eosinophilic fibrillary cytoplasm

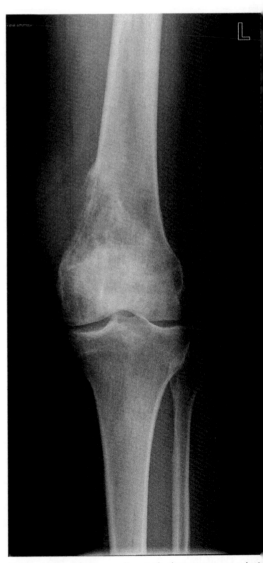

Fig. 1. LMS of bone: radiograph demonstrates a lytic lesion with cortical destruction and soft tissue infiltration.

variants exist, such as myxoid, epithelioid, giant cell–rich, and inflammatory LMS. Immunohisto-chemically, approximately 70% to 80% of cases stain with desmin whereas a vast majority stain with smooth muscle actin. H-caldesmon is positive in approximately 60% of cases. Approximately 30% of LMSs may exhibit multifocal positivity for epithelial membrane antigen (EMA) and/or cytoker-atin. LMS does not feature specific molecular aber-rations that can be used for diagnostic purposes.

Main differential diagnoses include classically fibroblastic osteosarcoma, spindle cell monopha-sic synovial sarcoma (SS) (discussed later) and malignant peripheral nerve sheath tumors (MPNST). The distinction of LMS from fibroblastic osteosarcoma can represent a real challenge. There exists significant immunophenotypic over-lap (both lesions can express desmin) and osteoid can be only focally present and, therefore, easily overlooked. Careful evaluation of imaging as well as extensive sampling is mandatory to avoid misclassification. Occurrence of MPNST as a pri-mary bone lesion represents an extremely rare condition and is most often associated with the presence of neurofibromatosis (NF)-1 syndrome. Morphologically, MPNST is most often composed of a markedly atypical, mitotically active, spindle cell proliferation exhibiting variation of cellularity and often a distinctive perivascular accentuation of cellularity. Pleomorphic RMS may occasionally metastasize to the bone; however, despite signifi-cant morphologic overlap with pleomorphic LMS, it can be recognized based on nuclear expression of myogenin. Because immunopositivity in

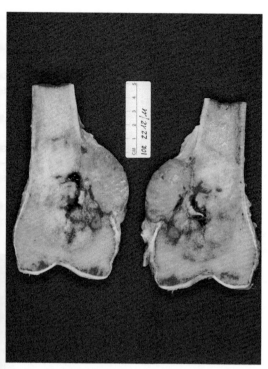

Fig. 2. LMS of bone: gross specimen showing a well-circumscribed, firm, gray-white mass with hemorrhag-ic and necrotic areas, extending in the surrounding soft tissues.

(Fig. 3). High-grade LMS may feature significant pleomorphism (Fig. 4) associated with numerous, often atypical, mitotic figures, and a variable amount of necrosis. Numerous morphologic

Fig. 3. Microscopically, LMS is composed of fasci-cles of spindle cells featuring distinctive eosinophilic fibrillary cytoplasm (H&E, original magnification, ×20).

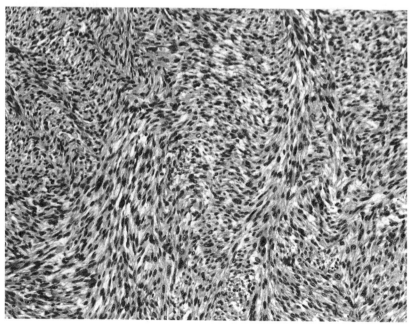

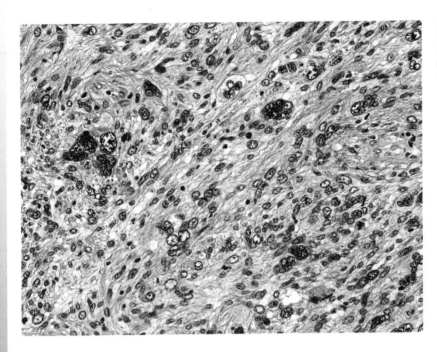

Fig. 4. In high-grade LMS, striking nuclear pleomorphism is often seen (H&E, original magnification, ×20).

pleomorphic RMS is most often limited to scattered neoplastic cells, careful examination of immunostains is mandatory.

A major diagnostic pitfall when dealing with LMS in bone is represented by the absence of complete clinical information. Metastatic LMS to the bone (most often from the uterus) is far more frequent than a primary LMS. It is, therefore, mandatory, particularly when dealing with female patients, to exclude a metastasic LMS from another primary LMS.

Primary LMS of bone represents an aggressive tumor with high rates of metastatic dissemination and tumor-related deaths.[9,10]

Key Features

- Occurrence in the long bones of adults
- Imaging: destructive, mostly lytic lesion invading the soft tissues
- Spindle cell proliferation featuring eosinophilic fibrillary cytoplasm and blunt-ended nuclei
- Variable pleomorphism: from none to extreme
- Immunohistochemical expression of smooth muscle differentiation markers
- Aggressive clinical behavior

Differential Diagnosis

- Osteosarcoma
  - Deposition of malignant osteoid
- Monophasic SS
  - Monomorphic spindle cell proliferation set in collagenous background
  - Hemangiopericytoma-like vascular pattern
  - Variable expression of cytokeratin and EMA
  - Expression of Transducin-Like Enhancer of Split 1 (TLE1)
  - Presence of SYT gene rearrangements
- MPNST
  - Possible association with NF1 syndrome
  - High-grade spindle cell proliferation featuring perivascular accentuation of cellularity
  - Focal expression of S100 protein in one-third of cases
- Pleomorphic RMS
  - Exceedingly rare in bone
  - Deeply eosinophilic, glassy cytoplasm
  - Expression at least focally of myogenin

Pitfalls

! Metastatic LMS to bone is more frequent than primary LMS of bone: check clinical history

! Multifocal cytokeratin expression can be observed in up to one-third of LMS

! The immunohistochemical profile of LMS can overlap with osteosarcoma (which can display focal desmin positivity and special AT-rich sequence-binding protein 2 (SATB2) is not always helpful in the distinction)

UNDIFFERENTIATED PLEOMORPHIC SARCOMA

As discussed previously, UPS represents the current denomination for the now abandoned label MFH[1] and represents less than 2% of all primary bone malignancies.[2-4] Primary bone UPS can occur at any age and predominates in the long bones. Imaging overlaps with that of LMS and SS, featuring large lytic lesions extending through the cortex and invading the soft tissues (Fig. 5).

Macroscopically, UPS exhibits a fleshy, often hemorrhagic and necrotic cut surface (Fig. 6). Morphologically, it is composed of a combination of spindle cell and pleomorphic mesenchymal cells (Fig. 7) most often featuring the presence of atypical mitoses as well as abundant necrosis (Fig. 8). By definition UPS must lack any evidence (both morphologic and immunophenotypical) of a specific line of differentiation.

Differential diagnosis is broad. The use of a panel of smooth muscle differentiation markers (namely desmin, smooth muscle actin, and h-caldesmon) allows recognition of both primary LMS and metastatic LMS. High-grade osteosarcoma may feature significant pleomorphism; however, both the presence of malignant osteogenic matrix and the immunoexpression of SATB2 represent important diagnostic clues.

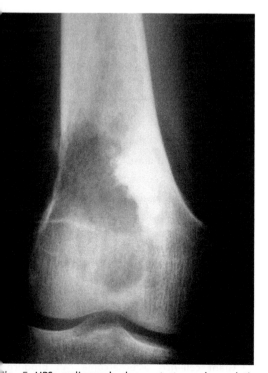

Fig. 5. UPS: radiograph demonstrates a large lytic lesion associated with periosteal reaction.

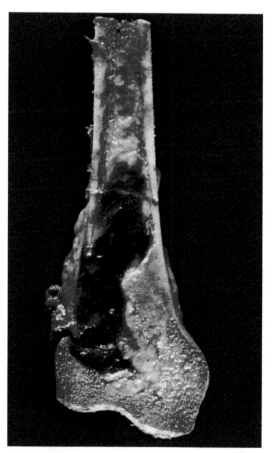

Fig. 6. UPS: macroscopically, a large necrotic-hemorrhagic mass is seen. In this case, cortical destruction and bone fracture are observed.

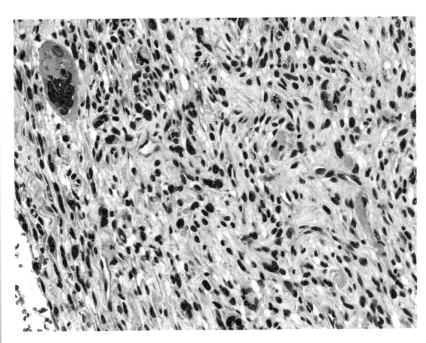

Fig. 7. UPS is composed of a combination of undifferentiated spindle and pleomorphic cells (H&E, original magnification, ×20).

Metastases also represent a potential pitfall, particularly when dealing with sarcomatoid carcinoma and melanoma. Abundant expression of cytokeratin and/or EMA should raise suspicion of sarcomatoid carcinoma and a widespread immunopositivity for S100 protein (both HMB-45 and Melan-A tend to be negative in sarcomatoid melanoma) should prompt considering metastatic melanoma. There are no recurrent cytogenetic alterations of help in the diagnosis of UPS.[3]

 Differential Diagnosis

- Pleomorphic LMS
  - Presence of at least small foci of spindle cells featuring eosinophilic fibrillary cytoplasm and blunt-ended nuclei
  - Expression of smooth muscle differentiation markers
- Pleomorphic RMS
  - Exceedingly rare in bone
  - Deeply eosinophilic, glassy cytoplasm
  - Expression at least focally of myogenin
- High-grade osteosarcoma
  - Presence of malignant osteoid
  - Immunohistochemical expression of SATB2

 Key Features

- Occurrence in the long bones; no age predilection
- Imaging: destructive, mostly lytic lesion invading the soft tissues
- Spindle cell and pleomorphic proliferation featuring atypical mitoses and necrosis
- Absence of expression of specific differentiation markers
- Aggressive clinical behavior

 Pitfalls

! Metastatic sarcomatoid melanoma and carcinoma may mimic UPS: check clinical history

! Giant cell–rich osteosarcoma can produce minimal amount of osteogenic matrix

Fig. 8. The presence of numerous atypical mitoses is a characteristic finding of UPS (H&E, original magnification, ×40).

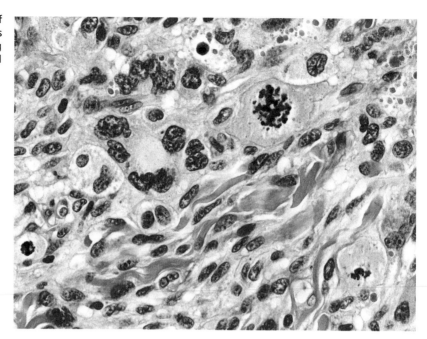

MYXOFIBROSARCOMA

Myxofibrosarcoma represents a well-defined entity in the soft tissue whereas in bone it has been reported only occasionally. It seems likely that until recently myxofibrosarcoma has been under-recognized and lumped within the now abolished category of MFH.[1,2] Myxofibrosarcoma in soft tissue occurs predominantly superficially (two-thirds of cases) in elderly patients. Multinodularity is most often observed. In bone, most cases arise in the long bones with a peak incidence in the fourth decade.[4]

Radiologically, myxofibrosarcoma presents as a centrally located lytic lesion, associated with cortex destruction and extension in the surrounding soft tissues (Fig. 9).

Microscopically, myxofibrosarcoma of bone overlaps entirely with its soft tissue counterpart and features a spindle cell and pleomorphic cell population set in a myxoid background and featuring the presence of capillary-sized archiform blood vessels (Fig. 10). Whereas in soft tissue there exists a spectrum of lesions (from low grade to high grade), in bone it seems like most lesions tend to be high grade. This may represent a bias, however, generated by the difficulty of recognizing low-grade forms of myxofibrosarcoma in bone. Immunohistochemically,

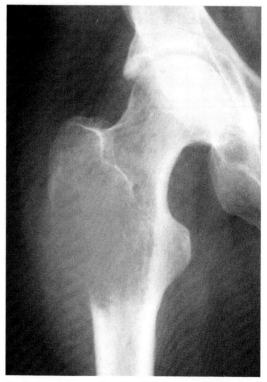

Fig. 9. On radiograph, myxofibrosarcoma appears as a lytic lesion, more often associated with cortex destruction.

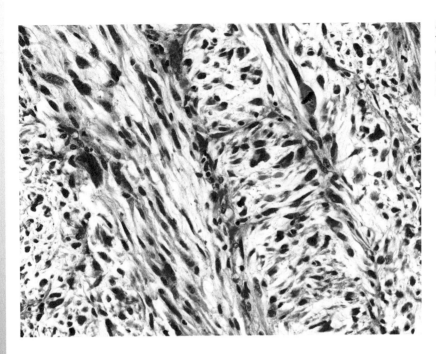

Fig. 10. High-grade myxo-fibrosarcoma is composed of spindle and pleomorphic cells set in abundant myxoid matrix (H&E, original magnification, ×20).

myxofibrosarcoma may exhibit focal smooth muscle actin positivity.

The outcome of primary myxofibrosarcoma of bone seems to be less aggressive than that of UPS both in terms of local recurrence and of metastatic spread. In consideration of the small numbers of cases reported, however, any conclusion seems to be premature.

Key Features

- Occurrence in the long bones of adults

- Imaging: destructive, mostly lytic lesion invading the soft tissues

- Spindle cell and pleomorphic proliferation set in a myxoid background and associated with archiform, thin-walled blood vessels

- Absence of expression of specific differentiation markers

Differential Diagnosis

- UPS
  - No myxoid stroma

Pitfall

! Myxoid areas may be focal and therefore overlooked if specimen is undersampled.

SYNOVIAL SARCOMA

SS represents a mesenchymal malignancy characterized by the capacity of undergoing epithelial differentiation. It seems likely that SS arising primarily in bone has been under-recognized until recently, due to the extensive use of the now abandoned label, hemangiopericytoma.[5] In bone, SS seems to occur predominantly in the long bones. The femur is affected most frequently, followed by the tibia and the pelvic bones.[4,11,12] Age distribution tends to be broader than in soft tissue, wherein occurrence is mostly observed in young adults.

Radiologically, SS often present as large, mostly lytic lesion that may, however, feature sclerotic areas. Cortex breakage is almost invariably observed and is associated with variable extension into the soft tissues (**Figs. 11** and **12**).

Macroscopically, most cases exhibit a fleshy appearance associated with the presence of cystic and hemorrhagic areas (**Fig. 13**).

Morphologically, 3 main morphologic variants of SS are described: spindle cell monophasic, biphasic, and undifferentiated. Monophasic spindle cell SS is composed of a cytologically uniform spindle cell population, organized in cellular sheets and fascicles, and set in a variably collagenous background often featuring a pericellular distribution as well as the presence of a hemangiopericytoma-like vascular network (Fig. 14). Extensive stromal hyalinization with calcifications, myxoid changes, bone metaplasia, and rarely chondroid changes can be variably observed. Biphasic SS is defined by the presence of variable amounts of epithelial differentiation in context with a spindle cell component that exhibits the same morphologic features of monophasic spindle cell SS (Fig. 15). Epithelial differentiation may be overt with formation of true glandular structures or be less obvious and represented by solid cluster of plump, epithelioid neoplastic cells (so-called incipient epithelial differentiation). The poorly differentiated variant (which is associated with more aggressive behavior) accounts for approximately 20% of all SSs and may exhibit 3 main cytomorphologies: large cell, spindle cell, and, most often, round cell (Fig. 16). In bone cases, the presence of multinucleated osteoclast-like giant cells can be observed (Fig. 17).

SS shows variable immunoreactivity for EMA and cytokeratins, EMA being far more sensitive than cytokeratins, particularly when dealing

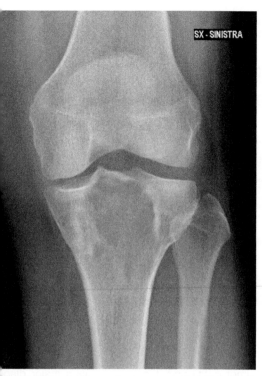

Fig. 11. SS: on radiograph a large, mostly lytic lesion is observed. Small areas of sclerosis are present.

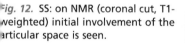

Fig. 12. SS: on NMR (coronal cut, T1-weighted) initial involvement of the articular space is seen.

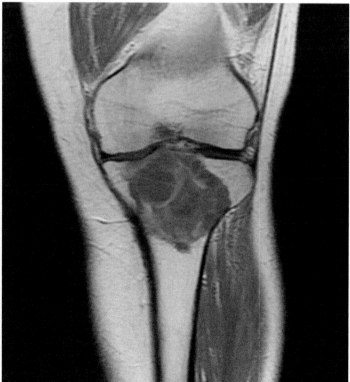

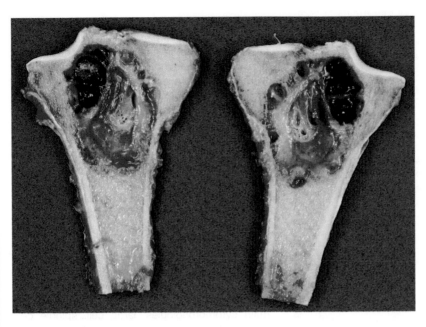

Fig. 13. SS: gross specimen shows the presence of a well-circumscribed mass featuring cystic and hemorrhagic areas.

with the poorly differentiated variant. CD99 immunopositivity is also seen in most cases, TLE1 represents a recently reported transcription factor that seems to sensitive albeit not entirely specific.

Genetically, SS is characterized by the presence of a t(X;18) translocation that fuses the *SYT* gene with *SSX1*, *SSX2*, and more rarely *SSX4*. This genetic aberration has proved unique to this tumor entity and, therefore, plays a major diagnostic role whenever dealing with challenging cases.

As discussed previously, the differential diagnosis includes LMS and MPNST. At times SS may feature a bland morphology that makes (also because of the presence of HPC-like vasculature) the differential diagnosis with solitary fibrous tumor (SFT) rather challenging

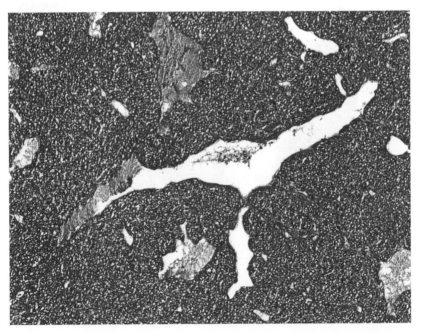

Fig. 14. The presence of an HPC-like vascular pattern is common in SS (H&E, original magnification, ×10).

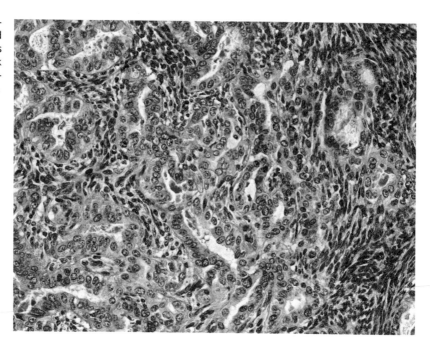

Fig. 15. The combinations of spindle cells and glandular structures is the diagnostic hallmark of biphasic SS (H&E, original magnification, ×20).

Negativity for STAT6, expression of epithelial markers, and presence of *SYT* gene rearrangement all represent extremely useful diagnostic findings.

The most relevant potential diagnostic pitfall is represented by the differential diagnosis with Ewing sarcomas, and this most often happens when dealing with the undifferentiated, round cell variant of SS. CD99 immunopositivity represents a further source of diagnostic confusion, because it tends to be present on both lesions. In SS, however, the pattern of staining tends to

Fig. 16. Round cell poorly differentiated SS enters the differential diagnosis with most round cell sarcoma, mostly Ewing sarcoma (H&E, original magnification, ×20).

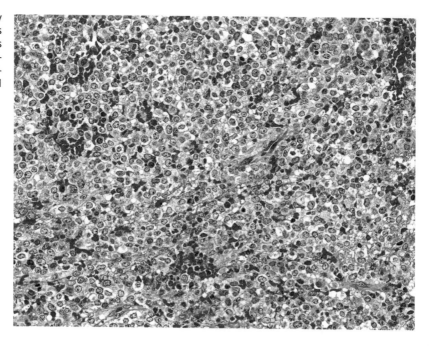

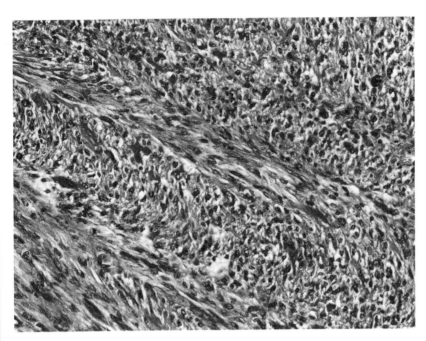

Fig. 17. The presence of scattered osteoclast-like giant cells can be observed in SS of bone (H&E, original magnification, ×20).

be diffuse, in stark contrast with the thick-membrane pattern, typically observed in Ewing sarcoma. Molecular genetics plays a major diagnostic role by demonstrating the presence of *SYT* gene rearrangements in SS and *EWSR1* gene rearrangements in Ewing sarcoma. Small cell osteosarcoma also enters the differential diagnosis. Identification of malignant osteoid (that may be only focal, therefore requiring extensive sampling) represents a key diagnostic clue, as is immunohistochemical expression of SATB2.[13] Another potential pitfall is represented by the differentiation between biphasic SS and a metastasis, most often from carcinoma of the breast, prostate, and kidney. Clinical history plays a major role as well as the application of a pertinent panel of immunostains.

A rare but important as well as challenging differential diagnosis is with adamantinoma. Adamantinoma occurs almost exclusively in the cortex of the tibia (and more rarely in the fibula) of adults with a peak incidence in the fourth decade. Morphologically, the main issue is represented by adamantinoma also featuring a biphasic pattern represented by a combination of spindle cells and cluster of epithelial cells. Overt squamous cell differentiation is frequently observed. Both lesions share expression of cytokeratins. Whereas TLE-1 expression seems limited to SS, p63 is instead observed in

adamantinoma. Molecular analysis demonstrating *SYT* gene rearrangement is also helpful in the differentiation between the 2 tumor entities. Most examples of adamantinoma feature a distinctive radiologic appearance represented by the presence of intracortical mixed sclerotic and lytic lesions.

With the limitations of the low numbers observed, there exists the impression that primary bone SS exhibits higher aggressiveness than its soft tissue counterpart.

Key Features

- Occurrence on the long bones of adults
- Imaging: destructive, mostly lytic lesion invading the soft tissues
- Monomorphic spindle cell proliferation featuring abundant pericellular collagen and HPC-like vascularization
- Epithelial differentiation in biphasic SS
- Immunohistochemical expression of cytokeratin, EMA, and TLE-1
- Presence of SYT-SSX gene fusions

Differential Diagnosis

- SFT
  - Patternless spindle cell proliferation set in collagenous background with cellular variation
  - Hemangiopericytoma-like vascular pattern
  - Expression of STAT6
  - Presence of NAB2-STAT6 gene fusion
- MPNST
  - Possible association with NF1 syndrome
  - High-grade spindle cell proliferation featuring perivascular accentuation of cellularity
  - Focal expression of S100 protein in one-third of cases
- Small cell osteosarcoma
  - Presence of malignant osteoid (may be very focal)
  - SATB2 immunopositivity

(!) **Pitfalls**

! Round cell poorly differentiated SS may closely mimic Ewing sarcoma

! Metastatic carcinoma to the bone is far more frequent than primary biphasic SS of bone

! Pericellular collagen may mimic osteoid

SOLITARY FIBROUS TUMOR

In soft tissues, SFT represents a ubiquitous (any anatomic site has been reported) fibroblastic neoplasm showing a distinctive hemangiopericytoma-like vascular network. In bone SFT tends to occur in the long bones, followed by the pelvic bones. Age range is broad; however, approximately 50% of cases, similar to what is observed in soft tissues, are diagnosed in late adulthood with a peak incidence between the fifth and the sixth decades. SFT encompasses a large majority of the once extremely popular mesenchymal lesion labeled with the now abandoned term, hemangiopericytoma.[4,5]

Imaging shows a solitary, centrally located lytic lesion that may erode the cortex and extend into the soft tissues (**Fig. 18**).

Microscopically, classic SFT is characterized by a variably cellular spindle cell proliferation (often with a distinctive combination of hypocellular and hypercellular areas), organized in a short storiform pattern (so-called patternless pattern). A characteristic hemangiopericytoma-like vascular pattern, characterized by thin-walled, gaping, branching blood vessels is almost invariably present (**Fig. 19**). In classic examples, neoplastic cells tend to exhibit mild atypia and are set in an abundant stromal collagen. Perivascular hyalinization is also frequently seen (**Fig. 20**).

Malignant SFT refers to cases in which mitotic activity is greater than 4 mitoses/10 high-power field (HPF) is observed. Increased mitotic activity is often associated with higher cellularity (**Fig. 21**), to the extent that the distinctive alternation between hypocellular and hypercellular areas may be lost. Also the presence of significant nuclear pleomorphism and necrosis, even in absence of high mitotic activity, should be regarded as unfavorable prognostic features.

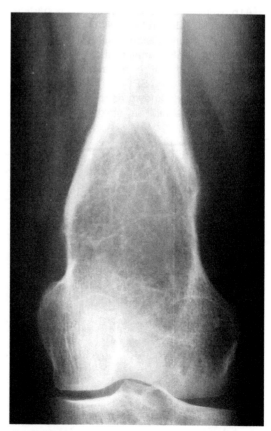

Fig. 18. Radiograph of SFT shows a centrally located lytic lesion.

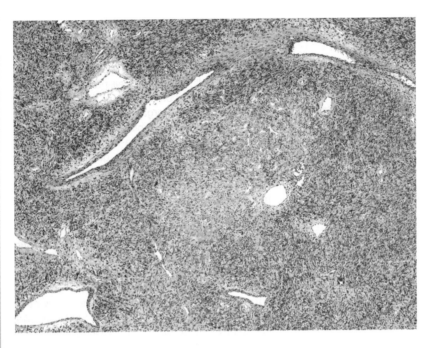

Fig. 19. A spindle cell proliferation showing variation of cellularity associated with HPC-like blood vessels is typically seen in SFT (H&E, original magnification, ×10).

Immunohistochemically, SFT is characterized by the expression in most cases of CD34 and STAT6. Nuclear expression of STAT6 is particularly valuable and correlates with the presence of *NAB2-STAT6* gene fusion (**Fig. 22**).

Similarly to LMS, a major pitfall is represented by the possibility of a metastasis. Malignant SFT in general and SFT of the meninges in particular (formerly known as meningeal hemangiopericytoma) exhibit a striking tendency to spread to the bone and soft tissue. As discussed previously, the presence of a hemangiopericytoma-like vascularization can be observed also in half of SS. Moreover, SS rarely exhibits a blander cytomorphology, generating significant overlap with SFT. The combination of immunomorphologic and molecular findings, however, allows distinction in most cases. A rare benign condition that also enters the differential diagnosis is represented by myofibroma/

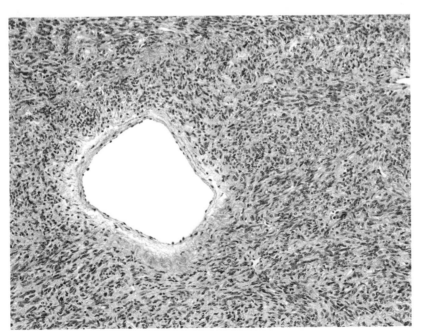

Fig. 20. Perivascular hyalinization is frequently observed in SFT (H&E, original magnification, ×20).

Fig. 21. Malignant SFT features higher atypia and presence of mitotic figures (H&E, original magnification, ×20).

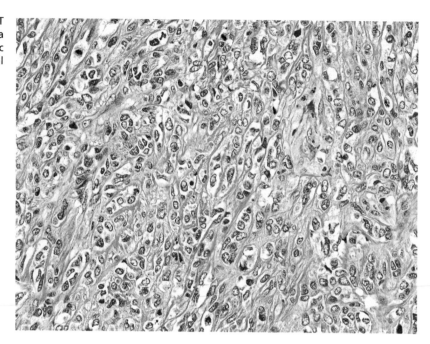

myofibromatosis. Both solitary and multiple forms of this distinctive myofibroblastic lesion (formerly known as infantile hemangiopericytoma) may occur primarily in bone. It is now clear that this condition can occur both in children (wherein multifocality is far more common) and in adults. At variance with SFT, myofibroma seems to predominate in the bones of the head and neck region but has been reported also in the long bones.[14] Morphologically, it is characterized by a distinct biphasic appearance generated by the presence of immature areas (in which hemangiopericytoma-like vessels are seen) merging with mature hypocellular, myoid areas (**Figs. 23** and **24**). The presence of a hemangiopericytoma-like vascular network

Fig. 22. Nuclear expression of STAT6 is of great help in the diagnosis of SFT (H&E, original magnification, ×20).

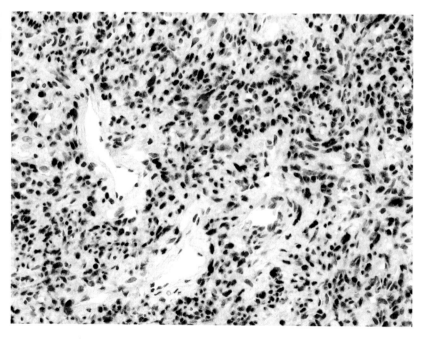

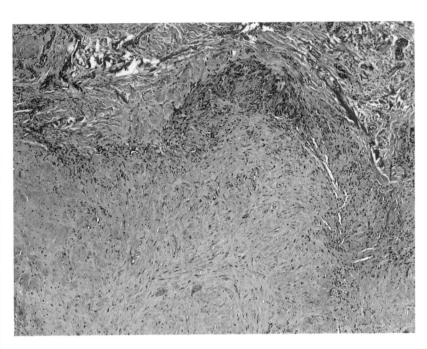

Fig. 23. Myofibroma is characterized by a distinctive biphasic appearance (H&E, original magnification, ×10).

greatly contributes to generate a potential diagnostic confusion with SFT. Immunohistochemically, myofibroma/myofibromatosis consistently expresses smooth muscle differentiation markers whereas STAT6 is consistently negative.

In consideration of its rarity to assess the clinical behavior of primary bone, SFT does not represent an easy task. Two of the reported cases reported by Verbeke and colleagues[5] developed distant metastases. Personal experience of the authors indicates higher aggressiveness than SFT of soft tissue.[4]

Key Features

- Occurrence in long bones of adult
- Imaging: solitary, centrally located lytic lesion that extends into the soft tissues
- Patternless spindle cell proliferation set in collagenous background with cellular variation
- Hemangiopericytoma-like vascular pattern
- Mitotic activity exceeding 5 mitoses/HPF associated with malignancy
- Nuclear expression of STAT6
- Presence of NAB2-STAT6 gene fusion

Differential Diagnosis

- Monophasic SS
  - Monomorphic spindle cell proliferation set in collagenous background
  - Hemangiopericytoma-like vascular pattern
  - Variable expression of cytokeratin and EMA
  - Expression of TLE1
  - Presence of SYT gene rearrangements

Pitfalls

! Metastatic SFT to the bone (most often from the meninges) is more common than primary SFT of the bone

! Myofibroma/myofibromatosis may occur in the bone and if immature areas predominate may mimic SFT

SCLEROSING EPITHELIOID FIBROSARCOMA

SEF represents an exceedingly rare mesenchymal fibroblastic malignancy that can easily be confused with metastatic carcinoma. First

Fig. 24. High-power view of the richly vascularized immature areas of myofibroma (H&E, original magnification, ×20).

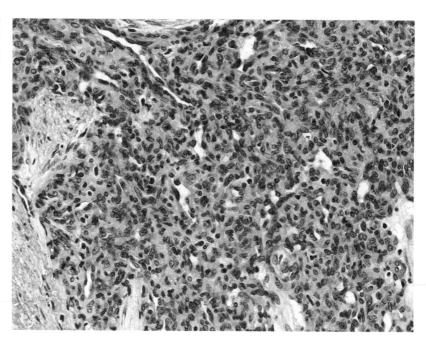

reported by Enzinger and coworkers in 1995, in soft tissue it tends to occur in middle-aged and elderly patients (median age 45 years) with no gender predilection.[15] In bone, SEF seems to occur most often in the long bones of the limbs and in the pelvic bones of adult patients.[15,16]

Radiologically, most cases presents as destructive, intramedullary, lytic lesions with occasional foci of sclerosis.

Microscopically, SEF is composed of an infiltrative proliferation of epithelioid cells, often featuring a clear cytoplasm organized in cords, strands, and nests set in a distinctively prominent sclerotic collagen background (Fig. 25). Some cases may exhibit areas indistinguishable from LGFMS, an entity morphologically as well as genetically closely related to SEF. Immunohistochemically, SEF exhibits EMA positivity in

Fig. 25. The presence of cellular epithelioid proliferation set in sclerotic stroma is the typical morphologic presentation of SEF (H&E, original magnification, ×20).

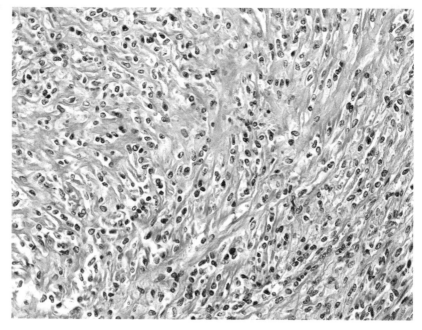

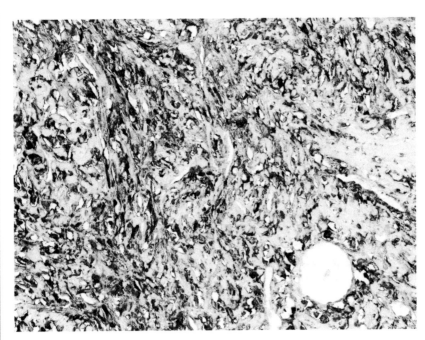

Fig. 26. Cytoplasmic expression of MUC4 is observed in the majority of SEF (H&E, original magnification, ×20).

approximately 50% of cases. Most importantly, more than two-thirds of cases show strong cytoplasmic immunoreactivity for Mucin 4 (MUC4) (**Fig. 26**), a finding that further supports the relationship between LGFMS and SEF. Genetically, in contrast to the marked predominance of FUS-CREB3L2 t(7;16) (q33;p11) in LGFMS, the genetics of SEF is more heterogeneous, showing more often FUS-CREB3L1 t(11;16) and EWSR1-CREB3L1 t(11;22) gene fusions.

The major diagnostic pitfall is represented by the differential diagnosis with osteosarcoma. This represents a true challenge because the sclerotic collagenous background of ESF may closely mimic the lacelike appearance of malignant osteoid. The combination of MUC4 and SATB2 immunostaining plays a key diagnostic role. With a single reported exception[16] MUC4 seems restricted to SEF whereas SATB2 (positive in osteosarcoma) has never been reported in SEF. In consideration of striking epithelioid morphology combined with EMA positivity, metastatic carcinoma always needs to be ruled out.

SEF in soft tissue is characterized by aggressive clinical behavior, with 10% to 20% of patients presenting with metastatic disease at diagnosis. In the few bone cases reported, approximately half of patients developed metastastic spread within 2 years from the diagnosis.

Key Features

- Occurrence in the long bones of adults
- Imaging: destructive, intramedullary, lytic lesions with occasional foci of sclerosis
- Epithelioid cell proliferation associated with collagenized, sclerotic background
- Immunohistochemical expression of MUC4
- Presence of FUS-CREB3L1 t(11;16) and EWSR1- CREB3L1 t(11;22) gene fusions
- Aggressive clinical behavior

Pitfalls

! Expression of EMA by an epithelioid cell malignancy overlaps with metastatic carcinoma

! The sclerotic stroma can be easily mistaken for osteogenic matrix leading to an erroneous diagnosis of osteosarcoma

PSEUDOMYOGENIC HEMANGIOENDOTHELIOMA

Pseudomyogenic hemangioendothelioma (PHE) is a recently described, rarely metastasizing vascular tumor of intermediate biological potential. Fully characterized for the first time by Hornick and Fletcher in 2011,[17] PHE most likely overlaps with both epithelioid sarcoma-like hemangioendothelioma[18] and the "fibroma-like, fibrohistiocytic/myxoid variant" of epithelioid sarcoma described by Mirra and colleagues[19] in 1992. PHE exhibits a male predominance with a male-to-female ratio of 4:1 associated with peak of incidence in the third decade. PHE exhibits a tendency to arise in the soft tissue of the extremities, especially on the lower limb, often involving multiple tissue planes with bone involvement occurring in 20% to 25% of cases.[17] More recently, cases of PHE arising primarily in the bone have been reported with a similar clinical behavior to its soft tissue counterpart.[20–22] Primary bone PHE arises predominantly in the lower limb with a predilection for the distal tibia and the foot.

Radiologically, most cases observed present with well-circumscribed, lytic, often multiple homogeneous lesions (**Fig. 27**).

Morphologically, PHE is composed of sheets and loose fascicles of plump spindle (**Fig. 28**) and/or epithelioid cells with abundant brightly eosinophilic cytoplasm, sometimes mimicking rhabdomyoblasts (**Fig. 29**). Tumor cells contain vesicular nuclei with small nucleoli and may feature the presence of scattered neutrophils. Mitoses tend to be rare. Immunohistochemistry plays a relevant diagnostic role. Neoplastic cells typically exhibit coexpression of endothelial (ERG and CD31) and epithelial (cytokeratin AE1/AE3) markers. Intact INI-1 nuclear immunoreactivity is observed in all cases. Recently, a recurrent balanced translocation t(7;19) (q22;q13) has been reported, which results in fusion of the *SERPINE1* and *FOSB* genes.[23,24] Immunohistochemical nuclear expression of FOSB has been shown to represent a highly sensitive and diagnostically useful marker.[25] The coexpression of epithelial and vascular differentiation markers, in association with FOSB expression represents extremely helpful diagnostic clues.

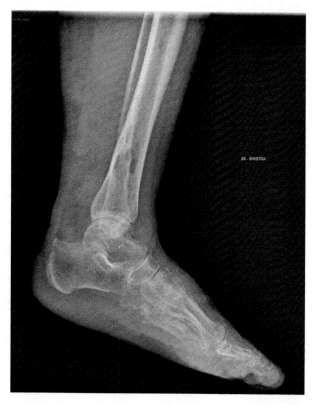

Fig. 27. Multiple well-circumscribed lytic lesions are seen in this example of PHE.

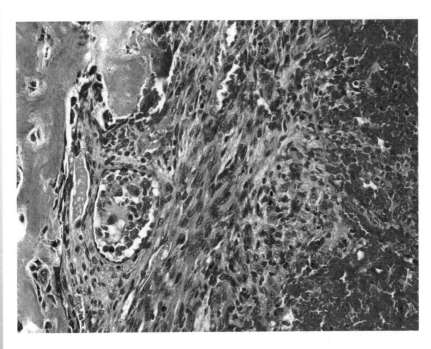

Fig. 28. A spindle cell, myoid proliferation is seen infiltrating between the bone lamellae (H&E, original magnification, ×20).

The major pitfall is represented by that PHE lacking overt vasoformative features, entering the differential diagnosis mostly with spindle cell and epithelioid neoplasm. Main differential diagnosis is with metastatic carcinoma (in which expression of vascular markers is never observed) and with epithelioid sarcoma that can express ERG but virtually always exhibits loss of nuclear expression of INI1.

Although the majority of PHE pursues an indolent clinical course with a tendency to recur or progress locally in absence of systemic spread, some cases of PHE with aggressive clinical behavior resulting in metastatic spread to the lungs have been reported.[26]

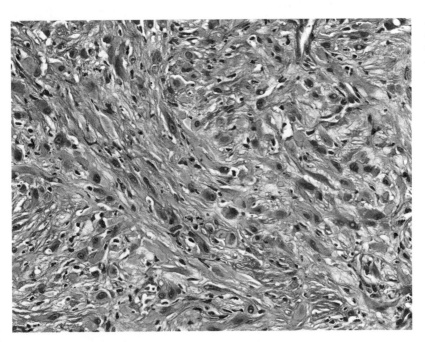

Fig. 29. In PHE, neoplastic cells may assume a striking epithelioid morphology almost mimicking rhabdomyoblasts (H&E, original magnification, ×20).

Key Features

- Occurrence in the bones of the lower limbs of young adults
- Involvement of multiple tissue planes
- Imaging: well circumscribed, often multiple lytic lesions
- Composed of plump spindle and/or epithelioid cells featuring abundant brightly eosinophilic cytoplasm
- Immunohistochemical expression of cytokeratin AE1/AE3, CD321, ERG, and FOSB
- Presence of a *SERPINE1* and *FOSB* gene fusion
- Indolent clinical course

Differential Diagnosis

- Epithelioid sarcoma
  - Composed of spindle and epithelioid cells
  - Presence of geographic necrosis
  - Loss of nuclear expression of INI1
  - No expression of CD31 (ERG and CD34 can be both positive)

Pitfalls

! Multifocality may be misinterpreted as expression of metastatic spread

! Expression of cytokeratin may lead to the diagnosis of metastatic carcinoma

! Coexpression of ERG and cytokeratin is observed also in epithelioid sarcoma

MYOEPITHELIAL NEOPLASM

Myoepithelial tumors of the soft tissue and bone represent a spectrum of lesions morphologically similar to myoepithelial neoplasms of salivary gland. Malignant forms are generally identified with the labels myoepithelial carcinoma or malignant myoepithelioma. Myoepitheliomas are definitely rare, particularly those arising as primary bone lesion.[27] Most frequent locations seems to be represented by the humerus followed by the pelvic bones and the tibia of adults; however, isolated cases have been reported at any location.[27,28]

Radiologically, whereas benign forms tend to be well circumscribed and associated with sclerotic margins, malignant forms tends to be lytic and to invade the surrounding soft tissue (**Fig. 30**).

Macroscopically, malignant myoepithelioma may feature solid gray to white areas often alternating with hemorrhagic foci (**Fig. 31**). Microscopically, most cases are composed of a proliferation of spindled to epithelioid cells (**Fig. 32**). Neoplastic cells organize in cords, strands, and trabeculae, often set in a myxoid or myxochondroid stroma (**Figs. 33** and **34**). Those cases featuring a prominent cytoplasmic vacuolization (somewhat

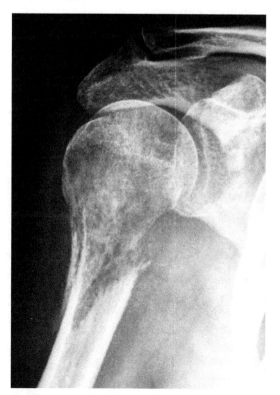

Fig. 30. Myoepithelial neoplasm: a destructive lytic lesion is observed associated with fracture.

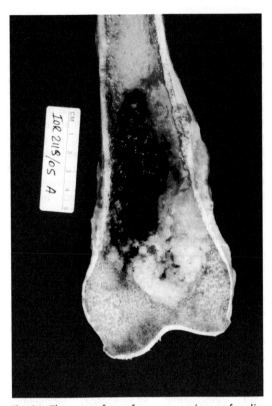

Fig. 31. The cut surface of a gross specimen of malignant myoepithelioma shows a solid gray mass with hemorrhagic areas.

mimicking a chordoma) in the past have been most likely diagnosed under the label parachordoma. Malignant myoepithelioma exhibits overt features of malignancy, including severe nuclear atypia, high mitotic activity, and necrosis (**Fig. 35**). High-grade cytology remains the best predictor of aggressiveness, whereas the significance of mitotic count as well as of infiltrative pattern of growth is unclear. Immunohistochemically, up to 90% of cases express pancytokeratins and S100 protein. EMA is also seen in two-thirds of cases, whereas glial fibrillary acidic protein (GFAP) is detected in approximately 50% of tumors. Smooth muscle actin is seen in one-third of cases whereas desmin stains no more than 10% of cases. In soft tissues, loss of INI1/SMARCB1 is observed in approximately one-third of malignant myoepitheliomas; however, in bone, data are still limited.

The genetics of myoepithelial neoplasm is rapidly evolving. *EWSR1* rearrangement occurs with a variety of fusion partners (*PBX1, PBX3, ZNF444, POU5F,* and *ATF1*) in approximately 50% of cases. Recently a small subset of EWSR1-negative soft tissue myoepitheliomas harboring *FUS* rearrangement has been identified and confirmed also in a primary bone case.[29]

Because myoepithelial neoplasm lays in between epithelial and mesenchymal neoplasms the differential diagnosis is broad. Metastatic carcinoma represents the major diagnostic pitfall with

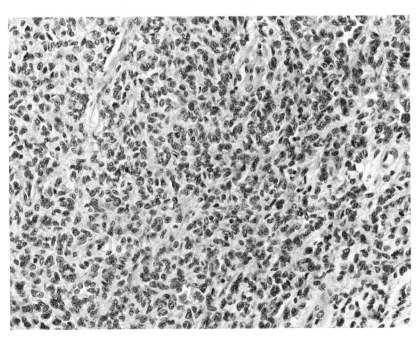

Fig. 32. Histologically, myoepithelioma is composed of spindle and epithelioid cells set in a stroma that can be both myxoid and fibrous, as in this example (H&E, original magnification, ×20).

Fig. 33. Sometimes the neoplastic myoepithelial cells are organized in cords and intersecting clusters set in an abundant myxochondroid stroma (H&E, original magnification, ×20).

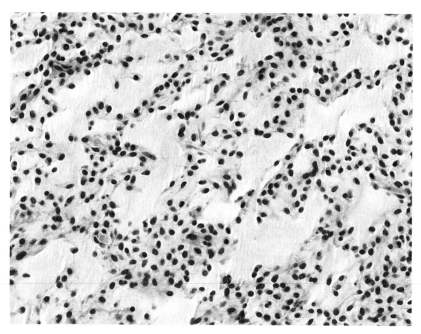

the further challenge that in both situations cytokeratins and EMA are consistently expressed. The expression of S100 and, less frequently, of smooth muscle markers, may help in the differential diagnosis. A challenging differential diagnosis is with those exceptional examples of extraskeletal myxoid chondrosarcoma (EMC) arising primarily in the bone. They both exhibit *EWRSR1* gene rearrangement (in EMC most often fusing with *NR4A3*); however, the expression of epithelial differentiation marker seems to be limited to myoepithelial neoplasms.[30]

In absence of overt features of malignancy, myoepithelioma of bone seems to pursue a benign clinical course. Malignant myoepithelioma tends to recur and may metastasize to the lungs and lymph nodes, even many years from initial diagnosis.

Fig. 34. In this myoepithelioma, the neoplastic cells show epithelioid morphology and large eosinophilic cytoplasm (H&E, original magnification, ×20).

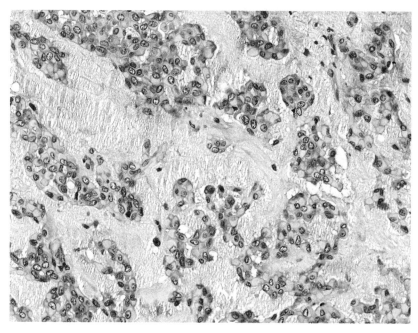

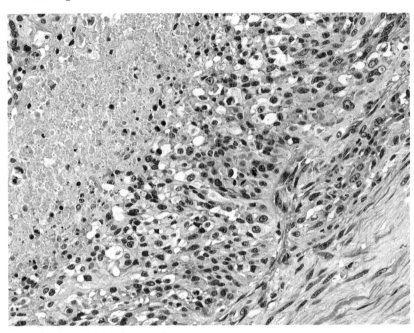

Fig. 35. Malignant myoe-pithelioma shows atypical epithelioid cells, featuring macronucleolation and necrosis (H&E, original magnification, ×20).

Key Features

- Occurrence in the bones of the lower limbs of adults

- Imaging: well circumscribed and confined to the bone when benign. Malignant forms tend to be lytic and destructive.

- Composed of spindle and/or epithelioid cells set in a myxoid or fibrous stroma.

- Immunohistochemical expression of cytokeratin, EMA, and S100

- Presence of *EWSR1* gene rearrangements

- Malignant forms behave aggressively

⚠ Differential Diagnosis

- EMC primary of bone
  - Multinodular pattern of growth
  - Epithelioid cells organized in cords and strands and set in a myxoid matrix
  - Areas of hemorrhage
  - Nonexpression of cytokeratin
  - Presence of *EWSR1-NR4A3* gene fusion

⊘ Pitfalls

! Metastatic carcinoma to the bone is far more frequent than primary myoepithelioma

! Presence of a *EWSR1* gene rearrangements may lead to an erroneous diagnosis of atypical Ewing sarcoma

SUMMARY

Soft tissue malignancies may rarely occur as primary bone lesions. A majority of these lesions tend to be under-recognized and, until recently, they have been lumped within the now abolished categories of both MFH/fibrosarcoma and hemangiopericytoma. After a profound conceptual reappraisal, and in consideration of the presence of a broader range of therapeutic options, currently pathologists have achieved a higher diagnostic accuracy.

Proper recognition of rare lesions arising at exceptional anatomic site certainly requires a carefully integrated evaluation of all the clinical, radiologic, immunomorphologic, and molecular findings. In consideration of their complexity, bone sarcomas should be mandatorily evaluated by a multidisciplinary team, in the context of an expert center.

REFERENCES

1. Fletcher CDM, Bridge JA, Hogendoorn PCW, et al, editors. WHO Classification of Tumours of Soft Tissue and Bone. Lyon (France): IARC Press; 2013. p. 153–4.
2. Romeo S, Bovée JV, Kroon HM, et al. Malignant fibrous histiocytoma and fibrosarcoma of bone: a re-assessment in the light of currently employed morphological, immunohistochemical and molecular approaches. Virchows Arch 2012;461: 561–70.
3. Mertens F, Romeo S, Bovee JVMG, et al. Reclassification and subtyping of so-called malignant fibrous histiocytoma of bone: comparison with cytogenetic features. Clin Sarc Res 2011;1:10.
4. Dei Tos AP, Righi A, Gambarotti M, et al. Reappraisal of primary spindle/pleomorphic sarcomas of bone. Mod Pathol 2014;27(Suppl 2):15A.
5. Verbeke SL, Fletcher CD, Alberghini M, et al. A reappraisal of hemangiopericytoma of bone; analysis of cases reclassified as synovial sarcoma and solitary fibrous tumor of bone. Am J Surg Pathol 2010;34:777–83.
6. Antonescu CR, Erlandson RA, Huvos AG. Primary leiomyosarcoma of bone: a clinicopathologic, immunohistochemical, and ultrastructural study of 33 patients and a literature review. Am J Surg Pathol 1997;21:1281–94.
7. Adelani MA, Schultenover SJ, Holt GE, et al. Primary leiomyosarcoma of extragnathic bone: clinicopathologic features and reevaluation of prognosis. Arch Pathol Lab Med 2009;133: 1448–56.
8. Myers JL, Arocho J, Bernreuter W, et al. Leiomyosarcoma of bone. A clinicopathologic, immunohistochemical and ultrastructural study of five cases. Cancer 1991;67:1051–6.
9. Mori T, Nakayama R, Endo M, et al. Forty-eight cases of leiomyosarcoma of bone in Japan: a multicenter study from the Japanese muscoloskeletal oncology group. J Surg Oncol 2016;114: 495–500.
10. Brewer P, Sumathi V, Grimer RJ, et al. Primary leiomyosarcoma of bone: analysis of prognosis. Sarcoma 2012;2012:636849.
11. Zulkarnaen M, Pan K, Shanmugam P, et al. Intraosseous synovial sarcoma of the proximal femur: case report. Malays Orthop J 2012;6: 49–52.
12. Kim KW, Park SY, Won KY, et al. Synovial sarcoma of primary bone origin arising from the cervical spine. Skeletal Radiol 2013;42:303–8.
13. Righi A, Gambarotti M, Longo S, et al. Small cell osteosarcoma: clinicopathologic, immunohistochemical, and molecular analysis of 36 cases. Am J Surg Pathol 2015;39:691–9.
14. Shemesh S, Kosashvili Y, Sidon E, et al. Solitary intraosseous myofibroma of the tibia in an adult patient: a case report. J Bone Oncol 2014;30: 80–3.
15. Meis-Kindblom JM, Kindblom LG, Enzinger FM. Sclerosing epithelioid fibrosarcoma. A variant of fibrosarcoma simulating carcinoma. Am J Surg Pathol 1995;19:979–93.
16. Wojcik JB, Bellizzi AM, Dal Cin P, et al. Primary sclerosing epithelioid fibrosarcoma of bone: analysis of a series. Am J Surg Pathol 2014;38: 1538–44.
17. Hornick JL, Fletcher CD. Pseudomyogenic hemangioendothelioma: a distinctive, often multicentric tumor with indolent behavior. Am J Surg Pathol 2011; 35:190–201.
18. Billings SD, Folpe AL, Weiss SW. Epithelioid sarcoma-like hemangioendothelioma. Am J Surg Pathol 2003;27:48–57.
19. Mirra JM, Kessler S, Bhuta S, et al. The fibroma-like variant of epithelioid sarcoma. A fibrohistiocytic/myoid cell lesion often confused with benign and malignant spindle cell tumors. Cancer 1992; 69:1382–95.
20. Sheng WQ, Wang J. Primary pseudomyogenic haemangioendothelioma of bone. Histopathology 2012; 61:1219–24.
21. Righi A, Gambarotti M, Picci P, et al. Primary pseudomyogenic haemangioendothelioma of bone: report of two cases. Skeletal Radiol 2015; 44:727–31.
22. Inyang A, Mertens F, Puls F, et al. Primary pseudomyogenic hemangioendothelioma of bone. Am J Surg Pathol 2016;40:587–98.
23. Trombetta D, Magnusson L, von Steyern FV, et al. Translocation t(7;19)(q22;q13)–a recurrent chromosome aberration in pseudomyogenic hemangioendothelioma? Cancer Genet 2011;204: 211–5.
24. Walther C, Tayebwa J, Lilljebjörn H, et al. A novel SERPINE1-FOSB fusion gene results in transcriptional up-regulation of FOSB in pseudomyogenic haemangioendothelioma. J Pathol 2014;232: 534–40.
25. Hung YP, Fletcher CD, Hornick JL. FOSB is a useful diagnostic marker for pseudomyogenic hemangioendothelioma. Am J Surg Pathol 2017;41(5): 596–606.
26. Shah AR, Fernando M, Musson R, et al. An aggressive case of pseudomyogenic haemangioendothelioma of bone with pathological fracture and rapidly progressive pulmonary metastatic disease: case report and review of the literature. Skeletal Radiol 2015;44:1381–6.

27. Kurzawa P, Kattapuram S, Hornicek JH, et al. Primary myoepithelioma of bone. Am J Surg Pathol 2013;37:960–8.

28. Rekhi B, Joshi S, Panchwagh Y, et al. Clinicopathoaloigc features of fine unusual cases of intraosseous myoepithelial carcinomas, mimicking conventional primary bone tumors, including EWSR1 rearrangement in one case. APMIS 2016;124:278–90.

29. Puls F, Arbajian E, Magnusson L, et al. Myoepithelioma of bone with a novel FUS-POU 5F1 fusion gene. Histopathology 2014;65: 917–22.

30. Kilpatrick SE, Inwards CY, Fletcher CD, et al. Myxoid Chondrosarcoma (chordoid sarcoma) of bone: a report of two cases and review of the literature. Cancer 1997;15:1903–10.

Conditions Simulating Primary Bone Neoplasms

Jodi M. Carter, MD, PhD[a], Benjamin Matthew Howe, MD[b], Carrie Y. Inwards, MD[a],*

KEYWORDS

- Osteonecrosis • Osteomyelitis • Sarcoidosis • Subchondral cyst • Amyloidosis
- Heterotopic ossification • Stress fracture

ABSTRACT

A number of nonneoplastic conditions can mimic tumors of bone. Some of the more common mimics of primary bone tumors include infectious, inflammatory, periosteal, and degenerative joint disease-associated lesions that produce tumorlike bone surface-based or intraosseous lesions. This article considers a spectrum of reactive and nonreactive processes including stress fracture, subchondral cysts, osteonecrosis, heterotopic ossification, osteomyelitis, sarcoidosis, and amyloidoma that can present in such a way that they are mistaken for a tumor arising primary in bone.

OVERVIEW

Conditions simulating primary bone neoplasms are encountered on a regular basis by those caring for patients with musculoskeletal abnormalities. In many of these scenarios, lesions with classic radiologic and clinical findings typically pose little diagnostic or patient management challenges. In contrast, lesions with unusual or inconclusive radiologic features are biopsied to exclude neoplasm. In these situations, the most common pitfall for the pathologist is to under-recognize the non-neoplastic lesional tissue and misinterpret the biopsy as nondiagnostic, leading to an unnecessary repeat biopsy. Alternatively, the lesion may be surgically removed without a preoperative diagnosis, and the pathologist runs into diagnostic difficulties by assuming it represents a neoplasm. These pitfalls can be avoided by gaining a better

understanding of the histologic, clinical, and radiologic features of these non-neoplastic mimics.

STRESS FRACTURES

Stress fractures are subclassified into fatigue fractures caused by excessive, repetitive load bearing onto normal bone (eg, long-distance running) and insufficiency fractures, caused by normal load bearing upon structurally compromised bone (eg, osteoporotic bone). Unlike pathologic fractures, this terminology generally refers to bones that are not involved by tumor.

Key Points
STRESS FRACTURE

- Subclassification includes 2 types—fatigue and insufficiency
- Affected bones are not involved by tumor
- Radiologic findings can mimic benign and malignant tumors. MRI (correlating T1- and T2-weighted images) is most helpful in making the distinction
- Histologic findings vary with lesional age. Early lesions—woven bone, immature cartilage, myofibroblastic cell proliferation, and fibrovascular tissue. More mature lesions—longer interconnecting trabeculae of woven bone with osteoblastic rimming.
- Can be mistaken for osteosarcoma, but lacks the disorganized growth pattern, cytologic atypia, and lace-like osteoid matrix seen in osteosarcoma.

---

[a] Division of Anatomic Pathology, Department of Laboratory Medicine and Pathology, Mayo Clinic, Hilton 11, 200 First Street South West Rochester, MN 55905, Rochester, MN, USA; [b] Division of Anatomic Pathology, Department of Radiology, Mayo Clinic, Hilton 11, 200 First Street South West Rochester, MN 55905, Rochester, MN, USA
* Corresponding author. Division of Anatomic Pathology, Department of Laboratory Medicine and Pathology, Mayo Clinic, Hilton 11, 200 First Street South West Rochester, MN 55905, Rochester, MN, USA.
E-mail address: inwards.carrie@mayo.edu

Surgical Pathology 10 (2017) 731–748
http://dx.doi.org/10.1016/j.path.2017.04.012

RADIOLOGIC FEATURES

Plain radiographs may demonstrate a visible fracture line, or localized osteopenia, periosteal reaction, sclerosis, or callus formation depending on the stage of healing at the time of presentation. These features are better demonstrated on computed tomography (CT), particularly in locations such as the pelvis and sacrum that are difficult to evaluate on radiographs given overlying structures. MRI is a highly sensitive and specific imaging tool for making the diagnosis of a stress fracture. It is critical to correlate the T1- and fluid-sensitive T2-weighted images, since the signal abnormality is frequently exaggerated on T2 and disproportionate to the findings on T1 images. Stress fractures can be confused with many benign and malignant processes in the bone, including osteomyelitis, metastases, and primary sarcoma. However, all of the other entities can usually be distinguished from stress fracture on MRI since they all result in confluent replacement of the marrow fat signal on T1-weighted images (Fig. 1).

MICROSCOPIC FEATURES

The histologic features of stress fracture depend on the chronologic age of the fracture and the degree of structural compromise to the bone. Following fracture, there may be an initial inflammatory component, followed by woven bone formation and then a chronic phase of bone remodeling (Fig. 2).[1] The abnormality is characterized by only minimal callus formation. Small biopsies of these fractures can be challenging to diagnose, and the most important pitfall for the pathologist is to not recognize that lesional tissue, albeit non-neoplastic tissue with reactive changes, is present in the biopsy. Tissue received in the later stages of healing shows a more organized pattern created by interconnected trabeculae of immature bone rimmed by osteoblasts.

DIFFERENTIAL DIAGNOSIS

Stress fractures, composed of abundant woven bone surrounded by a bland spindle cell stroma, bring fibrous dysplasia and low-grade osteosarcoma into the differential diagnosis. The distinction can be made by recognizing a reactive loose, fibrovascular proliferation containing slender, myofibroblastic spindled cells and several thin-walled dilated blood vessels in the setting of a fracture.[2] This contrasts with fibrous dysplasia, in which the cells contain oval- to spindle-shaped nuclei embedded in a more collagen-rich stroma containing only scattered thin-walled blood vessels. Once again, radiologic correlation is important, because the imaging features of fibrous dysplasia and low-grade osteosarcoma do not resemble those of a stress fracture.

When imaging findings of a stress fracture lead radiologists to be worried about a high-grade sarcoma such as Ewing sarcoma or osteosarcoma, pathologists can help avoid unnecessary repeat biopsy by recognizing the reactive histologic findings devoid of cytologic atypia, and thus suggest the possibility of a stress fracture. In these situations, it is important to be sure the biopsy tissue clearly represents the radiologic abnormality in question.

SUBCHONDRAL (SUBARTICULAR) CYSTS

Subchondral cysts refer to a group of non-neoplastic, intraosseous cysts located immediately below the articular cartilage. They occur in the setting of osteoarthritis, most commonly in degenerative joint disease (osteoarthritic cyst), but occasionally in inflammatory arthritides such as rheumatoid arthritis. These cysts are often referred to as geodes by radiologists and surgeons. Subchondral cysts may also arise as a result of trauma (post-traumatic cysts).

Intraosseous ganglion cysts are another type of subchondral cyst that can mimic a primary bone tumor. Intraosseous ganglia often present as incidentally detected juxta-articular lesions in asymptomatic adult patients. Unlike a true synovial cyst, they do not have a connection with adjacent synovial structures. They most often involve the subchondral aspect of bones in the regions of the foot and ankle, knee and hip.[3–5]

> ### Key Points
> #### SUBCHONDRAL CYSTS
>
> - Subclassification includes degenerative (osteoarthritic) and intraossesous ganglion cysts.
>
> - They are located immediately below articular cartilage.
>
> - Unlike intraosseous ganglions, radiologic features of advanced degenerative joint disease are always seen with osteoarthritic cysts.
>
> - Imaging features of large cysts can be mistaken for epiphyseal-based primary bone tumors.
>
> - Histologically, subchondral cysts contain loose myxoid material surrounded by a fibrous cyst wall.

Fig. 1. Axial T1 (*A*) and fat-saturated postgadolinium (*B*) MR images demonstrate an abnormality in the right sacral ala (*A, B* – *arrowheads*). A follow-up positron emission tomography (PET)/CT CT image demonstrates linear sclerosis which parallels the sacroiliac joint (*C* – *arrow*) consistent with an insufficiency fracture.

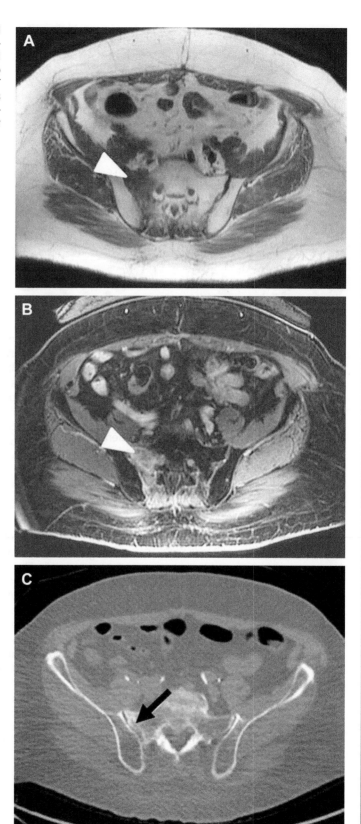

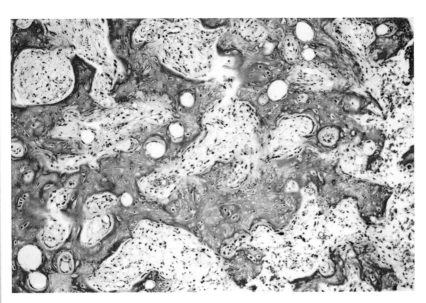

Fig. 2. Fatigue stress fracture involving the tibia of a marathon runner. Biopsy tissue shows interconnected trabeculae of woven bone with prominent osteoblastic rimming surrounded by hypocellular fibrovascular tissue.

RADIOLOGIC FEATURES

In the setting of advanced degenerative arthritis of the joint, degenerative subchondral cysts pose no diagnostic difficulty. However, large cysts may raise concern for a primary bone tumor. Intraosseous ganglion cysts are juxta-articular lesions encountered in joints with minimal, or no identifiable degenerative arthritis. Plain radiographs show a lytic lesion with a narrow zone of transition often with a thin margin of peripheral sclerosis (**Fig. 3**A). Because of its epiphyseal location and imaging features, the x-ray differential diagnosis can include giant cell tumor of bone, chondroblastoma, and clear cell chondrosarcoma. CT and MRI may be able to detect a narrow neck extending through the subchondral bone plate, establishing an articular connection and confirming the diagnosis. MRI can most often establish the cystic and benign nature of these lesions either by confirming the narrow joint connection, or the cystic nature with thin peripheral enhancement on postgadolinium images (see **Fig. 3** B, C).

MICROSCOPIC FEATURES

In a resection specimen for joint replacement, subchondral osteoarthritic cysts are accompanied by pathologic changes of degenerative joint disease, so accurate classification is not problematic. The diagnosis may be less apparent when fragmented portions of tissue are submitted from a curettage or biopsy procedure. In this setting, the fibrous subchondral cyst wall may be mixed with portions of sclerotic or necrotic bone. The intra-cystic contents include pale eosinophilic, paucicellular, loose myxoid material admixed with variable amounts of fibrous tissue, histiocytes, and occasionally other chronic inflammatory cells (**Fig. 4**).

The histologic features of an intraosseous ganglion are identical to those of its soft tissue counterpart. The bland cyst wall lacks an epithelial lining, is composed of fibrous tissue, and is surrounded by loosely arranged fibrovascular tissue with areas of myxoid degeneration (**Fig. 5**).[3,4]

DIFFERENTIAL DIAGNOSIS

Microscopically, the cyst wall of subchondral cysts lacks the prominent myofibroblastic proliferation with scattered multinucleated giant cells characteristic of aneurysmal bone cysts, and the eosinophilic fibrinoid material commonly seen in simple (unicameral) bone cysts. Moreover, the imaging finding of ABC and simple cysts differs from those of subchondral cysts. In order to avoid under recognition and misclassification of a benign appearing subarticular cyst as a nondiagnostic biopsy, pathologists should look for scattered fragments of fibrous cyst wall and areas of myxomatous change. In cases with histologic overlap between an osteoarthritic subchondral cyst and intraosseous ganglion, the diagnosis is swayed by whether there is radiologic evidence of degenerative joint disease in the adjacent joint.

OSTEONECROSIS

Osteonecrosis, also referred to as avascular necrosis or bone infarct depending on its location within the bone, has myriad etiologies, including metabolic causes, functional, medication

Fig. 3. Lytic lesion in the middle cuneiform with a narrow zone of transition (*A – arrow*). On MR imaging, the lesion is juxta-articular with T2-weighted hyperintensity, adjacent edema (*B – arrow*), and thin peripheral enhancement (*C – arrowhead*, postgadolinium fat-saturated image), confirming the cystic nature of this intraosseous ganglion cyst.

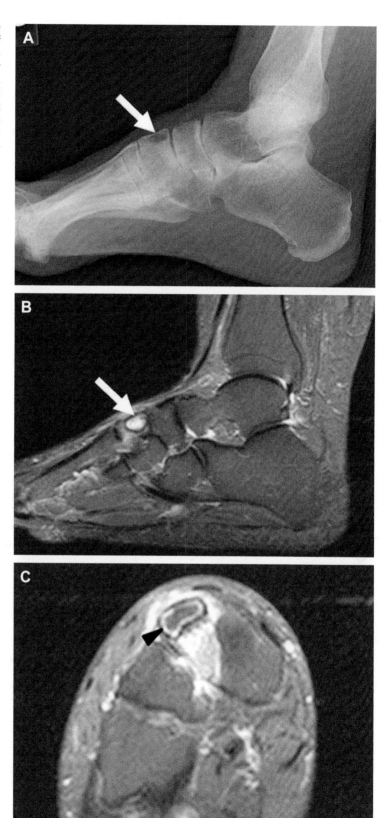

Key Points
OSTEONECROSIS

- The X-ray features of a metaphyseal and serpiginous sclerotic lesion may mimic cartilaginous tumors, in which case the MRI may be helpful.
- Histologically, osteonecrosis contains necrotic bone, marrow fibrosis, and fat necrosis with dystrophic calcification.
- Histologic differential diagnosis includes intraosseous lipoma. Radiologic findings are helpful in making the distinction.

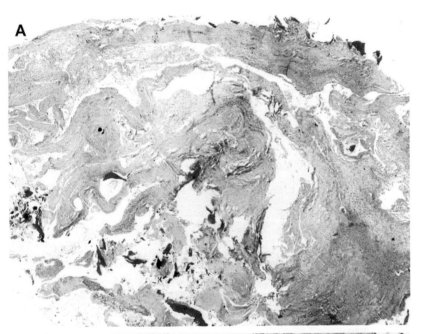

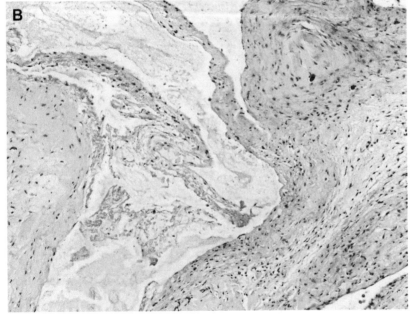

Fig. 4. Degenerative subchondral cyst. (*A*) Low-magnification showing multiple fragments of fibrous cyst wall admixed with shards of bone, myxoid material, and chronic inflammation. (*B*) Higher-magnification illustrating bland fibrous cyst wall and myxoid material. Radiologic imaging showed marked degenerative joint disease.

Fig. 5. Intraosseous ganglion. (*A*) Multiple strips of thin fibrous cyst wall associated with paucicellular myxomatous tissue. (*B*) Curetted tissue from an intraosseous ganglion demonstrating fragmented non-neoplastic bone and soft tissue admixed with fragments of fibrous cyst wall and myxoid material. Without radiologic correlation, the lesional tissue may be overlooked.

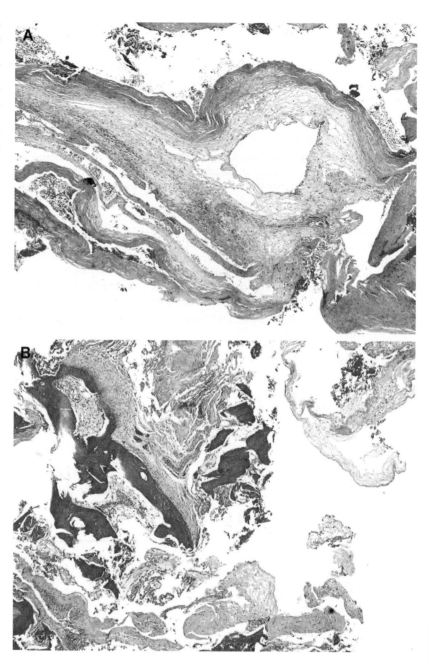

associated and hemoglobinopathies. Irrespective of the underlying etiology, the affected bone suffers ischemic injury from compromised blood supply. When the clinicoradiologic picture is straightforward (eg, a subchondral wedge infarct in the setting of femoral neck fracture), the radiologic features are often diagnostic, obviating the need for biopsy. However, a spectrum of imaging findings can be seen with bone infarcts that may lead to concern for a neoplasm.

RADIOLOGIC FEATURES

Bone infarcts are serpiginous sclerosis in the metaphyses of long bones. Often, bone infarcts are multifocal or associated with avascular necrosis of the epiphyses and the appearance and multifocal metaphyseal involvement allow for a confident diagnosis on plain radiographs. At times the sclerosis may mimic cartilage matrix formation, in which case MRI can be useful in distinguishing the 2 diagnoses. Bone infarcts can have a somewhat variable appearance on MRI, but typically demonstrate internal fat signal and a peripheral rim of decreased T1- and increased T2-weighted signal matching the serpiginous sclerosis seen on plain radiographs.[6]

MICROSCOPIC FEATURES

The histologic features of osteonecrosis reflect the ischemic injury to the bone. Due to osteocyte death, infarcted bone trabeculae have empty lacunae, and the medullary spaces show variable amounts of marrow fat necrosis with calcification, hyalinization, and occasionally cystic change (**Fig. 6**).[7,8] The best clues to considering a diagnosis of bone infarct are recognizing zones of fat necrosis containing fibrosis and dark blue dystrophic calcification intimately associated with fragmented trabeculae of infarcted bone.

DIFFERENTIAL DIAGNOSIS

As the radiologic differential diagnosis includes primary bone tumors, the most common pitfall for the pathologist is to under-recognize Osteonecrosis (ON) as the lesional tissue and misinterpret biopsy tissue as nondiagnostic. The histologic features of intraosseous lipoma (IOL) significantly overlap with those of ON, as both typically contain fat necrosis with calcification. However, IOLs contain broad zones of adipose tissue lacking hematopoietic elements, and the

bone should not be infarcted. In cases with significant histologic overlap, the distinction can usually be made with radiologic correlation, as bone infarct and IOL have differing imaging findings. Of note, osteonecrosis has a low, but well-established risk of malignant transformation to sarcoma.[9] In such cases, the imaging findings usually raise concern for the possibility of malignant transformation.[10] Microscopically, areas of bone infarct merge with zones of a high-grade sarcoma characterized by increased cellularity, frank cytologic atypia, and mitotic activity.

HETEROTOPIC OSSIFICATION

Heterotopic ossification (bone formation in extraskeletal tissue) is usually associated with a history of trauma or injury to the site involved, but rare genetic causes are also well described. Periosteum is a richly vascularized, thin connective tissue layer that envelops the surface of bone, and contains pluripotent mesenchymal cells that differentiate to chondrocytes or osteoblasts for repair following injury.[11] The periosteal repair response can be excessive, resulting in a soft tissue mass of heterotopic ossification (HO) associated with a variety of clinical and radiologic features. The lesion matures over time, and some cases spontaneously regress. Although the molecular mechanisms of HO remain unclear, cellular hypoxia-associated signaling cascades have been implicated in its development.[12]

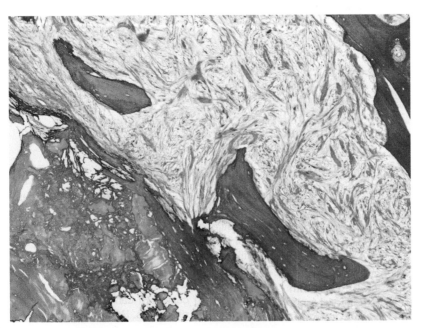

Fig. 6. Bone infarct containing necrotic trabeculae of bone devoid of viable osteocytes surrounded by fibrotic marrow with fat necrosis and dystrophic calcification.

RADIOLOGY

The differentiating feature of HO arising from the surface of bone is the characteristic zonal peripheral pattern of ossification. On MRI, the hallmark of early HO is marked edema and reactive enhancement, a finding that is more prominent than typically encountered with most sarcomas but can cause concern for malignancy. Early matrix during this initial phase can mimic a malignant pattern of osteoid formation. CT is the best modality to differentiate the developing zonal calcifications of HO from neoplastic matrix formation. As HO matures, the peripheral calcifications become more distinct, allowing for a more confident imaging diagnosis.[13] (Fig. 7).

MICROSCOPY

The central zone of HO is composed of a variably cellular and mitotically active myofibroblastic proliferation forming intersecting fascicles. As the lesion matures, a complex pattern of immature woven bone with cartilage formation (endochondral ossification) merges into more mature, longer seams of cancellous bone radiating toward the periphery of the mass where a rim of compact bone may develop (Fig. 8). In late stages with complete maturation, the fibrous tissue is replaced by adipose tissue with hematopoietic marrow.

DIFFERENTIAL DIAGNOSIS

The histologic differential diagnosis varies depending on the amount of tissue available for review and the chronologic stage of the lesion. The diagnosis is usually apparent when the mass is completely excised. However, oftentimes pathologists are faced with needle biopsy tissue in situations where the imaging findings are not straightforward (Fig. 9). The lack of cytologic atypia and the presence of immature woven bone with osteoblastic rimming within the lesional central zone aid in ruling out a high-grade osteosarcoma. Tissue obtained from more peripheral zones or mature lesions can raise concern for parosteal osteosarcoma (POGS), a tumor oftentimes included in the radiologic differential diagnosis as well.

Microscopically, POGS is composed of spindled cells with minimal atypia admixed with long, parallel trabeculae of woven bone. Hyaline cartilage forming a peripheral cap, or, less frequently, within the central portion of the tumor, is seen in approximately 50% of POGS. All of these findings can overlap with HO, creating a diagnostic challenge with a small amount of tissue. In general, the stroma of POGS has a more monotonous appearance than HO and contains more collagen fibers than the reactive fibroblastic stroma of HO. Radiologic correlation is essential, and at times it may not be possible to make the distinction purely based on the Hematoxylin and eosin (H&E) findings. In these situations, molecular genetic testing can be invaluable to arrive at a definitive diagnosis. POGS frequently contain supernumerary ring chromosomes with amplified material from 12q13-15, including the *MDM2* and *CDK4* loci.[14] As benign mimics, including HO, do not contain these genetic changes, testing for *MDM2* amplification can be a useful diagnostic adjunct.[15,16] Care should be taken to make sure the biopsy tissue is not decalcified in an organic acid solution, which can compromise molecular testing.

Subungual exostosis (SE) and bizarre parosteal osteochondromatous proliferation (BPOP) are surface-based osteochondromatous lesions that can be mistaken for heterotopic ossification. Subungual exostosis typically presents in young patients as an exophytic growth located beneath the nail bed of a digit, usually the great toe, and a history of trauma is common.[17,18] They are composed of a fibrocartilaginous cap containing a cytologically bland myofibroblastic proliferation, with progressive maturation to bone formation. In limited biopsies or in curettage specimens, the maturation pattern may not be readily apparent. A misdiagnosis can be avoided by recognizing the reactive-appearing osteocartilaginous proliferation in context with the anatomic location. SE contains a recurrent chromosomal translocation, t(X;6) (q13–14;q22), suggesting it is a neoplastic process rather than a reactive one.[19,20]

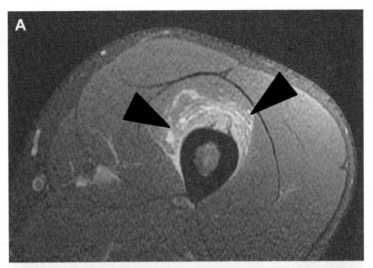

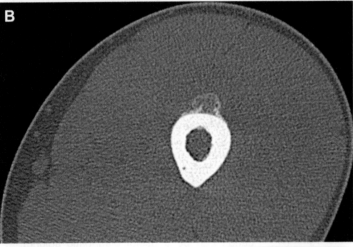

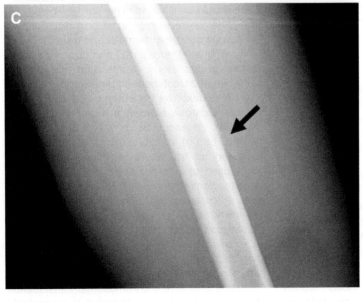

Fig. 7. Axial proton density fat saturated MRI. (*A*) of the thigh demonstrates a heterogeneous lesion arising from the anterior cortex of the femoral diaphysis, with prominent surrounding edema (*A – arrowheads*). CT (*B*) and radiograph (*C*) demonstrate a zonal pattern of calcification (*arrow*) consistent with heterotopic ossification.

Fig. 8. Heterotopic ossification. (*A*) Low-magnification demonstrating zonation phenomenon with peripheral zone of ossification (*left*) and central immature proliferation of fibrous tissue (*right*). (*B*) Fibrous tissue mixed with early bone formation merging into trabeculae of woven bone with prominent osteoblastic rimming.

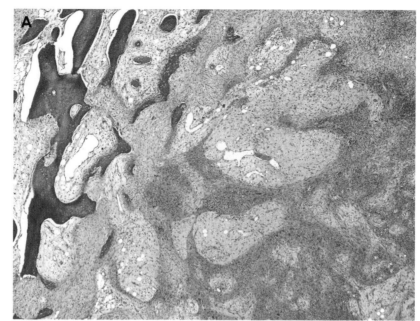

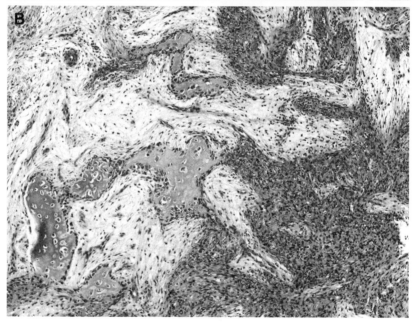

BPOP typically involves the small bones of the hands and feet, although approximately 25% of cases occur in long bones. In BPOP, the lesional components including bone, cartilage, and fibrous tissue are usually more disorganized than those of subungual exostosis (SUE) or HO. As with SUE, the cartilage is characteristically hypercellular with marked enlargement of the chondrocytes, which can raise concern for a chondrosarcoma. A key histologic clue is the distinctive basophilic blue quality to the calcification and woven bone in BPOP.[21] Recurrent genetic events, including translocation t(1;17) (q32;q2) and inversion of chromosome 7, have been identified in BPOP, suggesting its neoplastic nature.[22–25]

OSTEOMYELITIS

Osteomyelitis (OM) can be defined pathophysiologically into bacterial OM, granulomatous OM,

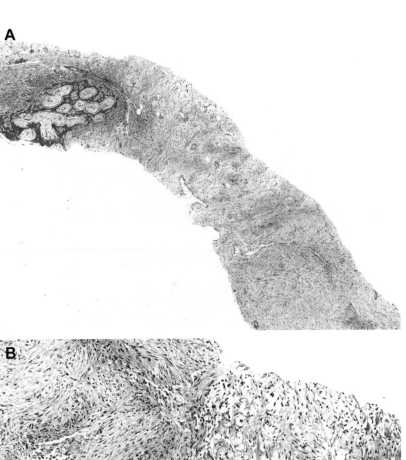

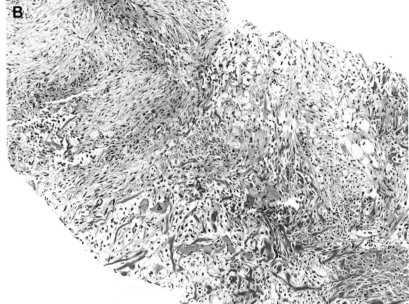

Fig. 9. Heterotopic ossification. (*A, B*) Needle biopsy tissue from an early phase of HO can be difficult to recognize as a reactive proliferation of fibroblastic tissue and immature bone. At higher magnification, it may be mistaken for osteosarcoma.

microangiopathic OM, neuropathic OM, and fibrocystic OM. Among these subtypes, bacterial OM and granulomatous OM most often mimic primary bone tumors or osseous involvement by metastasis or lymphoproliferative disorders.

Bacterial osteomyelitis can be defined temporally as acute, subacute, or chronic OM. Most often, the radiologic features of OM, particularly the permeative pattern, mimic Ewing sarcoma,

metastatic disease, or bone involvement by lymphoma. Subacute osteomyelitis (SAM) is an insidious, chronic low-grade infection of bone, often associated with *Staphylococcus* species.[26] In children, SAM often presents as a Brodie abscess, most often involving the tibia or distal femur, with imaging characteristics that virtually always include primary bone-forming tumors, particularly osteoid osteoma.[27–31]

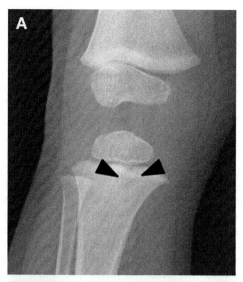

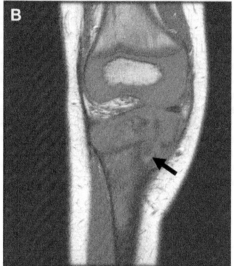

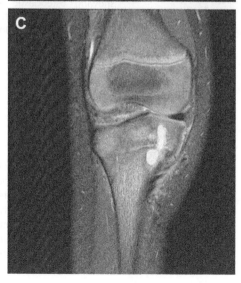

> **Key Points**
> OSTEOMYELITIS
>
> - Radiolologic features, particularly MRI, can mimic benign and malignant (sarcoma, lymphoma) tumors.
>
> - Radiologic features of Brodie abscess overlap with osteoid osteoma.
>
> - Histologic differential diagnosis includes Langerhans cell histiocytosis (LCH) and Rosai-Dorfman disease (RDD).
>
> - Langerhans cells in LCH are positive for CD1a and langerin.
>
> - HIstiocytes in RDD are positive for S100 protein, and emperipolesis is typically present.

RADIOLOGIC FINDINGS

Hematogenous osteomyelitis more commonly presents a diagnostic dilemma on imaging examinations. It is most common in the metaphysis in children. Radiographs may be negative in acute disease, with progression to an aggressive-appearing lytic process with ill-defined margins. MRI most often demonstrates confluent replacement of normal T1-weighted bone marrow signal, with signal intensity that is isointense to skeletal muscle. This area of abnormal signal should have corresponding T2-weighted hyperintensity in the absence of sclerosis and postgadolinium enhancement. Reactive edema in the adjacent soft tissues is common in acute osteomyelitis.

Brodie abscess often presents on radiographs as a lytic metaphyseal lesion (**Fig. 10**A), with a nonspecific appearance that prompts MRI to exclude a primary bone-forming tumor. MRI demonstrates a lesion with surrounding edema that may cross the growth plate in skeletally immature patients extending into the epiphysis. When present, the penumbra sign (rim of T1-weighted hyperintensity, lining an intraosseous abscess) is a relatively specific finding for an intraosseous abscess (see **Fig. 10** B, C).[32]

Fig. 10. Frontal radiograph of the knee in a skeletally immature patient (*A*) shows a lytic proximal tibial metaphyseal lesion (*A – arrowheads*) crossing into the epiphysis (T1 [*B*] and T2 fat saturated [*C*] MRI). Note the T1 hyperintense rim along the margin of the lytic lesion (*B – arrow*), which is a relatively specific MRI feature seen in subacute osteomyelitis.

MICROSCOPIC FEATURES

The histologic features of suppurative OM depend on the chronicity of the lesion. In acute OM, numerous polymorphonuclear leukocytes are intimately associated with host corticolamellar bone causing osteoclastic bone resorption, giving rise to a scalloped appearance (Fig. 11). Necrotic fragments of bone can be found lying within edematous marrow containing prominent blood vessels with endothelial hyperplasia and abundant acute inflammation. Brodie abscess contains a central abscess, often with a nidus of necrotic bone, surrounded by fibrosis, and the surrounding host bone will show sclerosis and remodeling changes. In chronic OM, the bone has a thickened, sclerotic appearance due to gradual reparative remodeling, creating numerous cement lines mimicking Paget disease. The marrow becomes replaced by fibrous tissue with scattered thin dilated vascular spaces and scattered chronic inflammatory cells. Gram stains rarely aid in identifying the causative microorganism, whereas tissue culture and molecular diagnostic techniques yield a much higher rate of positive testing.

Infectious granulomatous osteomyelitis, necrotizing and non-necrotizing, is caused by a variety of fungal and mycotic infections, including tuberculosis, brucellosis, blastomycosis, coccidioidomycosis, cryptococcosis, and aspergillosis.

Microscopically, bone marrow is replaced by fibrous tissue containing histiocytes and multinucleated giant cells forming either ill or well-defined granulomata surrounded by lymphocytes and plasma cells. Special stains for fungal or mycobacterial organisms, tissue cultures, and molecular genetic tests are helpful in identifying the infectious agent.

DIFFERENTIAL DIAGNOSIS

OM is a correlative diagnosis made with a combination of histologic, radiologic, clinical, and laboratory test information. Histologic features can suggest or be consistent with OM, but are rarely diagnostic on their own. The diagnosis is particularly challenging, and at times impossible, with a limited amount of tissue. Acute OM should be reserved for situations when prominent acute inflammation is intimately associated with bone undergoing architectural changes. Of note, both OM and bone-forming tumors, such as osteoid osteoma, will have remodeling changes of the host corticolamellar bone at the lesional interface. If these changes are the only component present on biopsy, a definitive diagnosis cannot be rendered. Osteoid osteoma contains anastomosing trabeculae of woven bone formation with prominent osteoblastic rimming surrounded by loose fibrovascular tissue, and unlike Brodie abscess, is devoid of acute inflammatory cells or necrotic bone.[33]

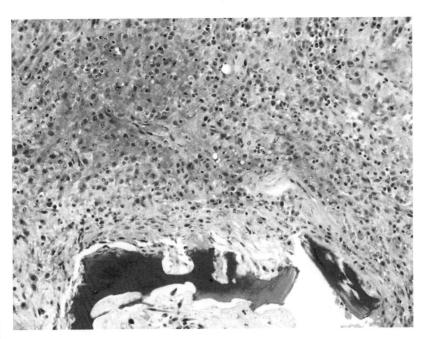

Fig. 11. Acute osteomyelitis. Fragments of bone showing osteoclastic resorption entrapped within abundant acute and chronic inflammation.

LCH is a diagnostic consideration in the differential diagnosis of OM due to its varying inflammatory components. When biopsies with abundant acute inflammation prompt concern for acute OM, one should always consider the possibility of LCH. In addition, some examples of LCH contain abundant chronic inflammatory cells and foamy histiocytes that mask the underlying diagnostic Langerhans cells. The presence of scattered eosinophils can be a helpful clue for LCH. The diagnosis is confirmed by recognizing the epithelioid-appearing Langerhans cells with indistinct cell membranes, oval nuclei, and irregular, grooved nuclear membranes.[34] Immunohistochemical stains for markers of Langerhans cells (eg, CD1a and langerin) are useful.[35,36]

The histologic features of Rosai-Dorfman disease (RDD) can be mistaken for chronic OM, because these lesions are characterized by a marked chronic inflammatory cell infiltrate, (predominantly plasma cells), admixed with foamy histiocytes and occasionally acute inflammatory cells. The diagnosis of RDD is made by identifying engulfed inflammatory cells and red blood cells, a feature termed emperipolesis, within S100-expressing histiocytes.[37]

SKELETAL SARCOIDOSIS

Approximately 10% of patients with sarcoidosis have osseous lesions. Typically, skeletal sarcoidosis involves the phalanges of the hands and feet, radiologically creating lace-like changes of the bone, with osteolysis and trabecular thickening. Occasionally, patients present with solitary lytic lesions of other bones, prompting biopsy to exclude a primary bone tumor.[38,39] Also, long-standing sarcoidosis can show multifocal lytic or sclerotic spine lesions, raising consideration of metastasis, hematolymphoid tumors, or infection.[40-42]

MICROSCOPIC FEATURES

Histologically, sarcoidosis is characterized by multiple noncaseating granulomata in a background of fibrotic tissue with chronic inflammation (**Fig. 12**). As with sarcoidosis at other anatomic sites, the microscopic features are indistinguishable from granulomatous inflammation secondary to an infectious etiology.

DIFFERENTIAL DIAGNOSIS

Pathologists should always consider the possibility of skeletal sarcoidosis before making a diagnosis of granulomatous OM, particularly in the setting of non-necrotizing granulomata. Clinicoradiologic correlation and appropriate laboratory testing to exclude infectious etiologies are required to diagnose skeletal sarcoidosis.

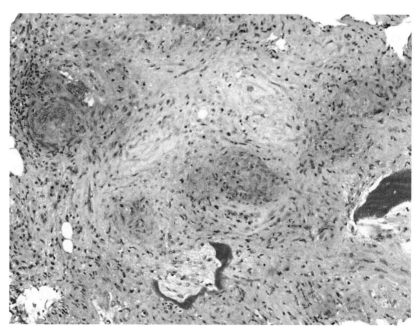

Fig. 12. Sarcoidosis. Non-necrotizing granulomatous inflammation involving needle biopsy tissue from a lumbar spine lesion in a 63-year-old woman clinically thought to have metastatic melanoma. Further clinical, laboratory, and radiologic work-up supported a diagnosis of sarcoidosis.

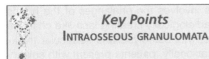

Key Points
INTRAOSSEOUS GRANULOMATA

Infectious

- Causative agents are primarily fungal and mycobacterial organisms

- Form necrotizing or non-necrotizing granulomata

- Special histochemical stains, cultures or molecular genetic testing required to identify infectious agent

Noninfectious

- Sarcoidosis and rarely neoplasm (eg, Hodgkin lymphoma)

- Non-necrotizing granulomatous inflammation

- Diagnosis of exclusion (rule out infectious etiology)

- Requires clinical, laboratory, radiologic correlation

Key Points
AMYLOIDOMA

- Amyloidoma is most common in patients with AL type amyloidosis, often associated with an underlying plasma cell dyscrasia.

- It is also seen in patients on longstanding hemodialysis (ABeta2M amyloidosis).

- Histologically, they are nodular masses of amorphous eosinophilic material resembling hyalinized fibrosis.

- Positive Congo red stain confirms diagnosis.

- Protein typing is best accomplished using mass spectrometry-based proteomic analysis.

AMYLOIDOMA

Amyloidosis is a group of diseases characterized by extracellular deposition of misfolded proteins. Osteoarticular amyloid deposition most commonly involves joints and periarticular soft tissues. However, amyloid proteins can deposit as mass-forming lesions in bone (amyloidoma or "amyloid tumor"), typically in the skull or spine.[43,44]

Massive focal deposition of amyloid in the bone can produce lytic lesions that may demonstrate aggressive features and present radiographically as worrisome for metastatic disease, myeloma, lymphoma, or primary osseous sarcoma.

Amyloid deposition is associated with a variety of clinical syndromes, and treatment depends on the underlying etiology.[45] Classification is based on the type of precursor protein involved, the most common of which include serum amyloid A (AA amyloidosis), transthyretin (ATTR amyloidosis), and immunoglobulin kappa or lambda light chains (AL amyloidosis). Amyloidomas of bone typically occur in patients with AL type amyloidosis, and most patients have an underlying plasma cell dyscrasia.

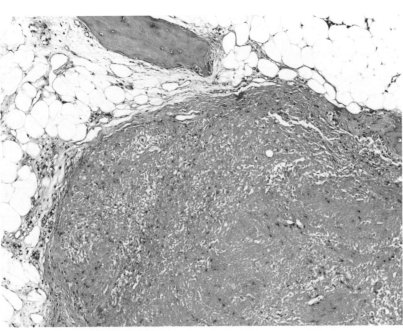

Fig. 13. Amyloidoma. Nodular mass of glossy eosinophilic material within the marrow space. A positive CR stain confirmed the diagnosis of amyloid. Mass spectrometry identified it as ABeta2M (beta-2 microglobulin)-type amyloid deposition. The patient had a history of longstanding renal dialysis.

such as multiple myeloma, monoclonal gammopathies, or light chain disease. Skeletal amyloidomas related to beta-2-microglobulin protein deposits (ABeta2M amyloidosis) are another well-described entity, most commonly occurring the setting of patients on longstanding hemodialysis.[45]

MICROSCOPIC FEATURES

Histologically, amyloid deposits are nodular masses or aggregates of amorphous eosinophilic material oftentimes associated with a limited number of monoclonal plasma cells and a few scattered foreign-body multinucleated giant cells (Fig. 13). These features may be mistaken for hyalinized fibrosis, particularly in limited tissue samples. Histochemical Congo red (CR) staining, demonstrating the characteristic apple green birefringence with polarized light, confirms the diagnosis of amyloid. Once the diagnosis of amyloidosis has been established by CR staining, typing of the protein is required for patient management. This is best accomplished using mass spectrometry-based proteomic analysis due to the relatively low specificity and sensitivity rates associated with immunohistochemistry as performed in most laboratories.[46]

SUMMARY

A variety of non-neoplastic conditions can present with clinical, radiologic, and histologic features resembling a primary surface-based or intramedullary bone tumor. It is important for pathologists to be aware of the microscopic findings and differential diagnosis of these mimics in order to avoid diagnostic pitfalls. Radiologic correlation is essential, but at times misleading. Therefore, pathologists play an important role in guiding appropriate treatment for patients with these lesions.

REFERENCES

1. Klein MJ, Bonar SF, Freemont T, et al. Non-neoplastic diseases of bones and joints. Washington, DC: The American Registry of Pathology; 2011.
2. Currey JD. Bone architecture and fracture. Curr Osteoporos Rep 2005;3(2):52–6.
3. Schajowicz F, Clavel Sainz M, Slullitel JA. Juxta-articular bone cysts (intra-osseous ganglia): a clinico-pathological study of eighty-eight cases. J Bone Joint Surg Br 1979;61(1):107–16.
4. Bauer TW, Dorfman HD. Intraosseous ganglion: a clinicopathologic study of 11 cases. Am J Surg Pathol 1982;6(3):207–13.
5. Rozbruch SR, Chang V, Bohne WH, et al. Ganglion cysts of the lower extremity: an analysis of 54 cases and review of the literature. Orthopedics 1998;21(2): 141–8.
6. Lafforgue P, Trijau S. Bone infarcts: unsuspected gray areas? Joint Bone Spine 2016;83(5):495–9.
7. Sissons HA, Nuovo MA, Steiner GC. Pathology of osteonecrosis of the femoral head. A review of experience at the Hospital for Joint Diseases, New York. Skeletal Radiol 1992;21(4):229–38.
8. Fondi C, Franchi A. Definition of bone necrosis by the pathologist. Clin Cases Miner Bone Metab 2007;4(1):21–6.
9. Domson GF, Shahlaee A, Reith JD, et al. Infarct-associated bone sarcomas. Clin Orthop Relat Res 2009;467(7):1820–5.
10. Stacy GS, Lo R, Montag A. Infarct-associated bone sarcomas: multimodality imaging findings. AJR Am J Roentgenol 2015;205(4):W432–41.
11. Colnot C, Zhang X, Knothe Tate ML. Current insights on the regenerative potential of the periosteum: molecular, cellular, and endogenous engineering approaches. J Orthop Res 2012;30(12):1869–78.
12. Agarwal S, Loder S, Brownley C, et al. Inhibition of Hif1alpha prevents both trauma-induced and genetic heterotopic ossification. Proc Natl Acad Sci U S A 2016;113(3):E338–47.
13. Walczak BE, Johnson CN, Howe BM. Myositis ossificans. J Am Acad Orthop Surg 2015;23(10):612–22.
14. Szymanska J, Mandahl N, Mertens F, et al. Ring chromosomes in parosteal osteosarcoma contain sequences from 12q13-15: a combined cytogenetic and comparative genomic hybridization study. Genes Chromosomes Cancer 1996;16(1):31–4.
15. Yoshida A, Ushiku T, Motoi T, et al. Immunohistochemical analysis of MDM2 and CDK4 distinguishes low-grade osteosarcoma from benign mimics. Mod Pathol 2010;23(9):1279–88.
16. Dujardin F, Binh MB, Bouvier C, et al. MDM2 and CDK4 immunohistochemistry is a valuable tool in the differential diagnosis of low-grade osteosarcomas and other primary fibro-osseous lesions of the bone. Mod Pathol 2011;24(5):624–37.
17. Landon GC, Johnson KA, Dahlin DC. Subungual exostoses. J Bone Joint Surg Am 1979;61(2):256–9.
18. Miller-Breslow A, Dorfman HD. Dupuytren's (subungual) exostosis. Am J Surg Pathol 1988;12(5):368–78.
19. Dal Cin P, Pauwels P, Poldermans LJ, et al. Clonal chromosome abnormalities in a so-called Dupuytren's subungual exostosis. Genes Chromosomes Cancer 1999;24(2):162–4.
20. Zambrano E, Nose V, Perez-Atayde AR, et al. Distinct chromosomal rearrangements in subungual (Dupuytren) exostosis and bizarre parosteal osteochondromatous proliferation (Nora lesion). Am J Surg Pathol 2004;28(8):1033–9.
21. Nora FE, Dahlin DC, Beabout JW. Bizarre parosteal osteochondromatous proliferations of the hands and feet. Am J Surg Pathol 1983;7(3):245–50.

22. Nilsson M, Domanski HA, Mertens F, et al. Molecular cytogenetic characterization of recurrent translocation breakpoints in bizarre parosteal osteochondromatous proliferation (Nora's lesion). Hum Pathol 2004;35(9):1063–9.

23. Endo M, Hasegawa T, Tashiro T, et al. Bizarre parosteal osteochondromatous proliferation with a t(1;17) translocation. Virchows Arch 2005;447(1):99–102.

24. Sakamoto A, Imamura S, Matsumoto Y, et al. Bizarre parosteal osteochondromatous proliferation with an inversion of chromosome 7. Skeletal Radiol 2011;40(11):1487–90.

25. Broehm CJ, M'Lady G, Bocklage T, et al. Bizarre parosteal osteochondromatous proliferation: a new cytogenetic subgroup characterized by inversion of chromosome 7. Cancer Genet 2013;206(11):402–5.

26. Hayes CS, Heinrich SD, Craver R, et al. Subacute osteomyelitis. Orthopedics 1990;13(3):363–6.

27. Lindenbaum S, Alexander H. Infections simulating bone tumors. A review of subacute osteomyelitis. Clin Orthop Relat Res 1984;(184):193–203.

28. Juhn A, Healey JH, Ghelman B, et al. Subacute osteomyelitis presenting as bone tumors. Orthopedics 1989;12(2):245–8.

29. Abril JC, Castillo F, Casas J, et al. Brodie's abscess of the hip simulating osteoid osteoma. Orthopedics 2000;23(3):285–7.

30. Schlur C, Bachy M, Wajfisz A, et al. Osteoid osteoma mimicking Brodie's abscess in a 13-year-old girl. Pediatr Int 2013;55(2):e29–31.

31. Gulati Y, Maheshwari AV. Brodie's abscess of the femoral neck simulating osteoid osteoma. Acta Orthop Belg 2007;73(5):648–52.

32. McGuinness B, Wilson N, Doyle AJ. The "penumbra sign" on T1-weighted MRI for differentiating musculoskeletal infection from tumour. Skeletal Radiol 2007;36(5):417–21.

33. Klein MH, Shankman S. Osteoid osteoma: radiologic and pathologic correlation. Skeletal Radiol 1992;21(1):23–31.

34. El Demellawy D, Young JL, de Nanassy J, et al. Langerhans cell histiocytosis: a comprehensive review. Pathology 2015;47(4):294–301.

35. Emile JF, Wechsler J, Brousse N, et al. Langerhans' cell histiocytosis. Definitive diagnosis with the use of monoclonal antibody O10 on routinely paraffin-embedded samples. Am J Surg Pathol 1995;19(6):636–41.

36. Valladeau J, Ravel O, Dezutter-Dambuyant C, et al. Langerin, a novel C-type lectin specific to Langerhans cells, is an endocytic receptor that induces the formation of Birbeck granules. Immunity 2000;12(1):71–81.

37. Demicco EG, Rosenberg AE, Bjornsson J, et al. Primary Rosai-Dorfman disease of bone: a clinicopathologic study of 15 cases. Am J Surg Pathol 2010;34(9):1324–33.

38. Aptel S, Lecocq-Teixeira S, Olivier P, et al. Multimodality evaluation of musculoskeletal sarcoidosis: Imaging findings and literature review. Diagn Interv Imaging 2016;97(1):5–18.

39. Chang JC, Sakurai H, Jagirdar J. Symptomatic rib lesions as the primary presentation of sarcoidosis. Report of two cases and review of literature. Sarcoidosis 1992;9(2):130–3.

40. Mangino D, Stover DE. Sarcoidosis presenting as metastatic bony disease. A case report and review of the literature on vertebral body sarcoidosis. Respiration 2004;71(3):292–4.

41. Packer CD, Mileti LM. Vertebral sarcoidosis mimicking lytic osseous metastases: development 16 years after apparent resolution of thoracic sarcoidosis. J Clin Rheumatol 2005;11(2):105–8.

42. Valencia MP, Deaver PM, Mammarappallil MC. Sarcoidosis of the thoracic and lumbar vertebrae, mimicking metastasis or multifocal osteomyelitis by MRI: case report. Clin Imaging 2009;33(6):478–81.

43. Pambuccian SE, Horyd ID, Cawte T, et al. Amyloidoma of bone, a plasma cell/plasmacytoid neoplasm. Report of three cases and review of the literature. Am J Surg Pathol 1997;21(2):179–86.

44. Prokaeva T, Spencer B, Kaut M, et al. Soft tissue, joint, and bone manifestations of AL amyloidosis: clinical presentation, molecular features, and survival. Arthritis Rheum 2007;56(11):3858–68.

45. Wechalekar AD, Gillmore JD, Hawkins PN. Systemic amyloidosis. Lancet 2016;387(10038):2641–54.

46. Vrana JA, Gamez JD, Madden BJ, et al. Classification of amyloidosis by laser microdissection and mass spectrometry-based proteomic analysis in clinical biopsy specimens. Blood 2009;114(24):4957–9.

Tumor Syndromes That Include Bone Tumors
An Update

Maria Gnoli, MD*, Francesca Ponti, BSB,
Luca Sangiorgi, MD, PhD (Clinical Genetics)

KEYWORDS

- Tumor syndromes • Bone neoplasms • Bone cancer • Osteosarcoma
- Genetic syndromes with bone cancer predisposition

Key points

- Tumor syndromes, which include bone neoplasias, are genetic predisposing conditions characterized by the development of a pattern of malignancies with early onset within a family.

- Occurrence of bilateral, multifocal, or metachronous neoplasias and specific histopathologic findings can suggest a genetic predisposition syndrome. Moreover, additional clinical features not related to the neoplasia can be an hallmark of specific genetic syndromes.

- Mostly, those diseases have an autosomal dominant pattern of inheritance with variable percentage of penetrance.

- On the other hand, some syndromic disorders with an increased tumor risk may show an autosomal recessive transmission or are related to somatic mosaicism.

- To date many genetic tumor syndromes are known. This update is specifically focused on syndromes predisposing to osteosarcoma (OS) (Li-Fraumeni syndrome [LFS], retinoblastoma [Rb], Rothmund-Thomson syndrome [RTS], and Werner syndrome [WS]) and to chondrosarcoma (multiple osteochondromas [MO] and enchondromatosis).

ABSTRACT

Tumor syndromes, including bone neoplasias, are genetic predisposing conditions characterized by the development of a pattern of malignancies within a family at an early age of onset. Occurrence of bilateral, multifocal, or metachronous neoplasias and specific histopathologic findings suggest a genetic predisposition syndrome. Additional clinical features not related to the neoplasia can be a hallmark of specific genetic syndromes. Mostly, those diseases have an autosomal dominant pattern of inheritance with variable percentage of penetrance. Some syndromic disorders with an increased tumor risk may show an autosomal recessive transmission or are related to somatic mosaicism. Many genetic tumor syndromes are known. This update is specifically focused on syndromes predisposing to osteosarcoma and chondrosarcoma.

OVERVIEW

Tumor syndromes are genetic conditions predisposing to developing malignancies, including a single primary tumor or multicentric neoplasms, with an early age of onset.[1]

Disclosure Statement: The authors have nothing to disclose.
Department of Medical Genetics and Skeletal Rare Diseases, Rizzoli Orthopedic Institute, Via Pupilli 1, Bologna 40136, Italy
* Corresponding author.
E-mail address: maria.gnoli@ior.it

It is well known that genetic alterations play a major role in cancer pathogenesis[2,3] and approximately 5% to 10% of all cancers arise from a background of genetic predisposition.[1] A suggestion of a genetic predisposition syndrome is given by onset of a certain cancer type at an earlier age than in the general population; occurrence of bilateral, multifocal, or metachronous neoplasias; specific histopathologic findings. Moreover, additional clinical features not related to the neoplasia can be a hallmark of specific genetic syndromes.[4] In a majority of cases, those diseases have an autosomal dominant pattern of inheritance with a complete or incomplete penetrance.[1]

Clinical expression – number or type of neoplasias and age of onset – can be extremely variable within the same family.[1] On the other hand, some syndromic disorders with an increased tumor risk, like Rothmund-Thomson syndrome (RTS) or Werner Syndrome (WS), may be inherited in an autosomal recessive way.[5–7] In addition, nonhereditary somatic mosaicism has been described for polyostotic fibrous dysplasia and McCune-Albright syndrome and for enchondromatosis (Ollier disease [OD] and Maffucci syndrome [MS]).[7]

So far, many genetic tumor syndromes are known.[1] This review focuses on tumor syndromes that include OS (Table 1) and chondrosarcoma (Table 2).

TUMOR SYNDROMES AND OSTEOSARCOMA

OS is the most common primary bone tumor, histologically characterized by the presence of malignant mesenchymal cells and the production of osteoid[8]; multiple somatic mutations and chromosomal aberrations have been described in sporadic OS.[9] Some hereditary genetic syndromes confer genetic predisposition to developing OS (see Table 1).

LI-FRAUMENI SYNDROME

LFS (Online Mendelian Inheritance in Man [OMIM] #151623), is an autosomal dominant cancer predisposition syndrome, resulting from germline heterozygous mutations of the tumor suppressor gene TP53 located on chromosome 17p13.1 (OMIM*191170).[7,10]

Tp53 gene product, the tumor protein p53, plays an important role in determining the fate of cells with damaged DNA, delaying cell cycle progression, and addressing DNA repair or apoptosis. When the wild-type p53 protein is absent, cells containing damaged DNA can survive and proliferate, contributing to malignant transformation.[11]

Therefore, the involvement of the p53 protein becomes a determinant aspect when considering the wide tumor spectrum in LFS. Its high variability regarding age of onset and cancer types between individuals, even within the same family, makes it difficult to suggest surveillance for early diagnosis and to have a full understanding of pathogenic mechanism involved in cancer development.[12] Since its first description in 1969 by Frederick Li and Joseph Fraumeni, the classic clinical definition of LFS was first established almost 20 years later.[12] The tumor spectrum was subsequently widened in 1988 and these malignancies still represent the majority of LFS-related tumors (Box 1).[12] Over time, more patients were described sharing only some of the characteristics previously identified; then, new sets of criteria for clinical diagnosis and for selecting patients for genetic testing were added. The Chompret criteria, developed in 2001 from a French cohort of TP53 mutation carriers showed the highest predictive value[13] and its more recent version (Bougeard and colleagues[12]) had an estimated sensitivity of 82% to 95% and specificity of 47% to 58%. Fig. 1 summarizes the different diagnostic criteria for LFS

Table 1
Main genetic syndromic conditions associated with osteosarcoma

Disease	Main Cancer Types	Bone Cancer Type	Gene	Transmission
LFS OMIM #151623	Breast cancer, soft tissue sarcoma, OS, CNS tumor, ACC, leukemia, bronchoalveolar lung cancer	OS	TP53	AD
RTS OMIM #268400	OS; skin cancer	OS	RECQL4	AR
Rb OMIM #180200	Retinoblastoma, retinoma, pinealoblastoma	OS	RB1	AD
WS OMIM #277700	Thyroid neoplasms, malignant melanoma and meningioma; leukemia; other neoplasms	OS	WRN	AR

Abbreviations: ACC, adrenal cortical carcinoma; AD, autosomal dominant; AR, autosomal recessive; CNS, central nervous system; OS, osteosarcoma.

Table 2
Syndromes characterized by lesions with risk of chondrosarcoma transformation

Disease	Main Clinical Features	Bone Cancer Type	Gene	Transmission
Multiple Osteochondromas, Exostoses, multiple (multiple cartilaginous exostoses, HME, diaphyseal aclasis, MO, osteochondromatosis) OMIM #133700, OMIM#133701	MO	CSP	EXT1; EXT2	Autosomal dominant (AD)
Multiple enchondromatosis, Maffucci type (MS) OMIM #614569) Enchondromatosis, multiple, Ollier type (OD) OMIM #166000	Multiple enchondromas (associated with angiomas in MS) Note: also other (not skeletal) neoplasias risk	CSC	IDH1, IDH2, PTHR1 (less common) (mosaic, not in all cases of OD or MS)	Sporadic

Within this tumor spectrum, the most frequent cancer types in childhood are OS (with incidence as high as 30% in affected children), adrenocortical carcinoma, central nervous system (CNS) tumor, and soft tissue sarcoma.[14]

Recent studies evaluated the incidence and age of onset in LFS patients series: the cumulative cancer incidence is 50% by 31 years among TP53-positive female patients (mostly due to breast cancer incidence) and 46 years among male patients. OS occurs in 5% of female patients and 11% of male patients.[15]

LFS-specific mutations may have a prognostic value because they have been related to OS predisposition at a young age and to metastasis.[16,17]

A few TP53 mutations are also found in sporadic OS, especially translocations involving intron 1 of TP53.[9,18]

Next-generation sequencing and commercially available inherited cancer panels will likely increase the number of identified germline or

somantic Tp53 mutation. Most of these mutations are missense mutations occurring in the DNA-binding region (exons 5–8).[10] Big deletions and duplications are rare events. These accomplishments, however, do not likely explain all scenarios and are challenged by atypical cases. Families with few or no characteristics of LFS with mutation in TP53 or families complying with the 2015 Chompret criteria and negative for TP53 mutations are reported, so the presence of a TP53 mutation should be considered a discriminating factor in the classification of LFS patients.[19] Moreover, none of the alternative LFS susceptibility genes investigated has proved to play a pivotal role in the disease.[20] Therefore, single nucleotide polymorphisms (SNPs) may contribute to alter the predisposition to cancer development[12] or modify cancer age of onset.[20] Several studies explored 3 SNPs: one on the TP53 gene, Pro72Arg TP53 Pro72Arg (NM_000546.5: c.215C > G, p.Pro72Arg, Chr17(GRCh37): g.7579472G > C, rs1042522); the other two both located in the MDM2 gene promoter region MDM2 SNP285 (NM_002392.3:c.14?285G > C, Chr12(GRCh37): g.69202556G > C, rs117039649); and SNP309 (NM_002392.3:c.14?309T > G, Chr12 (GRCh37): g.69202580T > G: rs2279744), which have been investigated as modifiers of cancer predisposition largely in TP53 mutation carriers.[20] Recently, a study performed by Ponti and colleagues[20] evaluated a correlation between these SNPs and cancer risk, age of onset, and cancer type also in LFS-suggestive patients (negative for TP53 mutation). In particular, a strong association emerged in the

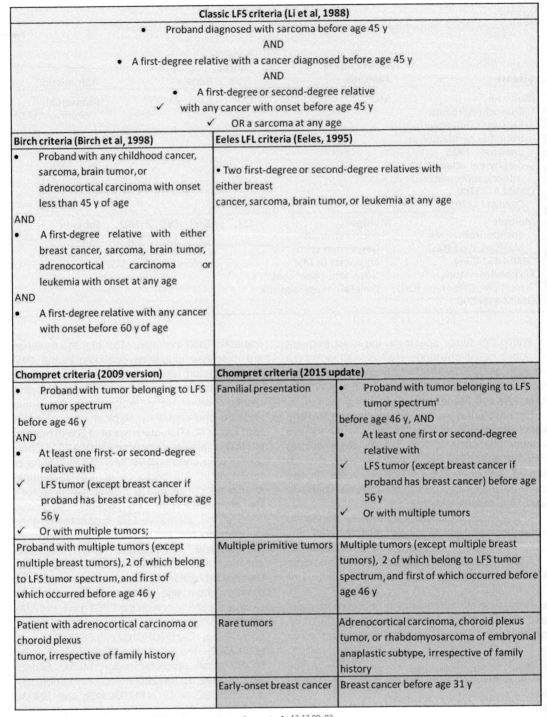

Classic LFS criteria (Li et al, 1988)		
• Proband diagnosed with sarcoma before age 45 y AND • A first-degree relative with a cancer diagnosed before age 45 y AND • A first-degree or second-degree relative ✓ with any cancer with onset before age 45 y ✓ OR a sarcoma at any age		

Birch criteria (Birch et al, 1998)	Eeles LFL criteria (Eeles, 1995)	
• Proband with any childhood cancer, sarcoma, brain tumor, or adrenocortical carcinoma with onset less than 45 y of age AND • A first-degree relative with either breast cancer, sarcoma, brain tumor, adrenocortical carcinoma or leukemia with onset at any age AND • A first-degree relative with any cancer with onset before 60 y of age	• Two first-degree or second-degree relatives with either breast cancer, sarcoma, brain tumor, or leukemia at any age	

Chompret criteria (2009 version)	Chompret criteria (2015 update)	
• Proband with tumor belonging to LFS tumor spectrum before age 46 y AND • At least one first- or second-degree relative with ✓ LFS tumor (except breast cancer if proband has breast cancer) before age 56 y ✓ Or with multiple tumors;	Familial presentation	• Proband with tumor belonging to LFS tumor spectrum[a] before age 46 y, AND • At least one first or second-degree relative with ✓ LFS tumor (except breast cancer if proband has breast cancer) before age 56 y ✓ Or with multiple tumors
Proband with multiple tumors (except multiple breast tumors), 2 of which belong to LFS tumor spectrum, and first of which occurred before age 46 y	Multiple primitive tumors	Multiple tumors (except multiple breast tumors), 2 of which belong to LFS tumor spectrum, and first of which occurred before age 46 y
Patient with adrenocortical carcinoma or choroid plexus tumor, irrespective of family history	Rare tumors	Adrenocortical carcinoma, choroid plexus tumor, or rhabdomyosarcoma of embryonal anaplastic subtype, irrespective of family history
	Early-onset breast cancer	Breast cancer before age 31 y

Fig. 1. LFS diagnostic criteria. [a] See Box 1. *Data from* Refs.[12,13,90–92]

presence of the MDM2 SNP309G allele and predisposition to cancer development and with the combined effect of both the TP53 Pro72 variant and the MDM2 309G allele. These results are strengthened by biochemical studies[21]; when considering Pro72 reduced capacity in inducing apoptosis and the TP53 basal level decrease caused by higher 309G-induced MDM2 levels, patients with SNP309G and Pro72 have less efficient TP53-mediated tumor suppression and consequently higher susceptibility in cancer development. Furthermore, the recently identified

MDM2 SNP285C variant, which resides on the SNP309G allele, creates a distinct SNP285C/309G haplotype, typical of the white population, able to neutralize the 309G variation effect with reduced risk in patients carrying a TP53 mutation with different cancer types.[20] This effect did not emerge in a TP53 LFS-suggestive patient group, probably due to the limited number of patients. No significant differences were detected analyzing the combined effect of these SNPs with both age of tumor onset and cancer type in a *TP53*-negative population. Therefore, in an LFS-suggestive TP53-negative group, SNP309G could act not only as a modifier but also as a potential disease-causing factor by affecting the LFS phenotype regardless of the presence of a TP53 germline alteration. In conclusion, it would be interesting to further investigate in a wider data set the involvement of novel SNPs, potential causative genes, or additional functional modifiers of the TP53-MDM2 pathway, such as miR-605,[22] to justify an LFS phenotype in absence of a TP53 mutation.

RETINOBLASTOMA

Rb, also known as glioma retinae, is a malignant tumor of the retina and is the most common intraocular cancer in childhood (1 in 15,000–20,000 live births).[23] Neoplastic cells carry biallelic oncogenic variants in the *RB1* gene.[24]

Rb occurs unilaterally in approximately 60% of patients, with a mean age of 2 years at diagnosis, or bilaterally in approximately 40% of cases, with diagnosis at 15 months. In the latter, tumors are usually synchronous (both eyes affected at the time of diagnosis) and can be multiple (multifocal).

Approximately 15% of unilateral cases and all bilateral or multifocal forms are hereditary.[23]

A positive family history with unilateral or bilateral Rb occurs in approximately 10% of cases.

Hereditary Rb (OMIM #180200) has an autosomal dominant inheritance with increased risk of developing other nonocular neoplasias[7,24] and diagnosis is established if the proband has an Rb or retinoma (benign retinal tumors) and a Rb-positive family history.

The most common clinical sign of Rb is leukocoria (white pupillary reflex), alone or associated with strabismus, occurring before or at the same time.[25] Other manifestations are eye appearance changes and reduced visual acuity.[24]

When a pinealoblastoma (retina-like tissue in pineal gland, a rare and usually fatal disorder) occurs with bilateral Rb, this condition is called trilateral Rb.[24]

Many different diseases have a clinical presentation reminiscent of Rb, that is, persistent hyperplastic primary vitreous and Coats disease or other hereditary ocular disease (exudative vitreoretinopathy or Norrie disease)[7,24]; moreover, some genetic syndromes have an ocular involvement similar to Rb clinical presentation but also additional and various clinical features (ie, von Hippel-Lindau disease, incontinentia pigmenti, and tuberous sclerosis).[7]

Rb and *RB1* gene represent a model for tumorigenesis. Knudson[26] observed that Rb occurs either as a sporadic or hereditary disease. Because hereditary forms exist, he supposed that a germline predisposing mutation and a second somatic mutation in retinal cells are required to cancer development.

This so-called 2-hits model[26] is applicable to other cancers. Molecular studies confirmed that other events, in addition to *RB1* mutations, are necessary for tumorigenesis.[23,26]

Furthermore, Rb patients have an increased risk for other neoplasias, most commonly OSs, soft tissue sarcomas (leiomyosarcoma and rhabdomyosarcomas), or melanomas, occurring in adolescence or adulthood. Patients exposed to external beam radiation therapy[27] have an increased risk (more than 50%) of developing a second cancer and patients with hereditary Rb have a high risk of developing a cancer later in life.[24,28]

OS represent 25% to 30% of all secondary neoplasms in Rb patients. In some series in medical literature, OS incidence and mortality are increased as high as several hundred–fold compared with the general population[24] and have an overall survival estimated incidence of 7% at 20 years.[29] In addition, chondrosarcoma and Ewing sarcoma have been reported in Rb patients.[30,31]

This increased risk compared with the general population is due to both previous radiotherapy and *RB1* gene mutations. It has been suggested gene that *RB1* mutations can be related to the development and progression of primary OS and can represent a prognostic marker of the disease.[32] Experimental findings in mouse models confirm a role of the Rb1 pathway in the development of radiation-induced malignancies.[33]

RB1 (OMIM *614041) is the first molecularly defined tumor suppressor gene[34] and is located at 13q14.2 region, encoding for a 110-kD nuclear phosphoprotein. Retinoblastoma protein (Rb protein or pRB) has a key role in regulating the exit from the cell cycle, in particular in the retinal cell and during rod development.[7]

Most of the *RB1* mutations result in a premature termination codon and are located throughout exon 1 to exon 25. Some mutations are recurrent (at methylated CpG dinucleotide, splice site donor site of intron 12). Also complex rearrangements and deletions and mutations in the promoter region have been reported.[24] Pathogenic variants cause loss of its cell-cycle regulating function: when functionality is partly conserved, the disease shows a low penetrance.[24]

RB1 somatic mutations are also identified in OSs and small cell lung cancers and at lower frequencies in a variety of other tumor types.[34]

ROTHMUND-THOMSON SYNDROME

RTS (OMIM #268400) is a rare genodermatosis with predisposition to cancer.[7]

Originally the disease was described by a German ophthalmologist, Auguste Rothmund, in 1868.[35] The true prevalence is not known, but fewer than 400 cases have been reported to date.[35,36]

The hallmark of the disease is a characteristic facial rash (poikiloderma). If an atypical rash occurs, RTS can be suspected in presence of at least 2 of the major clinical signs reported in Table 3.[5]

The diagnosis is generally on clinical basis or by molecular analysis of *RECQL4* gene.[5]

Some investigators distinguish 2 RTS forms: the RTS type II form (poikiloderma, congenital bone defects), in particular, has an increased risk of malignancies (OS in childhood and skin cancer later in life).[35]

OS is the most common cancer in RTS patients. The estimated prevalence is 30%[37] occurring in childhood (14 years mean age of onset) and in more than 1 sibling in some families.[37,38] More common location (femur and tibia) and histologic subtype (osteoblastic) of OS are similar to patients with sporadic OS, but developing at a younger age (14 vs 17 years).[5] At least 10 cases (3 considered metachronous) of multicentric OS have been reported, with higher incidence in RTS compared with sporadic OS.[35,39]

Cutaneous epithelial neoplasias occur in 5%, with mean age of onset 34.4 years. Other neoplasias are occasionally described in RTS patients. A second malignancy has been reported in few RTS patients: non-Hodgkin lymphoma and Hodgkin lymphoma, in both cases after therapy for OS.[37,40] RTS patients also have recurrence of the neoplastic disease.[35,39,41]

Table 4 summaries differential diagnosis for RTS.[35]

Remarkably, OS is a common finding in RTS and WS but not in this group of genodermatosis.

RTS is allelic with 2 disorders, RAPADILINO Syndrome (OMIM #266280) and Baller-Gerold syndrome (BGS) (OMIM #218600) (Table 5). The development of OSs and lymphomas has been reported in some RAPADILINO Syndrome patients.[42] Lymphoma has been reported in a BGS patient,[42,43] instead OS or lymphoma are not described in *RECQL4*-related BGS in a large series.[42]

RTS is an autosomal recessive disorder, related to biallelic mutations in *RECQL4* gene.

Table 3
Major clinical features in Rothmund-Thomson syndrome

Clinical Features	Details
Facial rash (poikiloderma) typical	Acute phase (between ages 3 mo and 6 mo) with erythema on the cheeks and face and extensor surfaces of the extremities typically, sparing of the trunk and abdomen Chronic phase: reticulated hyperpopigmentation and hypopigmentation, poikiloderma
Sparse scalp hair, eyelashes, and/or eyebrows	In some cases alopecia
Small size, usually symmetric for height and weight	Low birth weight and length for gestational age; normal growth hormone
Gastrointestinal disturbance	Chronic vomiting and diarrhea, sometimes requiring feeding tubes
Skeletal abnormalities	Radial ray defects, ulnar defects, absent or hypoplastic patella, osteopenia, abnormal trabeculation
Dental abnormalities	Rudimentary or hypoplastic teeth, enamel defects, delayed tooth eruption, caries
Nail abnormalities	Dysplastic or poorly formed nails
Hyperkeratosis, particularly of the soles of the feet	
Cataracts	Usually juvenile, bilateral; incidence and onset variable in series
Cancers	Skin cancers (basal cell carcinoma and squamous cell carcinoma) and in particular bone cancer (osteosarcoma)

Table 4
Differential diagnosis for Rothmund-Thomson syndromes

Disease	OMIM Entries
Hereditary sclerosing poikiloderma	173700
Poikiloderma with neutropenia	604173
Dyskeratosis congenita, (Clericuzio type)	127550: DYSKERATOSIS CONGENITA, AUTOSOMAL DOMINANT 1; DKCA1 224230: DYSKERATOSIS CONGENITA, AUTOSOMAL RECESSIVE 1; DKCB1 305000: DYSKERATOSIS CONGENITA, X-LINKED; DKCX 609377: ACD, MOUSE, HOMOLOG OF; ACD 613987: DYSKERATOSIS CONGENITA, AUTOSOMAL RECESSIVE 2; DKCB2 613988: DYSKERATOSIS CONGENITA, AUTOSOMAL RECESSIVE 3; DKCB3 613989: DYSKERATOSIS CONGENITA, AUTOSOMAL DOMINANT 2; DKCA2 613990: DYSKERATOSIS CONGENITA, AUTOSOMAL DOMINANT 3; DKCA3 615190: DYSKERATOSIS CONGENITA, AUTOSOMAL RECESSIVE 5; DKCB5 616353: DYSKERATOSIS CONGENITA, AUTOSOMAL RECESSIVE 6; DKCB6 616553: DYSKERATOSIS CONGENITA, AUTOSOMAL DOMINANT 6; DKCA6
Bloom syndrome	210900
WS	277700
Ataxia telangiectasia	208900
Cockayne syndrome	133540: COCKAYNE SYNDROME B; CSB 216400: COCKAYNE SYNDROME A; CSA
Fanconi anemia	227645: FANCONI ANEMIA, COMPLEMENTATION GROUP C; FANCC 227646: FANCONI ANEMIA, COMPLEMENTATION GROUP D2; FANCD2 227650: FANCONI ANEMIA, COMPLEMENTATION GROUP A; FANCA 300514: FANCONI ANEMIA, COMPLEMENTATION GROUP B; FANCB 600901: FANCONI ANEMIA, COMPLEMENTATION GROUP E; FANCE 603467: FANCONI ANEMIA, COMPLEMENTATION GROUP F; FANCF 605724: FANCONI ANEMIA, COMPLEMENTATION GROUP D1; FANCD1 609053: FANCONI ANEMIA, COMPLEMENTATION GROUP I; FANCI 609054: FANCONI ANEMIA, COMPLEMENTATION GROUP J; FANCJ 610832: FANCONI ANEMIA, COMPLEMENTATION GROUP N; FANCN 613390: FANCONI ANEMIA, COMPLEMENTATION GROUP O; FANCO 613951: FANCONI ANEMIA, COMPLEMENTATION GROUP P; FANCP 614082: FANCONI ANEMIA, COMPLEMENTATION GROUP G; FANCG 614083: FANCONI ANEMIA, COMPLEMENTATION GROUP L; FANCL 614087: FANCONI ANEMIA, COMPLEMENTATION GROUP M; FANCM 615272: FANCONI ANEMIA, COMPLEMENTATION GROUP Q; FANCQ 616435: FANCONI ANEMIA, COMPLEMENTATION GROUP T; FANCT 617244: FANCONI ANEMIA, COMPLEMENTATION GROUP R; FANCR
Xeroderma pigmentosum	278700: XERODERMA PIGMENTOSUM, COMPLEMENTATION GROUP A; XPA 278720: XERODERMA PIGMENTOSUM, COMPLEMENTATION GROUP C; XPC 278730: XERODERMA PIGMENTOSUM, COMPLEMENTATION GROUP D; XPD 278740: XERODERMA PIGMENTOSUM, COMPLEMENTATION GROUP E 278750: XERODERMA PIGMENTOSUM, VARIANT TYPE; XPV 278760: XERODERMA PIGMENTOSUM, COMPLEMENTATION GROUP F; XPF 278780: XERODERMA PIGMENTOSUM, COMPLEMENTATION GROUP G; XPG

located at chromosome 8q24.3, encoding a protein of 1208 amino acids (OMIM *603780). This protein belongs to the RecQ helicase family with RECQ2 and RECQ3; mutations in these genes are related to 2 other cancer predisposition disorders, Bloom syndrome and WS, respectively.

RecQ helicases are involved in genome maintenance and stability.[44] Interaction with p53 has been demonstrated and accumulation of transcriptionally active nuclear p53 causes enhanced sensitivity to DNA-damaging agents in RTS patients.[45] An oncogenic role in sporadic breast cancers has been suggested.[46]

Table 5
Allelic disorder of Rothmund-Thomson syndrome

Disorder	Main Clinical Findings	OMIM
RAPADILINO syndrome	Irregular pigmentation with café au lait macules (but no poikiloderma), small stature, palate defects, radial ray defects, patellar hypoplasia, and gastrointestinal abnormalities	OMIM #266280
BGS	Radial ray defects, skeletal dysplasia, short stature, and craniosynostosis	OMIM #218600

In sporadic OS, no mutations in *RECQL4* have been detected, but elevated levels of RECQL4 have been reported, so the molecular mechanism and its role in bone abnormalities and cancer development are not known.[47] *RECQL4* gene sequence analysis identifies mutations in 66% of the RTS clinically affected.[5] This spectrum includes both missense mutations and small deletions in short introns affecting splicing.[5] Nevertheless, it has been demonstrated that loss-of-function mutations occur in two-thirds of 33 RTS patients and are associated with an increased risk of OS.[48]

RTS type I (poikiloderma and juvenile cataracts) is not related to mutations in *RECQL4*, suggesting genetic heterogeneity, but a responsible gene has not been identified.

Few studies have investigated genotype-phenotype correlations: a relation between mutations predicted to cause loss of protein function and risk of OS has been suggested.[48] Nevertheless, the phenotype cannot be predicted by the combination of 2 mutations. Cancer risk is increased in patients with *RECQL4* mutations, even if this risk is well known in RTS patients, but only few RAPADILINO patients developed cancer.[35]

WERNER SYNDROME

WS (progeria of the adult) (OMIM #277700) is a rare genetic disease characterized by premature aging signs and cancer predisposition.[6]

The prevalence (estimated at 1:380,000–1,000,000) varies in different populations: it is higher in Japan (from approximately 1:20,000 to 1:40,000)[6] and in Sardinia, with an estimated frequency of approximately 1:50,000,[49] although the frequency is not exactly known in the US population.[6]

Even though the male/female ratio is 1:1 in the University of Washington International Registry of Werner Syndrome, women are slightly more represented, but it could be an ascertainment bias.[6] Approximately 90% of WS patients have all 4 cardinal signs: premature graying and/or thinning of scalp hair (100%), bilateral ocular cataracts (present in 99%), characteristic dermatologic pathology (96%), and short stature (95%).[6] Biallelic mutations in *WRN* gene account for approximately 90% of WS patients.[6]

Epstein and colleagues[50] reviewed clinical, pathologic, and genetic features of the WS in 1966. Since 1988, the University of Washington International Registry of Werner Syndrome includes WS cases, defined by suggestive clinical findings.[51] Diagnostic guidelines were updated in 2013,[52] evaluating incidence and relevance at diagnosis of some clinical signs in a nationwide epidemiologic study, including genetic analysis (Box 2).

As in LFS, a subset of WS patients does not carry mutations in *WRN* gene but has a clinical overlap with patients who fulfill diagnostic criteria: these atypical WS patients have an early age of onset and faster progression of the disease and 15% of them have a de novo heterozygous pathogenic mutation in *LMNA*.[53]

In other patients initially diagnosed with WS, mutations in other genes were identified: in addition to *LMNA*, these include *POLD1, SPRTN,* and *SAMHD1*.[54]

WS patients are also at risk for other age-dependent diseases, for istance cardiovascular disease,[55] and the most common causes of death are myocardial infarction and cancer. Median life span is 54 years.[6]

In childhood no clinical features are present, but patients have lack of a growth spurt during the early teen years. Loss and graying of hair, hoarseness, and scleroderma-like skin changes occur usually in the second decade, followed by bilateral ocular cataracts, type 2 diabetes mellitus, hypogonadism, skin ulcers, and osteoporosis in the 30s. Indolent deep skin ulcer around the ankles associated with soft tissue calcifications is considered a pathognomonic sign (80% of cases).[52]

The disease predisposes to an unusual spectrum of cancers, which can be also multiple in the same individual[56] and encompasses several cancer types identical to other cancer-predisposing syndromes associated with DNA instability (ie, LFS).[56]

Box 2
Diagnostic criteria for Werner syndrome

Cardinal signs and symptoms

- Progeroid changes of hair

- Cataract bilateral

- Changes of skin, intractable skin ulcers (atrophic skin, tight skin, clavus, callus)

- Soft tissue calcification (Achilles tendon, etc)

- Birdlike face

- Abnormal voice

Other signs and symptoms

- Abnormal glucose and/or lipid metabolism

- Deformation and abnormality of the bone osteoporosis and so forth

- Malignant tumors, nonepithelial tumors, thyroid cancer and so forth

- Parental consanguinity

- Premature atherosclerosis, angina pectoris, myocardial infarction

- Hypogonadism

- Short stature and low body weight

Genetic analysis

Data From Takemoto M, Mori S, Kuzuya M, et al. Diagnostic criteria for Werner syndrome based on Japanese nationwide epidemiological survey. Geriatr Gerontol Int 2013;13(2):479.

In a large study (189 patients), 6 groups of neoplasia represent a majority of cancer in WS patients.[56]

Approximately 8% of the patients develop OS and 10% have a soft tissue sarcoma diagnosis. Thyroid neoplasms, malignant melanoma, and meningioma occur with a higher frequency, followed by leukemia and preleukemic conditions of the bone marrow (9%).[56] Other neoplasms have a lower frequency (ie, other skin cancers, gastrointestinal, uterine/ovarian, genitourinary, head and neck, breast, lung, CNS, and adrenal cortical neoplasms).

Compared with RTS, the median age at cancer diagnosis is higher in WS and the spectrum of tumor types is wider than in RTS, which is mainly characterized by OSs and lymphomas.

Age of onset and association of the typical clinical features differentiate WS from other disease: that is, early onset of bilateral cataract without hair graying and skin findings is likely not associated with WS. Main differential diagnosis are listed in Table 6.

WS is an autosomal recessive disorder, related to biallelic mutations in the *WRN* gene, located at chromosome 8p12, encoding a multifunctional nuclear protein of 1432 amino acids, for which no alternatively spliced forms are described so far[54] (OMIM *604611 RECQ protein-like 2 [RECQL2]).

Like the RTS gene, WRN is member of the RecQ DNA helicase family.

The mutational spectrum reported in the University of Washington International Registry of Werner Syndrome and Japanese Werner Consortium, has been recently updated for a total of 83 mutations.[54] One allele (c.1105C > T) accounts for approximately 20% of pathogenic alleles in the European and Japanese populations. The c.2089-3024A > G variant is a founder variant in the Sardinian population, with a heterozygous frequency of approximately 1 in 120.[49] A majority of pathogenic variants result in the truncation of the protein; instead, missense mutations are rarer.[6] The pathogenic mechanism of the investigated missense variants seem related to protein instability (ie, p.K125N or p.K135E) or alteration of helicase activity (ie, p.G574R).[54]

WS is considered a model for study of accelerated aging: specific *WRN* polymorphisms are related to longevity, cardiovascular risk factors,[54,57] and different cancers.[54] The p.C1367R variation seems to protect against soft tissue sarcomas and non-Hodgkin lymphoma.[54]

Even though the protein function and pathogenic mechanism of *WRN* mutations are not clear, it is known that it has a role in DNA repair, recombination, replication, and transcription.

As described previously, among the 5 RCQ human proteins, 3 have been related to syndromic disorders, but the molecular bases underlying different cancer risk and clinical signs of these syndrome are not known. Remarkably, Bloom syndrome patients develop similar cancers for type and frequencies to the general population[44] but at earlier age; moreover, OS is described, even though it does not represent the most common neoplasia in this disorder.[58] Further studies need to be conducted to elucidate molecular mechanisms in these syndromes and to explain their clinical differences.

SYNDROMES WITH INCREASED RISK FOR CHONDROSARCOMAS

Some skeletal disorders are characterized by multiple benign bone tumors, with an increased risk of malignant transformation toward secondary

Table 6
Differential diagnosis for Werner syndromes

Disease	Main Clinical Signs	Notes
Mandibuloacral dysplasia (OMIM #248370, #608612)	Short stature, type A lipodystrophy with loss of fat in the extremities but accumulation of fat in the neck and trunk, thin, hyperpigmented skin, partial alopecia, dysmorphisms (prominent eyes, convex nasal ridge, tooth loss, micrognathia, retrognathia), progeroid appearance, and short fingers.	
Hutchinson-Gilford syndrome (progeria of childhood) (OMIM #176670)	Short stature, low weight, early loss of hair, facial features (progeroid appearance) lipodystrophy, scleroderma, decreased joint mobility, osteolysis	Childhood onset of progeria in Hutchinson-Gilford syndrome
Myotonic dystrophy (OMIM #160900; #602668)	Young adult–onset cataracts, muscle weakness and wasting, myotonia and cardiac abnormalities	The diabetes mellitus and muscular symptoms not described in WS
Bloom syndrome (OMIM #210900)	Proportionate prenatal and postnatal growth deficiency; sun-sensitive, telangiectatic, hypopigmented and hyperpigmented skin	Childhood onset in Bloom syndrome
LFS (OMIM #151623)	Premenopausal breast cancer, soft tissue sarcoma, OS, central nervous system tumors adrenocortical carcinoma, leukemia, lung bronchoalveolar cancer	Cataracts or premature aging are not features of LFS

chondrosarcoma (see **Table 2**). Chondrosarcoma often develops within a benign precursor lesion, osteochondroma for peripheral chondrosarcoma (CSP), or enchondroma for central chondrosarcoma (CSC).

Chondrosarcoma is a malignant neoplasia producing cartilaginous matrix and represents approximately 25% of malignant bone tumors[59] and belongs mainly to 5 distinct subtypes (see details in de Andrea and Julian[60]).

MULTIPLE OSTEOCHONDROMAS

MO, also named hereditary multiple exostoses (OMIM #133700, #133701), is an autosomal dominant disorder characterized by multiple benign cartilage-capped bone tumors (osteochondromas) (**Fig. 2**) that develop during skeletal growth.

The first description of the disease was performed by John Hunter in 1786. The term, multiple exostoses, for designation of the disease was used first by Virchow in 1876.[61]

Many questions are still open about MO. For example, in medical literature a prevalence of at least 1 in 50,000 has been reported[62] but this value is probably underestimated, because individuals

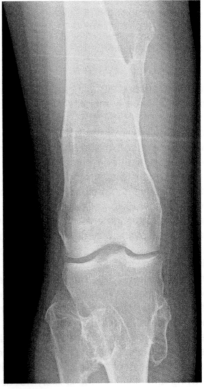

Fig. 2. Exostoses in MO.

with milder clinical expression are often not diagnosed as MO.[61]

The disease shows variable entity in clinical expression even in the same family, suggesting that additional factors, other than specific *EXT* genes mutation can modulate the expression of phenotype.[62]

Another issue concerns incidence of malignant transformation toward CSP in MO (that can occur in adulthood), related risk factors, and molecular bases of this event.

Most CSPs in MO occur in the third to fifth decades of life (in the past mean age 31 years)[61] but reports of recent and large series do not describe accurate detail about this.

Incidence of malignant transformation in MO seems higher than in cases of a solitary osteochondroma, occurring in 1% to 2% of patients[63]

Previous studies suggested a lifetime risk in MO of approximately 2% to 4%,[64,65] but reported prevalence can vary from less than 1% to 25% in different reports, with plausible bias due to the small series or to data collection in tertiary referral institutions.[65] Considering more recent and larger series, malignant transformation occurs in approximately 5% to 7%.[64–66] Further studies have to be performed to define the true prevalence of chondrosarcoma in MO and if a genotype-phenotype correlation exists.

Another challenge is the distinction of benign osteochondroma from low-grade malignant lesions, in particular in MO. The cartilaginous cap size (exceeding 1.5–2 cm) is the most reliable feature of suspecting malignant transformation,[67] and histology alone cannot distinguish an osteochondroma from low-grade CSP so diagnosis needs specialized bone tumor pathologists as well as a multidisciplinary approach.[68]

EXT1 and *EXT2* mutations account for a majority of MO cases.[7] In the past years, many studies focused on molecular biology of growth plate and on the roles of heparan sulfate (HS) deficiency on exostosis formation and MO pathogenesis in general.

Many advances came from different animal models (mice or zebrafish)[69]: osteochondroma development seems the effect of HS-dependent signaling pathways modifications.

Also, microRNA involvement has been advocated in development and malignant transformation[70] but the molecular mechanism has yet to be largely clarified.[71] These advances could point to therapeutic targets in the future.

ENCHONDROMATOSIS (OLLIER DISEASE AND MAFFUCCI SYNDROME)

Enchondromas are benign hyaline cartilage tumors of medullary bone and appear as radiolucent defects that originate in the metaphyses (**Figs. 3** and **4**).[60]

Enchondromas often occur as a solitary lesion, representing common benign bone tumors and accounting for a proportion as high as 15% of bone benign tumors,[72] and they are seen in more than 3% of the general population.

Multiple enchondromas characterize a group including several different conditions, named Multiple enchondromatosis. The original classification of 6 types by Spranger and colleagues in 1978 recently was reviewed in light of new insights into their molecular bases.[73,74]

The most known form is Ollier Disease (OD OMIM %166000) and the variant named Maffucci Syndrome (MS OMIM %614569), characterized by the association of angioma and multiple enchondromas,[73] whereas the other subtypes (ie, metachondromatosis, genochondromatosis) are extremely rare.[73,75] The first reported OD dates back to 1899. The prevalence is estimated at 1/100,000,[76] but true incidence can be higher, because mild case can be missed.

The incidence of malignant transformation in multiple enchodromatosis differs between studies; in a recent series, the incidence is as high as 40%,[77] depending on the location of the tumors. It usually occurs between 13 years and 69 years of age.[78] It is higher in MS, with a more severe prognosis than in OD.[76] Both diseases are nonhereditary and somatic mutations in different genes (*PTHR1*, *IDH1*, and *IDH2*) have been described.[79]

In a mice model, somatic mutations in the *IDH* genes are sufficient to induce enchondroma development.[80]

A role of *IDH* genes is described in glioma, glioblastoma, acute myeloid leukemia, T-cell lymphoma, and intrahepatic cholangiocarcinomas (OMIM *147700).[80] One report suggested a role of *IDH2* and *TP53* in gliomagenesis in a patient with MS,[81] and *IDH* genes mutations have been previously related to early stages of gliomagenesis.[81]

An increased risk for several other cancers have been reported in OD and MS; recently reports of these neoplasias are reviewed.[77,82]

Metachondromatosis (OMIM #156250) is an autosomal dominant disorder related to loss-of-function mutations in *PTPN11* gene and characterized by both multiple exostoses and multiple enchondromas; it can be expected that these lesions have a risk of malignant transformation as in MO and OD; moreover, malignant

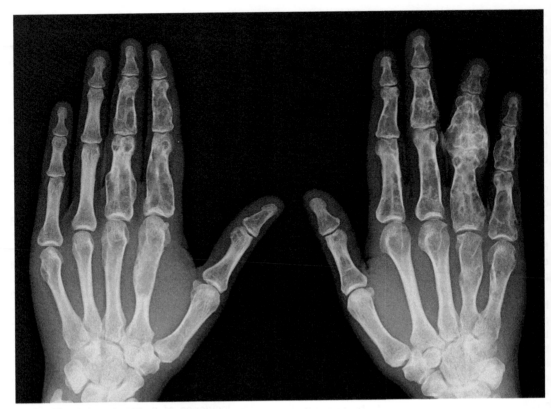

Fig. 3. Echondromas in MS.

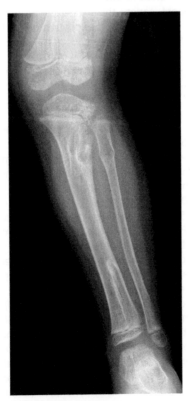

Fig. 4. Echondromas in OD.

transformation in metachondromatosis has been described in only 1 report to date.[83] Germline mutations in *PTPN11* gene cause dysmorphologic syndromes as Noonan syndrome (#163950) and LEOPARD syndrome (#151100) with a different molecular pathogenic mechanism (gain-of-function mutations).

PTPN11 has a role in modulating cellular proliferation, differentiation, migration, and apoptosis; promotes epidermal growth factor-mediated RAS/ERK/MAPK activation[84] and is also involved in terminal differentiation of growth plate chondrocytes.[85] This role is demonstrated by the finding of mutations in *PTPN11* in sporadic tumors (including leukemia and solid tumors) cells. In metachondromatosis, loss-of-function mutations is causative of the disorder and the different molecular pathways involved in MO, OD and metachondromatosis maybe can explain the different cancer transformation risk in the 2 diseases.

OTHER GENETIC SYNDROMES WITH OSTEOSARCOMA AND CHONDROSARCOMA

In **Table 7** other diseases with rare occurrence of bone tumors are listed.[86–89]

Table 7
Other genetic disorders with bone tumors

Disease	Clinical Signs	Bone Tumor and Reference	Gene	Transmission
Familial adenomatous polyposis 1 (FAP1) OMIM #175100	Hundreds to thousands of adenomatous polyps of the colon and rectum	Osteoma	APC	Autosomal dominant
McCune-Albright syndrome OMIM #174800	Polyostotic fibrous dysplasia, café au lait skin pigmentation, and peripheral precocious puberty	OS (2 cases) (Taconis,[86] [1988])	GNAS (mosaic)	Sporadic
Neurofibromatosis type 1 OMIM #162200	Café au lait spots, Lisch nodules in the eye, and fibromatous tumors of the skin; Freckling in the axillary or inguinal regions, optic glioma; tibial pseudoarthrosis; sphenoid dysplasia;	OS (Hatori et al,[87] 2006; Chowdhry et al,[88] 2009)	NF1	Autosomal dominant
Hutchinson-Gilford progeria syndrome OMIM #176670	Short stature, low body weight, early loss of hair, lipodystrophy, scleroderma, decreased joint mobility, osteolysis, and facial features that resemble aged persons; onset in first year	Tumor rate is not increased over that of the general population. One individual died of a chondrosarcoma of the chest wall at age 13 y (King et al,[89] 1978).	LMNA	Autosomal dominant, autosomal recessive
Trichorhinophalangeal syndrome, type II (TRPS2) OMIM #150230	Clinical features of trichorhinophalangeal syndrome type I (OMIM #190350) and multiple exostoses	No cases of malignant transformation of exostoses were identified, although the number of patients followed was low to define if there is a specific neoplasia risk.	Contiguous gene syndrome on 8q24.1, involving the TRPS1 and EXT1 genes.	Autosomal dominant, most de novo deletions

REFERENCES

1. Garber JE, Offit K. Hereditary cancer predisposition syndromes, [review]. Clin Oncol 2005;23(2):276–92.
2. Knudson AG. Cancer genetics, [review]. Am J Med Genet 2002;111(1):96–102.
3. Balmain A, Gray J, Ponder B. The genetics and genomics of cancer, [review]. Nat Genet 2003; 33(Suppl):238–44.
4. Lewis KM. Identifying hereditary cancer: genetic counseling and cancer risk assessment. Curr Probl Cancer 2014;38(6):216–25.
5. Wang LL, Plon SE. Rothmund-Thomson syndrome. In: Pagon RA, Adam MP, Ardinger HH, et al, editors. GeneReviews® [Internet]. Seattle (WA): University of Washington, Seattle; 1999. p. 1993–2016, [updated August 11, 2016].
6. Oshima J, Martin GM, Hisama FM. Werner syndrome. In: Pagon RA, Adam MP, Ardinger HH, et al, editors. GeneReviews® [Internet]. Seattle (WA): University of Washington, Seattle; 2002. p. 1993–2016, [updated September 29, 2016].
7. Available at: https://www.ncbi.nlm.nih.gov/omim/. Accessed December 15, 2016.
8. Morrow JJ, Khanna C. Osteosarcoma Genetics and Epigenetics: Emerging Biology and Candidate Therapies. Crit Rev Oncog 2015;20(3–4):173–97.
9. Chen X, Bahrami A, Pappo A, et al, St. Jude Children's Research Hospital–Washington University Pediatric Cancer Genome Project. Recurrent somatic structural variations contribute to tumorigenesis in pediatric osteosarcoma. Cell Rep 2014;7(1):104–12.
10. Schneider K, Zelley K, Nichols KE, et al. Li-Fraumeni syndrome. In: Pagon RA, Adam MP, Ardinger HH, et al, editors. GeneReviews® [Internet]. Seattle (WA): University of Washington, Seattle; 1999. p. 1993–2016, [updated April 11, 2013].
11. Reinhardt HC, Schumacher B. The p53 network: cellular and systemic DNA damage responses in aging and cancer. Trends Genet 2012;28(3): 128–36.
12. Bougeard G, Renaux-Petel M, Flaman JM, et al. Revisiting Li-Fraumeni syndrome from TP53 mutation carriers. J Clin Oncol 2015;33(21):2345–52.
13. Chompret A, Abel A, Stoppa-Lyonnet D, et al. Sensitivity and predictive value of criteria for p53 germline mutation screening. J Med Genet 2001; 38(1):43–7.
14. Ognjanovic S, Olivier M, Bergemann TL, et al. Sarcomas in TP53 germline mutation carriers: a review of the IARC TP53 database. Cancer 2012;118(5): 1387–96.
15. Mai PL, Best AF, Peters JA, et al. Risks of first and subsequent cancers among TP53 mutation carriers in the National Cancer Institute Li-Fraumeni syndrome cohort. Cancer 2016;122(23):3673–81.
16. Mirabello L, Yeager M, Mai PL, et al. Germline TP53 variants and susceptibility to osteosarcoma. J Natl Cancer Inst 2015;107(7), [pii: djv101].
17. Yao D, Cai GH, Chen J, et al. Prognostic value of p53 alterations in human osteosarcoma: a meta analysis, [review]. Int J Clin Exp Pathol 2014;7(10): 6725–33.
18. Ribi S, Baumhoer D, Lee K, et al. TP53 intron 1 hotspot rearrangements are specific to sporadic osteosarcoma and can cause Li-Fraumeni syndrome. Oncotarget 2015;6(10):7727–40.
19. Tinat J, Bougeard G, Baert-Desurmont S, et al. 2009 version of the Chompret criteria for Li Fraumeni syndrome. J Clin Oncol 2009;27(26):e108–9.
20. Ponti F, Corsini S, Gnoli M, et al. Evaluation of TP53 Pro72Arg and MDM2 SNP285-SNP309 polymorphisms in an Italian cohort of LFS suggestive patients lacking identifiable TP53 germline mutations. Fam Cancer 2016;15(4):635–43.
21. Dumont P, Leu JI, Della Pietra AC 3rd, et al. The codon 72 polymorphic variants of p53 have markedly different apoptotic potential. Nat Genet 2003; 33(3):357–65.
22. Said MD. A functional variant in miR-605 modifies the age of onset in Li-Fraumeni syndrome. Cancer Genet 2015;208(1–2):47–51.
23. Aerts I, Lumbroso-Le Rouic L, Gauthier-Villars M, et al. Retinoblastoma. Orphanet J Rare Dis 2006;1:31.
24. Lohmann DR, Gallie BL. Retinoblastoma. In: Pagon RA, Adam MP, Ardinger HH, et al, editors. Genereviews® [Internet]. Seattle (WA): University of Washington, Seattle; 2000. p. 1993–2016, [updated November 19, 2015].
25. Balmer A, Zografos L, Munier F. Diagnosis and current management of retinoblastoma. Oncogene 2006;25:5341–9.
26. Knudson AG Jr. Mutation and cancer: statistical study of retinoblastoma. Proc Natl Acad Sci U S A 1971;68:820–3.
27. Wong FL, Boice JD Jr, Abramson DH, et al. Cancer incidence after retinoblastoma. Radiation dose and sarcoma risk. JAMA 1997;278:1262–7.
28. Temming P, Viehmann A, Arendt M, et al. Pediatric second primary malignancies after retinoblastoma treatment. Pediatr Blood Cancer 2015;62(10): 1799–804.
29. Hawkins MM, Wilson LM, Burton HS, et al. Radiotherapy, alkylating agents, and risk of bone cancer after childhood cancer. J Natl Cancer Inst 1996;88: 270–8.
30. Cope JU, Tsokos M, Miller RW. Ewing sarcoma and sinonasal neuroectodermal tumors as second malignant tumors after retinoblastoma and other neoplasms. Med Pediatr Oncol 2001;36:290–4.
31. Moll AC, Imhof SM, Schouten-Van Meeteren AY, et al. Second primary tumors in hereditary

retinoblastoma: a register-based study, 1945–1997: is there an age effect on radiation-related risk? Ophthalmology 2001;108:1109–14.

32. Ren W, Gu G. Prognostic implications of RB1 tumour suppressor gene alterations in the clinical outcome of human osteosarcoma: a meta-analysis. Eur J Cancer Care (Engl) 2017;26(1):e.12401.

33. Gonzalez-Vasconcellos I, Domke T, Kuosaite V, et al. Differential effects of genes of the Rb1 signalling pathway on osteosarcoma incidence and latency in alpha-particle irradiated mice. Radiat Environ Biophys 2011;50(1):135–41.

34. Dyson NJ. RB1: a prototype tumor suppressor and an enigma. Genes Dev 2016;30(13):1492–502.

35. Larizza L, Roversi G, Volpi L. Rothmund-Thomson syndrome. Orphanet J Rare Dis 2010;5:2.

36. Larizza L, Roversi G, Verloes A. Clinical utility gene card for: Rothmund-Thomson syndrome. Eur J Hum Genet 2012;21(7):260.

37. Wang LL, Levy ML, Lewis RA, et al. Clinical manifestations in a cohort of 41 Rothmund-Thomson syndrome patients. Am J Med Genet 2001;102:11–7.

38. Lindor NM, Furuichi Y, Kitao S, et al. Rothmund-Thomson syndrome due to RECQ4 helicase mutations: report and clinical and molecular comparisons with Bloom syndrome and Werner syndrome. Am J Med Genet 2000;90:223–8.

39. Hicks MJ, Roth JR, Kozinetz CA, et al. Clinicopathologic features of osteosarcoma in patients with Rothmund-Thomson syndrome. J Clin Oncol 2007; 25:370–5.

40. Spurney C, Gorlick R, Meyers PA, et al. Multicentric osteosarcoma, Rothmund-Thomson syndrome, and secondary nasopharyngeal non-Hodgkin's lymphoma: a case report and review of the literature. J Pediatr Hematol Oncol 1998;20:494–7.

41. Stinco G, Governatori G, Mattighello P, et al. Multiple cutaneous neoplasms in a patient with Rothmund-Thomson syndrome: case report and published work review. J Dermatol 2008;35:154–61.

42. Siitonen HA, Sotkasiira J, Biervliet M, et al. The mutation spectrum in RECQL4 diseases. Eur J Hum Genet 2009;17(2):151–8.

43. Debeljak M, Zver A, Jazbec J. A patient with Baller-Gerold syndrome and midline NK/T lymphoma. Am J Med Genet 2009;15:755–9.

44. Croteau DL, Popuri V, Opresko PL, et al. Human RecQ helicases in DNA repair, recombination, and replication. Annu Rev Biochem 2014;83:519–52.

45. De S, Kumari J, Mudgal R, et al. RECQL4 is essential for the transport of p53 to mitochondria in normal human cells in the absence of exogenous stress. Cell Sci 2012;125(Pt 10):2509–22.

46. Arora A, Agarwal D, Abdel-Fatah TM, et al. RECQL4 helicase has oncogenic potential in sporadic breast cancers. J Pathol 2016;238(4):495–501.

47. Ng Walia MK, Smeets MF, Mutsaers AJ, et al. The DNA helicase recql4 is required for normal osteoblast expansion and osteosarcoma formation. PLoS Genet 2015;11(4):e1005160.

48. Wang LL, Gannavarapu A, Kozinetz CA, et al. Association between osteosarcoma and deleterious mutations in the RECQL4 gene in Rothmund-Thomson syndrome. J Natl Cancer Inst 2003;95:669–74.

49. Masala MV, Scapaticci S, Olivieri C, et al. Epidemiology and clinical aspects of Werner's syndrome in North Sardinia: description of a cluster. Eur J Dermatol 2007;17(3):213–6.

50. Epstein CJ, Martin GM, Schultz AL, et al. Werner's syndrome a review of its symptomatology, natural history, pathologic features, genetics and relationship to the natural aging process, [review]. Medicine (Baltimore) 1966;45(3):177–221.

51. Available at: www.wernersyndrome.org. Accessed December 15, 2016.

52. Takemoto M, Mori S, Kuzuya M, et al. Diagnostic criteria for Werner syndrome based on Japanese nationwide epidemiological survey. Geriatr Gerontol Int 2013;13(2):475–81.

53. Oshima J, Hisama FM. Search and insights into novel genetic alterations leading to classical and atypical Werner syndrome. Gerontology 2014;60: 239–46.

54. Yokote K, Chanprasert S, Lee L, et al. WRN mutation update: mutation spectrum, patient registries, and translational prospects. Hum Mutat 2017;38(1):7–15.

55. Goto M. Hierarchical deterioration of body systems in Werner's syndrome: implications for normal ageing. Mech Ageing Dev 1997;98(3):239–54.

56. Lauper JM, Krause A, Vaughan TL, et al. Spectrum and risk of neoplasia in Werner syndrome: a systematic review, [review]. PLoS One 2013; 8(4):e59709.

57. Sebastiani P, Bae H, Sun FX, et al. Meta-analysis of genetic variants associated with human exceptional longevity. Aging (Albany NY) 2013;5:653–61.

58. Savage SA, Mirabello L. Using epidemiology and genomics to understand osteosarcoma etiology. Sarcoma 2011;2011:548151.

59. Mosier SM, Patel T, Strenge K, et al. Chondrosarcoma in childhood: the radiologic and clinical conundrum. J Radiol Case Rep 2012;6(12):32–42.

60. de Andrea CE, Julian MS. JVMG bovee cartilagineous tumors. Surg Pathol Clinics 2017.

61. Hennekam RC. Hereditary multiple exostoses. J Med Genet 1991;28(4):262–6.

62. Schmale GA, Conrad EU 3rd, Raskind WH. The natural history of hereditary multiple exostoses. J Bone Joint Surg Am 1994;76(7):986–92.

63. Garrison RS, Unni KK, McLeod RA, et al. Chondrosarcoma arising in osteochondroma. Cancer 1982; 49:1890–7.

64. Goud AL, de Lange J, Scholtes VA, et al. Pain, physical and social functioning, and quality of life in individuals with multiple hereditary exostoses in the Netherlands: a national cohort study. J Bone Joint Surg Am 2012;94:1013–20.

65. Czajka CM, DiCaprio MR. What is the proportion of patients with multiple hereditary exostoses who undergo malignant degeneration? Clin Orthop Relat Res 2015;473(7):2355–61.

66. Pedrini E, Jennes I, Tremosini M, et al. Genotype-phenotype correlation study in 529 patients with multiple hereditary exostoses: identification of "protective" and "risk" factors. J Bone Joint Surg Am 2011;93(24):2294–302.

67. Bernard SA, Murphey MD, Flemming DJ, et al. Improved differentiation of benign osteochondromas from secondary chondrosarcomas with standardized measurement of cartilage cap at CT and MR imaging. Radiology 2010;255(3):857–65.

68. de Andrea CE, Kroon HM, Wolterbeek R, et al. Interobserver reliability in the histopathological diagnosis of cartilaginous tumors in patients with multiple osteochondromas. Mod Pathol 2012;25(9):1275–83.

69. de Andrea CE, Prins FA, Wiweger MI, et al. Growth plate regulation and osteochondroma formation: insights from tracing proteoglycans in zebrafish models and human cartilage J. Pathol 2011;224(2):160–8.

70. Zuntini M, Salvatore M, Pedrini E, et al. MicroRNA profiling of multiple osteochondromas: identification of disease-specific and normal cartilage signatures. Clin Genet 2010;78:507–16.

71. Huegel J, Sgariglia F, Enomoto-Iwamoto M, et al. Heparan sulfate in skeletal development, growth, and pathology: the case of hereditary multiple exostoses, [review]. Dev Dyn 2013 Sep;242(9):1021–32.

72. Herget GW, Strohm P, Rottenburger C, et al. Insights into enchondroma, enchondromatosis and the risk of secondary chondrosarcoma. Review of the literature with an emphasis on the clinical behaviour, radiology, malignant transformation and the follow up. Neoplasma 2014;61(4):365–78.

73. Superti-Furga A, Spranger J, Nishimura G. Enchondromatosis revisited: new classification with molecular basis, [review]. Am J Med Genet C Semin Med Genet 2012;160C(3):154–64.

74. Pansuriya TC, Kroon HM, Bovée JV. Enchondromatosis: insights on the different subtypes, [review]. Int J Clin Exp Pathol 2010;3(6):557–69.

75. Silve C, Juppner H. Ollier disease. Orphanet J Rare Dis 2006;1:37.

76. Verdegaal SH, Bovée JV, Pansuriya TC, et al. Incidence, predictive factors, and prognosis of chondrosarcoma in patients with Ollier disease and Maffucci syndrome: an international multicenter study of 161 patients. Oncologist 2011;16(12):1771–9.

77. Kumar A, Jain VK, Bharadwaj M, et al. Ollier disease: pathogenesis, diagnosis, and management. Orthopedics 2015;38(6):e497–506.

78. Pansuriya TC, van Eijk R, d'Adamo P, et al. Somatic mosaic IDH1 and IDH2 mutations are associated with enchondroma and spindle cell hemangioma in Ollier disease and Maffucci syndrome. Nat Genet 2011;43(12):1256–61.

79. Hirata M, Sasaki M, Cairns RA, et al. Mutant IDH is sufficient to initiate enchondromatosis in mice. Proc Natl Acad Sci U S A 2015 Mar 3;112(9):2829–34.

80. Moriya K, Kaneko MK, Liu X, et al. IDH2 and TP53 mutations are correlated with gliomagenesis in a patient with Maffucci syndrome. Cancer Sci 2014;105(3):359–62.

81. Yan H, Parsons DW, Jin G, et al. IDH1 and IDH2 mutations in gliomas. N Engl J Med 2009;360:765–73.

82. Prokopchuk O, Andres S, Becker K, et al. Maffucci syndrome and neoplasms: a case report and review of the literature. BMC Res Notes 2016;9:126.

83. Mavrogenis AF, Skarpidi E, Papakonstantinou O, et al. Chondrosarcoma in metachondromatosis: a case report. J Bone Joint Surg Am 2010;92(6):1507–13.

84. Tartaglia M, Kalidas K, Shaw A, et al. PTPN11 mutations in Noonan syndrome: molecular spectrum, genotype-phenotype correlation, and phenotypic heterogeneity. Am J Hum Genet 2002;70:1555–63.

85. Bowen ME, Ayturk UM, Kurek KC, et al. SHP2 regulates chondrocyte terminal differentiation, growth plate architecture and skeletal cell fates. PLoS Genet 2014;10(5):e1004364.

86. Taconis WK. Osteosarcoma in fibrous dysplasia Skeletal Radiol 1988;17(3):163–70.

87. Hatori M, Hosaka M, Watanabe M, et al. Tohoku Osteosarcoma in a patient with neurofibromatosis type 1: a case report and review of the literature. J Exp Med 2006;208(4):343–8.

88. Chowdhry M, Hughes C, Grimer RJ, et al. Bone sarcomas arising in patients with neurofibromatosis type 1. J Bone Joint Surg Br 2009;91(9):1223–6.

89. King CR, Lemmer J, Campbell JR, et al. Osteosarcoma in a patient with Hutchinson-Gilford progeria J Med Genet 1978;15(6):481.

90. Li FP, Fraumeni JF Jr, Mulvihill JJ, et al. A cancer family syndrome in twenty-four kindreds. Cancer Res 1988;48(18):5358–62.

91. Birch JM, Hartley AL, Tricker KJ, et al. Prevalence and diversity of constitutional mutations in the p53 gene among 21 Li-Fraumeni families. Cancer Res 1994;54:1298–304.

92. Eeles RA. Germline mutations in the TP53 gene Cancer Surv 1995;25:101–24.

Moving?

Make sure your subscription moves with you!

To notify us of your new address, find your **Clinics Account Number** (located on your mailing label above your name), and contact customer service at:

Email: journalscustomerservice-usa@elsevier.com

800-654-2452 (subscribers in the U.S. & Canada)
314-447-8871 (subscribers outside of the U.S. & Canada)

Fax number: 314-447-8029

Elsevier Health Sciences Division
Subscription Customer Service
3251 Riverport Lane
Maryland Heights, MO 63043

ELSEVIER

Printed and bound by CPI Group (UK) Ltd, Croydon, CR0 4YY

03/10/2024

01040384-0001